# Hemostasis in Dentistry

Richard P. Szumita • Paul M. Szumita
Editors

# Hemostasis in Dentistry

Springer

*Editors*
Richard P. Szumita
Department of Dentistry
St. Joseph's Regional Medical Center
Department of Dentistry
Paterson, NJ
USA

Paul M. Szumita
Department of Pharmacy Services
Brigham and Women's Hospital
Department of Pharmacy Services
Boston, MA
USA

ISBN 978-3-030-10033-9 ISBN 978-3-319-71240-6 (eBook)
https://doi.org/10.1007/978-3-319-71240-6



Printed on acid-free paper

This Springer imprint is published by the registered company Springer Nature Switzerland AG
The registered company address is: Gewerbestrasse 11, 6330 Cham, Switzerland

# Contents

# Introduction

Understanding hemostasis is essential for the safe management of patients undergoing dental treatment. The dental literature has consistently reviewed topics in hemostasis, particularly in management of patients with pathology of hemostasis and on medications altering hemostasis. The literature has detailed time-tested protocols to help with decision-making in the perioperative period. With this literature support and clinical experience, dental clinicians, along with their physician colleague input when appropriate, have been proficient in safely managing patients with disorders of hemostasis.

However, two major categories of changes related to hemostasis have surfaced in the recent past. First, evolution of the understanding of hemostasis, the pathology of hemostasis, and medical advances relating to hemostasis continue to occur. Second, the number of medications—especially oral medications—impacting upon hemostasis has been increasing rapidly. These additional medications are not simply clones of medications that we have all gained clinical experience in managing—but newer classes of medications with different pharmacodynamics and varying indications for clinical use. The "time-tested" clinical guidelines for which clinicians have relied may no longer be appropriate for the newer classes of medications now being prescribed. In order to safely manage patients, clinicians need to be familiar with important steps in the hemostatic process and with how the newer drugs impact hemostasis.

To standardize the information presented throughout this book, a few critical terms are reviewed. *Antithrombotic* medications refer to any medications that cause an effect on the formation and/or maintenance of a thrombus or clot. Antithrombotic medications include anticoagulants, antiplatelet, and fibrinolytic medications. *Anticoagulants* refer to medications reducing the formation of fibrin from fibrinogen. *Antiplatelet* medications affect formation of a platelet plug. *Fibrinolytic* mediations are "clot" busters used in the hospital environment for the emergency treatment of thromboembolic diseases—ischemic stroke, myocardial infarction, and acute pulmonary embolism [1]. Patients taking anticoagulant and antiplatelet agents are commonly presenting for dental care, and therefore, their review is a primary focus of this work. Since fibrinolytics are not encountered in dental practice, the discussion of these agents will be limited.

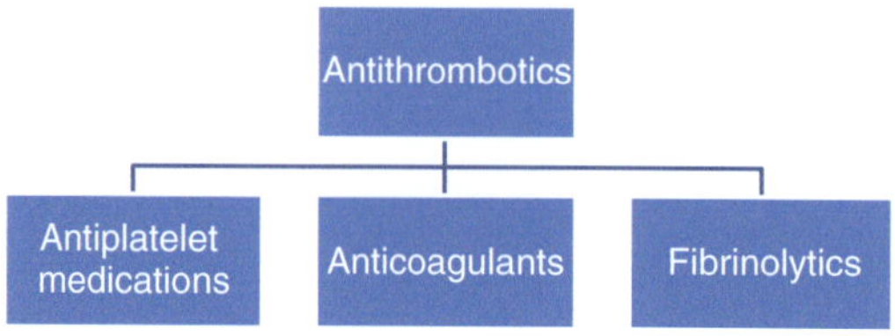


Although there are slight variations in the definition of hemostasis, a clinical definition that seems apropos for the climate in which we practice is reflected in the following: *Hemostasis* is the physiologic system of competent blood vessels, endothelial cells, platelets, and numerous plasma proteins that act in a finely controlled manner to preserve blood vessel integrity and prevent pathologic *hemorrhage* or *thrombosis* [2]. While surgical disciplines (including dentistry) strive to prevent excessive hemorrhage during and following procedures, medicine and pharmacology are increasing the number of medications used to alter hemostasis in order to decrease the morbidity and mortality associated with inappropriate thrombus formation. Dental clinicians should be familiar with contemporary treatment recommendations.

In this book, the physiology and pathophysiology of hemostasis will be reviewed with emphasis on updated topics. The physiology of hemostasis is complex. The review provided herein is intended to be of sufficient depth to allow students, residents, and practicing clinicians in dentistry and the dental specialties a thorough understanding of the updated models of hemostasis and the essential steps and reactions responsible for cessation of bleeding and prevention of excessive thrombus formation. A limited number of pathologic alterations in hemostasis will be reviewed in order to contrast normal physiology. This work will highlight pharmacologic agents that affect hemostasis with emphasis on the expanding number and role of direct oral antithrombotics which will be increasingly prevalent in dental practice. Finally, evidence-based guidelines are presented to assist the clinician in delivering safe dental treatment.

## References

1. Hamilton R. Tarascon pocket pharmacopoeia: 2015. Burlington, MA: Jones & Bartlett Publishing; 2015.
2. Macik BG. Hemostasis. In: Moylan JA, editor. Surgical critical care. St. Louis: Mosby-Year Book, Inc.; 1994. P. 697–718.

Paterson, NJ, USA — Paul M. Szumita
Boston, MA, USA — Richard P. Szumita

# Part I

# Review of Hemostasis

# 1 Local Tissues in Hemostasis and Platelet Review

Tiffany Kuang and Richard P. Szumita

**Abstract**

Hemostasis is a complex physiologic state able to change rapidly depending on the needs of the organism. The hemostatic system broadly consists of three essential elements: local (vascular) tissues, platelets, and biochemical factors. In health, these three elements maintain a state of neutrality (or mild antithrombosis) to prevent pathologic intravascular clotting. When needed to stop hemorrhage at a site of injury, the hemostatic system rapidly allows for a powerful prothrombotic response at the site of injury while maintaining neutrality throughout the remainder of the organism.

Maintaining the appropriate state of hemostasis begins with the very tissues in which the blood circulates—blood vessels. Endothelium, which lines the vessels, and subendothelial structures are physiologically active in hemostasis. When uninjured and in a non-pathologic state, the endothelium allows blood to remain in a fluid state, preventing pathologic intravascular thrombosis. With vessel injury, the endothelium and subendothelial tissues are responsible for initiating the explosion of pro-hemostatic responses culminating in clotting and cessation of bleeding.

The second component of hemostasis, the platelet, also fluctuates from neutral to prothrombotic states. With hemorrhage, platelets become the essential mediators that anchor the procoagulant reactions to the site of vascular injury, leading to local thrombus formation and the cessation of bleeding.

This chapter reviews the fundamental physiology and pathophysiology of local tissues and platelets in hemostasis. This knowledge is essential for understanding diseases and management of patients with bleeding disorders attributed to local tissues and platelets and the pharmacology of current and developing antiplatelet medications.

T. Kuang (✉)
Oral and Maxillofacial Surgery Resident, St. Joseph's University Medical Center, Paterson, NJ, USA

R. P. Szumita
Department of Dentistry/Oral and Maxillofacial Surgery, St. Joseph's University Medical Center, Paterson, NJ, USA

Private Practice, Little Falls, NJ, USA
e-mail: Szumita@northeastoralsurgerycenter.com

Hemostasis is a complex physiologic process that involves an intricate balance between the prothrombotic activity of platelets, enzymes, and coagulation factors and the antithrombotic activity of the fibrinolytic system and coagulation inhibitors. A critical component of this balance is the very tissues in which the blood circulates—blood vessels, endothelium, which lines the vasculature, and subendothelial structures. When uninjured



R. P. Szumita, P. M. Szumita (eds.), *Hemostasis in Dentistry*, https://doi.org/10.1007/978-3-319-71240-6_1

and in a non-pathologic state, the endothelium allows blood to remain in a fluid state, preventing pathologic intravascular thrombosis. On the contrary, with vessel injury, the endothelium and subendothelial tissues are responsible for initiating the explosion of pro-hemostatic responses culminating in clotting and cessation of bleeding. Physiologic hemostasis is often described as occurring in three phases: vascular (local tissues), platelet, and coagulation. Therefore, understanding hemostasis begins with understanding the basic physiology of the local tissues—blood vessels, endothelium, and subendothelium.

## 1.1 Blood Vessels

The initial vascular response to injury is to minimize blood loss followed by initiating the first phase of wound healing—inflammation [1]. When a blood vessel is injured, vasoconstriction of the vessel occurs immediately via neurogenic reflex mechanisms from pain and other afferent receptors in the injured tissue. Vasoconstriction is further supported by a number of endothelial cell and platelet-derived mediators released at the site of injury and interacting with the vessel wall smooth muscle. Vasoconstrictor endothelial mediators released include thromboxane $A_2$, endothelin, and endoperoxides ($PGH_2$) [2–5]. Platelet vasoconstrictor mediators include thromboxane $A_2$, serotonin (5-HT), and ADP [6, 7]. Blood vessel constriction initially diverts blood flow to the injured site limiting the amount of blood loss and increasing the ability of attachment of platelets to the injured vessel walls.

In dental procedures, epinephrine in local anesthetics has been shown to help in local hemostasis. The smaller blood vessels of the mucous membranes in the oral cavity primarily contain α-receptors. Epinephrine is an α-agonist and causes vasoconstriction of these local vessels [8]. Increased hemostasis has been demonstrated with the use of vasoconstrictors present in local anesthetics [8–10].

As part of the normal physiologic process, vessel dilation occurs following initial vasoconstriction as the initial response to wound healing. Wound healing is described in three phases: inflammatory, proliferative, and maturation. The inflammatory phase begins immediately following hemostasis and is characterized by local blood vessel dilation [11, 12]. The time from initial vessel constriction to physiologic vasodilation varies from seconds to several minutes or longer [11, 12]. The time to vasodilation is delayed after dental procedures when local anesthetics with vasoconstrictors are used. This is clinically significant in the dental patient, since delayed postoperative bleeding is seen clinically. It has been shown delayed bleeding can be seen approximately 6 h after a dental procedure [8]. In the absence of pathology, this "rebound" bleeding is usually minimal and controlled with local pressure (i.e., gauze pressure to the site).

## 1.2 Endothelium

Endothelium lines the vasculature system, is in perpetual contact with flowing blood, and provides the only barrier between blood and all other tissues. The endothelium is composed of approximately 1–6 × $10^{13}$ endothelial cells comprising a surface area of between 4000 and 7000 square meters [3, 4]. Aside from serving as a barrier, endothelial cells possess multiple metabolic and synthetic functions exerting their effects on vessel smooth muscle and components in circulating blood [4]. Endothelial cell function, then, is essential in maintaining the balance between blood circulating in the fluid state and initiating the rapid process of clotting when a vessel is injured. Endothelial functions promoting and inhibiting thrombosis are reviewed.

## 1.3 Endothelial Inhibition of Thrombosis

Intact endothelium functions to maintain blood flow and reduce the propensity for clotting. Several characteristics are present which help prevent intravascular clotting in intact endothelium and help to control and contain a developing thrombus in an injured vessel. The key elements supporting antithrombosis are smooth surface; mucopolysaccharide layer; membrane-bound thrombomodulin and antithrombin; and synthesis and secretion of tissue plasminogen activator (tPA), prostacyclin, and nitric oxide (NO).

The endothelium is smooth in the non-pathologic state. The smoothness helps prevent activation of platelets and the initiation of the intrinsic coagulation pathway [5]. A "blanket" layer of mucopolysaccharides is adherent to the surface of the endothelium and repels platelets and clotting factors. The mucopolysaccharide layer also serves as a binding site for antithrombin (also referred to as antithrombin III). Antithrombin is synthesized in the liver and circulates in plasma. Antithrombin is a natural anticoagulant which inactivates thrombin and activated factors IX, X, XI, and XII of the coagulation sequence [2, 3].

The endothelium also synthesizes and expresses thrombomodulin on its membrane. Thrombomodulin serves as an antithrombotic by binding thrombin (factor IIa). Binding of thrombin serves two functions. Thrombin is powerfully prothrombotic via several mechanisms including platelet activation and conversion of fibrinogen (factor I) to fibrin. Thrombin is neutralized when bound to thrombomodulin. In addition, the membrane-bound thrombomodulin-thrombin complex activates a natural anticoagulant, protein C. Protein C circulates in plasma and, when activated, neutralizes activated factors V and VIII (fVa and fVIIIa) of the coagulation sequence [2, 5, 13].

(Tissue-type) Tissue plasminogen activator (tPA), prostacyclin, and nitric oxide (NO) are synthesized by the endothelium. tPA is an enzyme which catalyzes the activation of circulating plasminogen into plasmin. Plasmin dissolves fibrin clots [2]. Prostacyclin and NO both inhibit platelet aggregation and are vasodilatory [4].

## 1.4 Endothelial Promotion of Thrombosis

Upon injury of the endothelium and exposure of subendothelium, an explosive prothrombotic response is initiated. Injury exposes highly thrombogenic components from *endothelial cells* and the *subendothelium*. One of the critical prothrombotic elements exposed from the endothelium after vessel injury is von Willebrand factor (vWF). The endothelium synthesizes two forms of vWF. The first are vWF dimers which are secreted into the plasma and subendothelium. The second form is stored as multimers in the Weibel-Palade bodies of the endothelium. With endothelial injury, the stored vWF is rapidly mobilized. vWF is an important adhesive protein aiding in platelet adhesion to the injured tissue by binding with collagen and with the platelet membrane receptor, GPIb/IX/V [4, 14].

The primary prothrombotic components exposed in the subendothelium upon vessel injury include tissue factor, collagen, and von Willebrand factor (vWF).

Tissue factor (TF) is factor III in the coagulation sequence and is also known as thromboplastin. TF initiates the coagulation process through the extrinsic pathway. The extrinsic pathway is activated when exposed TF at the site of injury binds activated factor VII (fVIIa). This binding then initiates coagulation by activating factor X of the common pathway [5, 13, 15–17].

Exposed collagen in the subendothelium of injured perivascular tissue serves two major functions. First, collagen is a potent platelet activator. Second, collagen serves as a binding site for platelet adhesion via vWF or as direct binding to platelet membrane receptor GPVI [13, 18, 19].

## 1.5 Local Tissues Upon Vessel Injury

See Fig. 1.1.

In summary, the impact injured vascular and perivascular (local) tissues have on the process of bleeding cessation are immediate vasoconstriction decreasing blood flow; platelet activation; providing substrate for platelet adhesion; and initiation of coagulation.

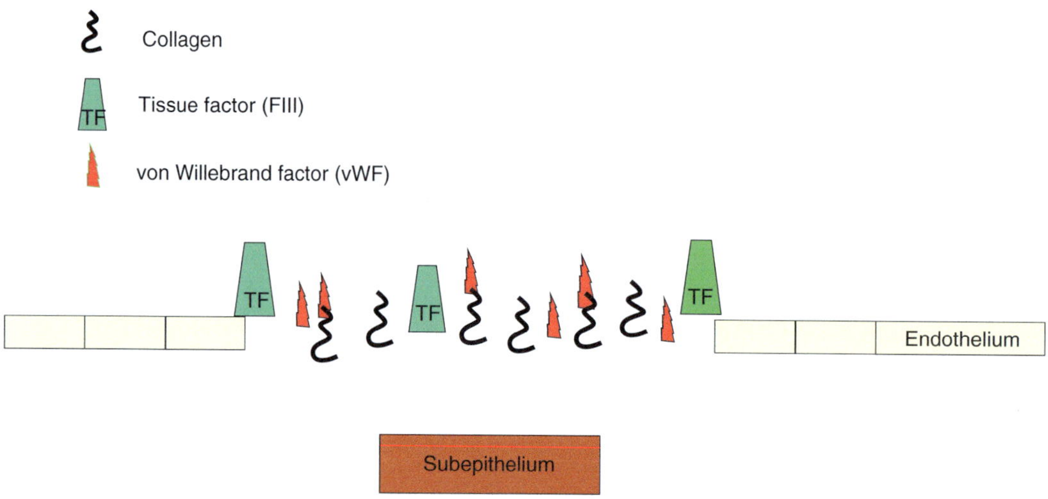


**Fig. 1.1** Exposed bioactive compounds upon damage to endothelium/subepithelium

> **Contribution of Local Tissues to Bleeding Cessation/Thrombus Formation**
>
> 1. Vasoconstriction with decreased blood flow to leaking vessel.
> 2. Platelet activation.
> 3. Exposure of substrates to allow platelet adhesion.
> 4. Initiation of coagulation.

## 1.6 Platelet Review

Knowledge of platelet physiology is essential for understanding hemostasis, antiplatelet medications, and management of patients with bleeding disorders. After vessel wall injury and the exposure of subepithelial elements (discussed above), platelets provide the critical platform which allows a thrombus to form. Platelets should be considered the "center" of thrombus formation and not simply a "pass-through" phase on the way to clot generation. The platelet's central role in hemostasis is reviewed.

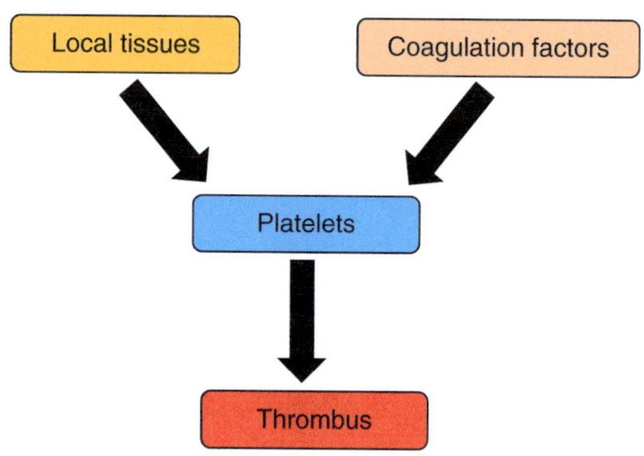


## 1.7 Platelet Anatomy

Platelets are derived from megakaryocytes in bone marrow. They are disc-shaped, anucleate cells approximately 2–3 μm in diameter [20]. By comparison, red blood cells are approximately

7 μm, lymphocytes are 6–10 μm, monocytes are 12–20 μm, and granulocytes are 8–14 μm in diameter [21].

In the adult, there are approximately one trillion platelets in circulation—two thirds in the general circulation and one third reversibly sequestered in the spleen. Their average life span is 8–10 days [20]. The primary sites for platelet removal appear to be the spleen, liver, and bone marrow [22]. Normal platelet counts are 150,000–400,000 per microliter (μl). To sustain a steady state of platelets, approximately 100 billion new platelets are produced daily [20].

Platelets are designed to circulate within intact vasculature and never interact with the endothelial surface [19, 23]. However, with disruption of a vessel wall, platelets rapidly respond through a complex of interactions with exposed subendothelial structures to initiate the adhesion of platelets to the site of injury and clumping together (aggregation).

Structural elements integral in the function of platelets are membrane, cytoplasm, and secretory granules. The platelet membrane is a phospholipid bilayer. Glycoproteins, cholesterol, and glycolipids are embedded within the platelet membrane and are exposed on the membrane's external surface [20]. These exposed membrane molecules, especially the glycoprotein receptors, serve as highly specific surface receptors involved in platelet activation, adhesion, aggregation, and intracellular signaling [20]. The transmembrane glycoprotein receptors are designated by the preface GP. Glycoprotein receptors have complex structures and have also been classified, and referred to, as integrins—cell adhesion receptors involved in physiologic and pathologic processes [24]. For purposes of this chapter, the receptors will be referred to by their glycoprotein (GP) designation. The receptors critical to platelet function include GPIa/IIa, GPIIb/IIIa, GPVI, and GPIb/IX/V (shortened to GPIb). Along with their roles in cellular adhesion, the platelet membrane glycoprotein receptors are also involved with intracellular signaling, important in regulating and coordinating the complex and numerous reactions required for proper platelet function [25, 26]. These functions are discussed below.

The platelet cytoplasm contains elements to form a cytoskeleton, organelles, and intracellular messaging systems. Platelet form is maintained via a cytoskeleton primarily via spectrin microtubules and actin filaments. Organelles in the platelet cytoplasm, including lysosomes and peroxisomes, contain a number of degradative enzymes used against material ingested via phagocytosis. Intracellular messaging is aided by canalicular and tubular systems within the cytoplasm [20].

A large number of biologically active molecules are stored in secretory granules within the platelet—α-granules and dense granules. The α-granules are more abundant. Their contents are involved in hemostasis, immunity, inflammation, and wound healing [27]. Pro-hemostatic substances contained in the α-granules are von Willebrand factor (vWF); factors I (fibrinogen), V, XI, and XIII; protein S; and platelet activator inhibitor (PAI-1). Dense granules contain serotonin (5-HT), ADP, ATP, and calcium (factor IV). These substances are secreted in an orchestrated fashion during critical steps and during the evolution of the thrombus [22, 27].

## 1.8 The Platelet

See Fig. 1.2.

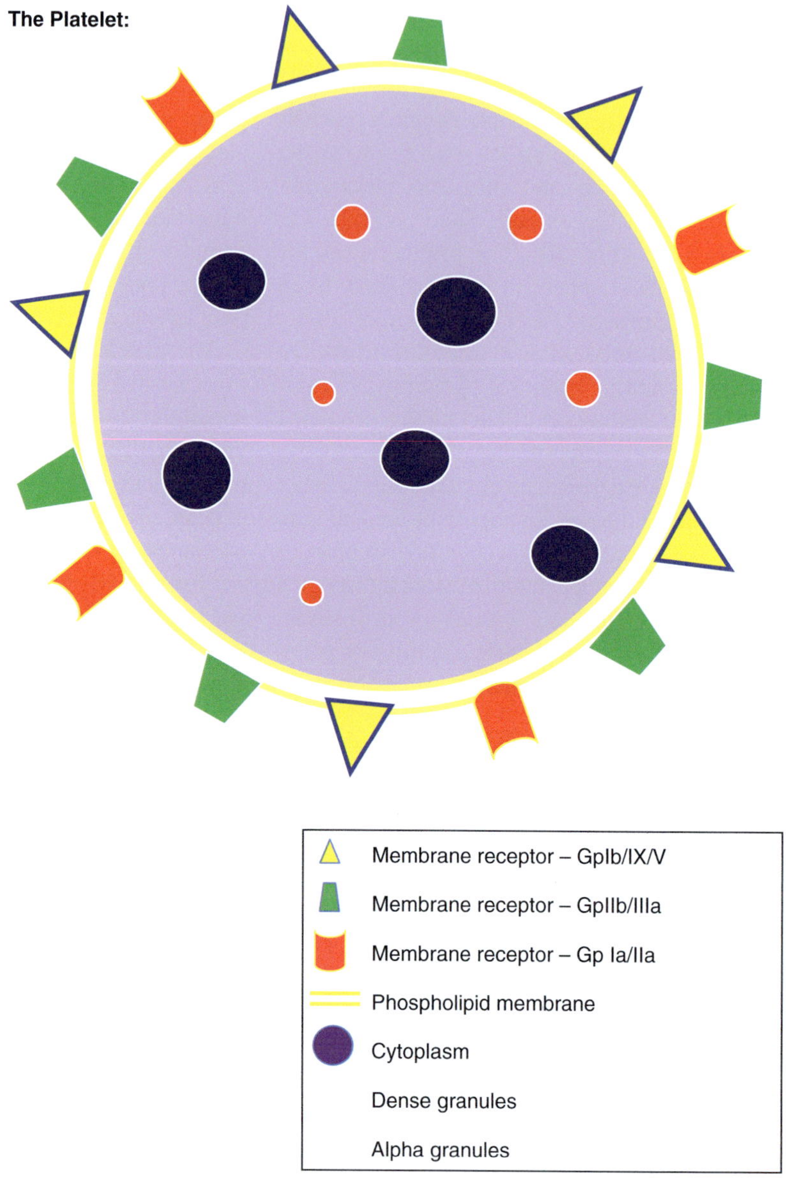


**Fig. 1.2** Functional elements of the platelet

## 1.9 Platelets and Clotting

Platelets are central to the formation of a clot. In physiologic hemostasis, platelets interact at the site of disruption of vessels (surgery or trauma) in the prevention of bleeding. Platelets also play a role in the formation of pathologic thrombi, mircothrombi, and emboli that are associated with myocardial infarction, stroke, pulmonary embolism, and end-organ damage. There are both similarities and differences in platelets' role in the physiologic and pathologic states.

In patient management, it will help the dental professional to understand the concept of physiologic and pathologic thrombi formation. Dental treatment of patients being managed with antiplatelet medications to reduce the risk of pathologic thrombus formation can often be accomplished with minimal impact on the physiologic formation of a wound thrombus (discussed further in chapters).

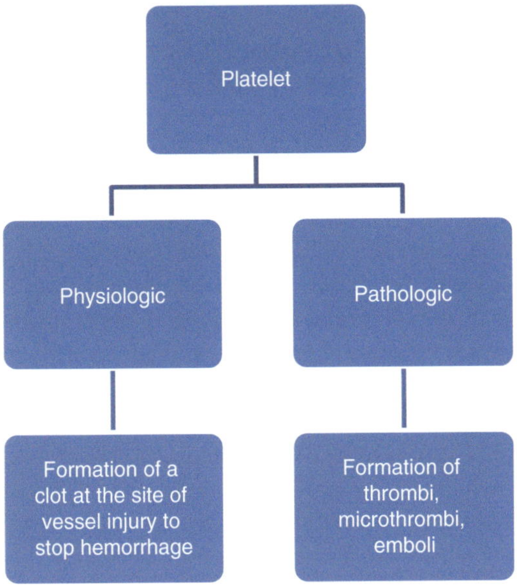


## 1.10 Platelets in Physiologic Hemostasis

Platelets perform several important functions in physiologic coagulation: control of thrombin generation, support of fibrin formation, and regulation of fibrin clot retraction [28]. Additionally, platelets anchor these functions directly at the site of tissue/vessel injury.

**Platelet Functions in Physiologic Hemostasis** [28]

1. Control of thrombin generation.
2. Support of fibrin formation.
3. Regulation of fibrin clot retraction.
4. Anchor the reactions at the site of tissue injury/hemorrhage.

To accomplish these functions, platelets go through well-coordinated and regulated processes: activation, adhesion, aggregation, and secretion.

Immediately after vessel injury from surgery or trauma, vessel vasoconstriction occurs and subendothelial substances are exposed: vWF, collagen, tissue factor (factor III), and others. Rapid interactions occur between these subendothelial structures and circulating platelets to initiate the hemostatic process [19]. These initial reactions activate the circulating platelets predisposing them to adhere to the damaged endothelium. Platelets then coalesce or aggregate. This "clump" of platelets is then able to focus and direct multiple biochemical reactions at the site of injury leading to the formation of fibrin. Research continues to reveal the central roles and complex nature platelets play in hemostasis. Recent findings suggest there may actually be different platelet populations, with distinct surface properties, each group designed to carry out different roles in coagulation [28].

## 1.11 Platelet Activation

Platelets circulate in a non-activated state. Upon vessel injury, platelet membrane receptors interact with the damaged endothelium and subendothelial substances leading to platelet activation. A major pathway in platelet activation is collagen binding to platelet membrane GPVI [17]. Additional activation occurs with the binding of vWF to platelet membrane GPIb [19, 23]. Other substances shown to promote platelet activation include thrombin, thromboxane A2, 5-HT, epinephrine, and ADP. With activation, several structural and physiologic changes occur to the platelet and include platelet shape change, expression of pro-inflammatory molecules, expression of platelet procoagulant activity, potentiation of aggregation by other prothrombotic factors (i.e., collagen), and conversion of platelet receptor GpIIb/IIIa into active form [29, 30]. Platelet activation "primes" the platelet to begin its pro-hemostatic and pro-healing functions.

## 1.12 Platelet Adhesion

Once activated, platelets are "primed" to adhere to the injured site—a critical step in formation of an effective thrombus. Platelet adhesion relies primarily on exposed collagen at the site of injury, vWF, and glycoprotein receptors in the platelet membrane. [It is important to note here that another substance is exposed after endothelial damage—tissue factor (factor III). As will be discussed shortly, tissue factor is responsible for initiating the process of thrombin and fibrin formation.]

The initial critical step in adhesion involves von Willebrand factor (vWF) and the platelet glycoprotein receptor Ib/V/IX (GPIb). von Willebrand factor (vWF) is a large glycoprotein found in several locations: in the circulation in an inactive form, in the subendothelial matrix of blood vessels, within Weibel-Palade bodies of endothelial cells, and in α-granules of platelets [25, 31]. Platelet receptor GPIb/IX/V is a complex of glycoproteins on the platelet membrane where the major binding site is on the glycoprotein (GP) Ib subunit. In hemostasis, GPIb binds vWF [14, 32]. GPIb also binds a leukocyte receptor (Mac-1) which plays a role in vessel wall inflammation in atherosclerosis, thrombosis, and restenosis [33].

Upon endothelial damage, collagen becomes exposed and binds vWF. Binding of vWF causes a conformational change in the molecule and exposes the binding site for the platelet membrane GPIb. vWF then acts as the link anchoring collagen at the site of vessel injury and the platelet via GPIb receptor [19, 32]. This interaction appears to be critical especially in high flow, high shear stresses in injured vessels—microvascular and stenotic arteries [34]. This initial bonding decelerates platelets and holds them in close contact with the exposed subendothelial matrix where additional interaction with platelet receptors leads to further activation and adhesion [17, 23].

Additional anchoring of platelets to the site of vessel injury is provided by direct collagen binding to platelet membrane receptor glycoproteins: GPIa/IIa and GPVI. GPIa/IIa binds directly to the collagen types I and IV found in the subendothelial matrix. This binding is thought to be limited to low shear stress conditions (veins and larger arteries) in the injured vessel. GPVI also likely binds directly to collagen but may have a greater role as an activator of GPIa/IIa via intracellular signaling [19, 34].

Other proteins in the subendothelial matrix have also been shown to play a role in platelet function: fibronectin, thrombospondin, laminin, and vitronectin. Fibronectin and thrombospondin are both stored in α-granules in platelets. Fibronectin binds to platelet membrane glycoprotein (GPIIb/IIIa) which is involved in platelet aggregation (discussed below). Thrombospondin release from the platelets with subsequent binding to the platelet membrane interacts with fibrinogen, fibrin, and collagen. These interactions appear to help overcome local antithrombotic activity by providing positive feedback, enhancing platelet adhesion and aggregation [19].

Laminin is a large glycoprotein in the subendothelial matrix. Laminin acts like collagen by binding to platelet membrane receptor GPVI leading to platelet activation. Laminin also interacts with the binding of vWF and platelet GPIb further enhancing platelet adhesion [19, 35].

Vitronectin is also found in the subendothelial matrix and, like fibronectin, binds to platelet membrane receptor GPIIb/IIIa enhancing platelet aggregation [19].

## 1.13 Platelet Aggregation

Aggregation of platelets to each other is the next step in the evolution of a thrombus. This "clumping" together of platelets occurs primarily between platelet membrane glycoprotein receptors (GPIIb/IIIa) and fibrinogen. Fibrinogen is the intermediary between GPIIb/IIIa receptors on adjacent platelets. GPIIb/IIIa can also bind vWF assisting in aggregation (Note: GPIIb/IIIa is also referred to in the literature as αIIbβ3 integrin.) [26]. Platelet aggregation results in concentrating a greater volume of platelets at the site of injury, providing membrane surfaces for the anchoring of the coagulation reactions terminating in the conversion of fibrinogen (factor I) to fibrin at the site of injury.

## 1.14 Platelet Quality: Secretion

Among its attributes, the platelet is a biochemical manufacturing and storage "warehouse." Dentistry has extensively studied and employed platelet concentrates in clinical practice for its positive effects on wound and bone healing [36–39]. Platelets store a multitude of substances that are important in hemostasis as well as in healing. These bioactive substances are contained in α-granules, dense granules, and the cytoplasm. The stored molecules involved in hemostasis are as follows. α-Granules contain vWF; factors I (fibrinogen), V, and XI; protein S; PAI-1; and HMWK. Dense granules contain serotonin, ADP, ATP, and calcium. The cytoplasm contains factor XIII. These substances are secreted during the evolution of the thrombus [22].

## 1.15 Platelets in Pathologic Hemostasis (Thrombotic Disease)

The formation of pathologic thrombi in both the arterial (myocardial infarction and stroke) and venous (deep vein thrombosis potentially leading to pulmonary emboli) vasculature is well documented. Even though pathologic clotting (within vessels with intact endothelium) shares similarities to physiologic clotting, many mechanisms for initiation and propagation exist that are unique to pathologic clotting. Mechanisms of pathologic clotting even differ between the arterial and venous systems. Arterial pathologic thrombi appear to be anchored to vessel walls by platelet interactions. In venous thromboembolism, fibrin appears to be the main mediator anchoring the clot to the vessel wall [40]. Clinically, this explains the need for antiplatelet medication in arterial disease and anticoagulants in venous disease.

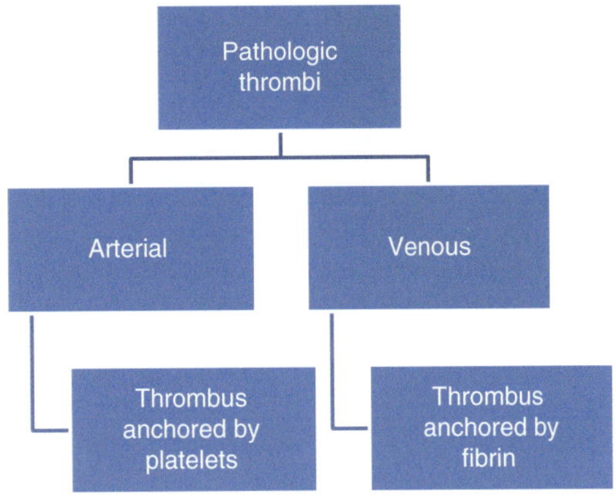


In the arterial system, mechanisms proposed to explain pathologic thrombi formation include rupture of atherosclerotic plaques, deformation of vWF in high shear stress arterial vessels, and systemic inflammatory states. When atherosclerotic lesions rupture, vWF and collagen can become exposed initiating platelet activation, adhesion, and coagulation. In partially occluded arteries, high sheer stress of the blood flow can alter ("unfold") vWF allowing it to bind to platelet receptor GPIb/IX/V and initiate clotting. Systemic inflammatory states are associated with many diseases including cardiovascular disease. Inflammatory states are known to activate platelets and promote endothelial cell dysfunction by making them more adhesive to circulating platelets.

Venous thromboembolism is less well understood but appears to be related to inflammation and stasis [40].

## References

1. Sabiston DC, Townsend CM. Sabiston textbook of surgery: the biological basis of modern surgical practice. 19th ed. Philadelphia, PA: Elsevier Saunders; 2012.
2. Shuman MA. Endothelial cell structure and function. In: Hoffman R, Benz Jr EZ, Edward J, Shattil SJ, Furie B, Cohen HJ, Silberstein LE, editors. Hematology: basic principles and practice. 2nd ed. New York: Churchill Livingstone Inc.; 1995. p. 1552–65.
3. Yau JW, Teoh H, Verma S. Endothelial cell control of thrombosis. BMC Cardiovasc Disord. 2015;15:130.

4. Sumpio BE, Riley JT, Dardik A. Cells in focus: endothelial cell. Int J Biochem Cell Biol. 2002;34(12):1508–12.
5. Guyton AC, Hall JE. Textbook of medical physiology. 11th ed. Philadelphia: Elsevier Inc.; 2006.
6. Schror K, Braun M. Platelets as a source of vasoactive mediators. Stroke. 1990;21(12 Suppl):IV32–5.
7. Goto S, Hasebe T, Takagi S. Platelets: small in size but essential in the regulation of vascular homeostasis – translation from basic science to clinical medicine. Circ J. 2015;79(9):1871–81.
8. Malamed SF. Handbook of local anesthesia. 5th ed. St. Louis, MO: Elsevier/Mosby; 2004.
9. Sisk AL. Vasoconstrictors in local anesthesia for dentistry. Anesth Prog. 1992;39(6):187–93.
10. Sisk AL. Long-acting local anesthetics in dentistry. Anesth Prog. 1992;39(3):53–60.
11. Leong M, Phillips LG. Wound healing. In: Townsend CM, Beauchamp RD, Evers BM, Mattox KL, editors. Sabiston textbook of surgery, the biological basis of modern surgical practice. 19th ed. Philadelphia: Elsevier Saunders; 2012. p. 151–77.
12. Stucki-McCormick SU, Santiago P. The metabolic and physiologic aspects of wound healing. In: Hudson JW, editor. Oral and maxillofacial surgery clinics of North America, wound healing, vol. 8. Philadelphia: W.B. Saunders Company; 1996. p. 467–76.
13. Versteeg HH, Heemskerk JW, Levi M, Reitsma PH. New fundamentals in hemostasis. Physiol Rev. 2013;93(1):327–58.
14. Andrews RK, Berndt MC. Platelet physiology and thrombosis. Thromb Res. 2004;114(5–6):447–53.
15. Furie B, Furie BC. Molecular and cellular biology of blood coagulation. N Engl J Med. 1992;326(12):800–6.
16. Furie B, Furie BC. Molecular basis of blood coagulation. In: Hoffman R, Benz Jr EZ, Shattil S, Furie B, Cohen H, Silberstein L, editors. Hematology: basic principles and practice. 2nd ed. New York: Churchill Livingstone Inc.; 1995. p. xxix. 1919 p., 1917 p. of plates.
17. Clemetson KJ. Platelets and primary haemostasis. Thromb Res. 2012;129(3):220–4.
18. Hall JE. Guyton and Hall textbook of medical physiology. 12th ed. Philadelphia: W.B. Saunders Company; 2011.
19. Lowenberg EC, Meijers JC, Levi M. Platelet-vessel wall interaction in health and disease. Neth J Med. 2010;68(6):242–51.
20. Thon JN, Italiano JE. Platelets: production, morphology and ultrastructure. Handb Exp Pharmacol. 2012;210:3–22.
21. Bailey FR, Kelly DE, Wood RL, Enders AC. Bailey's textbook of microscopic anatomy. 18th ed. Baltimore: Williams & Wilkins; 1984.
22. Calverly DCT, Christiane D. Platelet structure and function in hemostasis and thrombosis. In: Greer JP, Foerster J, Rodgers GM, et al., editors. Wintrobe's clinical hematology, vol. 1. Philadelphia: Lippincott Williams & Wilkins; 2009.
23. Broos K, Feys HB, De Meyer SF, Vanhoorelbeke K, Deckmyn H. Platelets at work in primary hemostasis. Blood Rev. 2011;25(4):155–67.
24. Barczyk M, Carracedo S, Gullberg D. Integrins. Cell Tissue Res. 2010;339(1):269–80.
25. Nuyttens BP, Thijs T, Deckmyn H, Broos K. Platelet adhesion to collagen. Thromb Res. 2011;127(Suppl 2):S26–9.
26. Nieswandt B, Pleines I, Bender M. Platelet adhesion and activation mechanisms in arterial thrombosis and ischaemic stroke. J Thromb Haemost. 2011;9(Suppl 1):92–104.
27. Jenne CN, Urrutia R, Kubes P. Platelets: bridging hemostasis, inflammation, and immunity. Int J Lab Hematol. 2013;35(3):254–61.
28. Heemskerk JW, Mattheij NJ, Cosemans JM. Platelet-based coagulation: different populations, different functions. J Thromb Haemost. 2013;11(1):2–16.
29. Angiolillo DJ, Capodanno D, Goto S. Platelet thrombin receptor antagonism and atherothrombosis. Eur Heart J. 2010;31(1):17–28.
30. Davi G, Patrono C. Platelet activation and atherothrombosis. N Engl J Med. 2007;357(24):2482–94.
31. Wagner DD, Ginsburg D. Structure, biology, and genetics of von Willebrand factor. In: Hoffman R, Benz Jr EZ, Edward J, Shattil SJ, Furie B, Cohen HJ, Silberstein LE, editors. Hematology: basic principles and practice. 2nd ed. New York: Churchill Livingstone Inc.; 1995. p. 1717–25.
32. Andrews RK, Gardiner EE, Shen Y, Whisstock JC, Berndt MC. Glycoprotein Ib-IX-V. Int J Biochem Cell Biol. 2003;35(8):1170–4.
33. Wang Y, Sakuma M, Chen Z, et al. Leukocyte engagement of platelet glycoprotein Ibalpha via the integrin Mac-1 is critical for the biological response to vascular injury. Circulation. 2005;112(19):2993–3000.
34. Rivera J, Lozano ML, Navarro-Nunez L, Vicente V. Platelet receptors and signaling in the dynamics of thrombus formation. Haematologica. 2009;94(5):700–11.
35. Inoue O, Suzuki-Inoue K, Ozaki Y. Redundant mechanism of platelet adhesion to laminin and collagen under flow: involvement of von Willebrand factor and glycoprotein Ib-IX-V. J Biol Chem. 2008;283(24):16279–82.
36. Marx RE. Platelet-rich plasma: evidence to support its use. J Oral Maxillofac Surg. 2004;62(4):489–96.
37. Marx RE, Carlson ER, Eichstaedt RM, Schimmele SR, Strauss JE, Georgeff KR. Platelet-rich plasma: growth factor enhancement for bone grafts. Oral Surg Oral Med Oral Pathol Oral Radiol Endod. 1998;85(6):638–46.
38. Freymiller EG, Aghaloo TL. Platelet-rich plasma: ready or not? J Oral Maxillofac Surg. 2004;62(4):484–8.
39. Slapnicka J, Fassmann A, Strasak L, Augustin P, Vanek J. Effects of activated and nonactivated platelet-rich plasma on proliferation of human osteoblasts in vitro. J Oral Maxillofac Surg. 2008;66(2):297–301.
40. Lopez JA, Chen J. Pathophysiology of venous thrombosis. Thromb Res. 2009;123(Suppl 4):S30–4.

# 2 Coagulation Enzymes Review and Review of Hemostasis: Putting It All Together

Richard P. Szumita

**Abstract**

Hemostasis is a well-coordinated interplay of cells and biochemical substrates which can quickly respond to vascular injury and form a local thrombus to stop hemorrhage. In addition, this prothrombotic response is balanced by endogenous antithrombotic elements to prevent excessive thrombus generation and to clear a clot once bleeding is controlled and tissue healing progresses. This first part of this chapter reviews the major biochemical mediators involved in thrombus formation (coagulation factors) and prevention and dissolution of thrombi (antithrombotic factors).

The second part of this chapter focuses on how the three components of hemostasis—local tissues and platelets (described in the previous chapter) and coagulation factors—interact in a well-orchestrated and tightly regulated explosion of reactions leading to thrombus formation and cessation of bleeding. Two models of hemostasis are reviewed. The first is the model by which the physiology of hemostasis has traditionally been taught and studied. This model is referred to as the *cascade or biochemical model.* This ubiquitously reported model elucidates the multiple reactions and sequencing of these reactions leading to formation of a thrombus. The second model is referred to as the *cell-based model* of hemostasis and is widely reported to more accurately describe in greater detail where reactions are occurring in vivo and how they relate to clinical hemostasis and better explain pathologies of hemostasis.

R. P. Szumita
Department of Dentistry/Oral and Maxillofacial Surgery, St. Joseph's University Medical Center, Paterson, NJ, USA

Private Practice, Little Falls, NJ, USA
e-mail: Szumita@northeastoralsurgerycenter.com

## 2.1 Coagulation Factors

With formation of the platelet plug, the next step in development of a clot is the formation of fibrin—referred to as secondary hemostasis. The formation of fibrin is the end result of a well-orchestrated and regulated sequence of enzymatic conversions of protein factors. The end products of these reactions are the production of thrombin and fibrin. In this chapter, the individual factors are reviewed. In the subsequent chapter, the sequencing will be reviewed.

The substances involved in the biochemical reactions leading ultimately to the formation of



R. P. Szumita, P. M. Szumita (eds.), *Hemostasis in Dentistry*, https://doi.org/10.1007/978-3-319-71240-6_2

fibrin are referred to as the clotting factors. In an effort to standardize the nomenclature of the blood clotting proteins, in 1954 the International Committee for the Standardization of the Nomenclature of Blood Clotting Factors was established. Then, in 1958, the Committee agreed the substances involved in blood clotting would be assigned Roman numerals [1]. Presently, there are 12 factors: I, II, III, IV, V, VII, VIII, IX, X, XI, XII, and XIII. By convention, factors are designated with the letter "F" followed by the Roman numeral. As an example, factor I would be reported as FI. As will be discussed in this and the subsequent chapter, most of the factors are proteins which will under proteolysis to an "active" form which will cause proteolysis of the next factor in the sequence. An activated factor is designated with a lower case "a" after the factor name. For example, activated factor VII would be FVIIa. Despite the international designation with Roman numerals, several factors are commonly referred to by names.

## 2.2 The Factors

Factor I is fibrinogen, a large protein synthesized in the liver and circulates in plasma [2]. Fibrinogen serves two critical functions. Firstly, fibrinogen plays an important role in platelet aggregation through binding to adjacent platelet membrane GPIIb/IIIa receptors. Secondly, fibrinogen is the precursor of fibrin. In the presence of thrombin, fibrinogen undergoes proteolysis to yield fibrin. Along with platelets, fibrin is an essential component of a thrombus.

Factor II is also commonly referred to as prothrombin. Factor II is converted to thrombin. Factor II is synthesized in the liver and is one of four factors (II, VII, IX, X) that contains carboxylated glutamic acid residues needed for function. These residues require vitamin K for synthesis. The activated form of FII is thrombin. Thrombin has many important functions including catalyzing the conversion of fibrinogen to fibrin; activating factors V, VIII, XI, and XIII; and activating platelets [3–5].

Factor III is commonly referred to as tissue factor (TF). TF is unique in that it is a membrane protein found in subendothelial cells of blood vessels and cells of perivascular tissue, i.e., fibroblasts [4, 6, 7]. Upon vessel disruption/injury, TF becomes exposed and initiates coagulation.

Factors IV, V, and VIII are cofactors. Without these cofactors, several of the proteolytic factor activations would not occur. Specifically, factor IV, which is calcium, is required as a cofactor in the activation of factors II, IX, X, and XI. Factor V is a cofactor with calcium to convert factor II (prothrombin) to thrombin. Factor VIII is also known as antihemophilic factor. Decreases in factor VIII levels are associated with classic hemophilia (hemophilia A). Factor VIII circulates in plasma bound to vWF. It is converted to an active form by thrombin and then serves as a cofactor with calcium for the activation of factor X [2, 4, 8].

Factor VII is a protein synthesized in the liver and circulates in the blood. Factor VII is also one of the four factors that require vitamin K to complete synthesis. When activated, FVIIa forms a complex with exposed tissue factor (FIII) at the site of injury. Factors III and VII and cofactor calcium (FIV) comprise the extrinsic pathway [9].

Factor IX is also known as Christmas factor. It is a protein and manufactured in the liver. Deficiencies in FIX are responsible for hemophilia B or Christmas disease [2].

Factor X is synthesized in the liver. Factor X, along with factors I and II, constitutes the common pathway. FXa is responsible for the activation of FII (prothrombin) into thrombin (FIIa).

Factors XI and XII are also proteins synthesized in the liver. Both are part of the intrinsic pathway.

Factor XIII is the fibrin-stabilizing factor. The fibrin monomers formed by proteolysis of fibrinogen are initially held together by weak noncovalent bonding. Factor XIII, after activation by thrombin, converts the fibrin linkages to strong covalent bonds and creates the fibrin mesh by cross-linking adjacent fibrin molecules [2].

## 2.3 Summary of Factors

| Factor | Synonym | Site of synthesis |
|---|---|---|
| I | Fibrinogen | Liver |
| II | Prothrombin | Liver |
| III | Tissue factor | Membrane protein in perivascular tissues |
| IV | Calcium | Absorbed from diet; stored in bones |
| V | Proaccelerin | Liver, megakaryocytes |
| VII | Prothrombin conversion factor | Liver |
| VIII | Antihemophilic factor | Liver |
| IX | Christmas factor | Liver |
| X | Stuart-Prower factor | Liver |
| XI | Plasma thromboplastin antecedent | Liver |
| XII | Hageman factor | Liver |
| XIII | Fibrin-stabilizing factor | Liver, megakaryocytes |

Adapted from Hall: Textbook of Medical Physiology [10]

## 2.4 Cofactors

| Factor | Synonym | Site of synthesis |
|---|---|---|
| IV | Calcium | |
| V | Proaccelerin | Liver, megakaryocytes |
| VIII | Antihemophilic factor | Liver |

## 2.5 Factors Requiring Vitamin K for Synthesis

| Factor | Synonym | Site of synthesis |
|---|---|---|
| II | Prothrombin | Liver |
| VII | Prothrombin conversion factor | Liver |
| IX | Christmas factor | Liver |
| X | Stuart-Prower factor | Liver |

## 2.6 Endogenous Antithrombotic Factors

In order to maintain proper flow of blood through the vasculature, prevent pathologic thrombosis, and to clear clots during healing, endogenous factors/systems are present to provide a "checks and balances" to the prothrombotic reactions. The antithrombotic systems are divided into *anticoagulants*, which decrease the formation of fibrin through inhibition of coagulation sequence enzymes, and the *fibrinolytic system* which lyses fibrin that thereby dissolves forming/formed thrombi (clots). The primary components of the endogenous anticoagulants are antithrombin, tissue factor pathway inhibitor, thrombomodulin, and protein C. The endogenous fibrinolytic enzyme is plasmin.

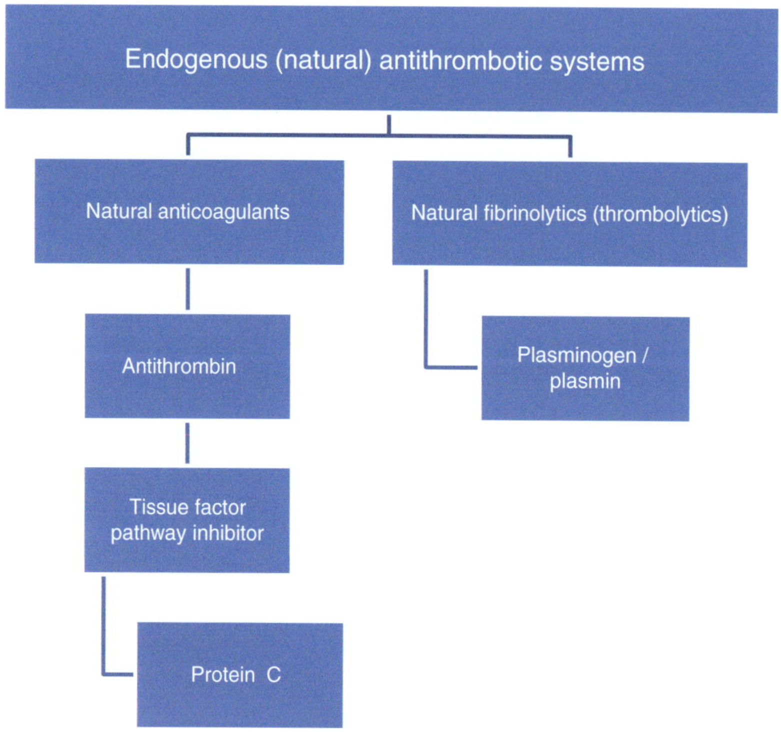


## 2.7 Antithrombin

Antithrombin is synthesized in the liver and circulates in plasma. Antithrombin is a natural anticoagulant which inactivates thrombin and activated factors IX, X, XI, and XII of the coagulation sequence [11, 12].

## 2.8 Tissue Factor Pathway Inhibitor

Tissue factor pathway inhibitor (TFPI) is present in endothelial cells and platelets. Upon endothelial injury, the enzyme is released. TFPI directly inhibits the enzymes of the extrinsic pathway by inhibition of the complex of tissue factor (TF)/factor VIIa/factor Xa. TFPI also inhibits free factor X. The result is a delay and reduction in thrombin and, subsequently, fibrin formation [12].

## 2.9 Thrombomodulin and Protein C

The endothelium also synthesizes and expresses thrombomodulin on its membrane surface. Thrombomodulin serves as an antithrombotic by binding thrombin (factor IIa). Thrombin is potently prothrombotic. However, once bound to thrombomodulin, thrombin is neutralized preventing thrombin-stimulated platelet activation and the conversion of fibrinogen (factor I) to fibrin. In addition, membrane-bound thrombomodulin-thrombin complex activates the natural anticoagulant, protein C. Protein C circulates in plasma and, when activated, neutralizes activated factors V and VIII (fVa and fVIIIa) of the coagulation sequence [13–15].

## 2.10 Fibrinolytic System

The formation of a thrombus is essential in bleeding cessation. The fibrinolytic system is responsible for removing thrombi in order to maintain blood flow to damaged tissues and to allow for tissue healing once bleeding has stopped and the clot is no longer needed. Fibrinolysis relies on the enzyme plasmin to dissolve fibrin. The dissolution of fibrin clots into fibrin degradation products is achieved by a protease called plasmin. Plasminogen, the proenzyme, is manufactured in the liver and released into circulation. Plasminogen binds to fibrinogen and fibrin and is incorporated into the forming blood clot. Plasminogen is cleaved to plasmin in the presence of tissue plasminogen activator (tPA) and urokinase. tPA is released from endothelial cells upon injury and is also stimulated by tissue occlusion, thrombin, epinephrine, vasopressin, and strenuous exercise [12, 15, 16].

Once plasminogen and plasmin are released, they are rapidly inactivated by their inhibitors. The main inhibitors include plasminogen activator inhibitor, which irreversibly inhibits tPA, thereby preventing widespread fibrinolysis [16].

## 2.11 Review of Hemostasis: Putting It All Together

Describing the interactions of the coagulaton enzymes in an attempt to explain the formation of fibrin during coagulation has for decades been provided by the biochemical model of coagulation. Although this model provides insight into the enzymatic reaction and sequencing, hematologists have known for years it does not accurately explain how bleeding is halted at the site in injury. More recently, the cell based model of hemostasis has been proposed as representative of how all of the cellular and enzymatic elements combine to efficiently stop hemorrhage. Both models are reviewed below.

### 2.11.1 Biochemical Model

Our understanding of coagulation has been evolving over the last century and continues to evolve through present day. A major contribution to our understanding of hemostasis occurred in 1964 when the article "Waterfall Sequence for Intrinsic Blood Clotting," in the journal *Science*, proposed a simple waterfall sequence of the clotting factor reactions leading to a fibrin clot [17, 18]. This article was the summation of years of extensive research by a number of scientists in many institiutions [19]. The coagulation "cascade" was then established and has been divided into three interrelated sequences: extrinsic, intrinsic, and common pathways. The extrinsic pathway is also referred to as the initiator and tissue factor pathways since studies suggest coagulation is initiated by tissue factor (factor III) complexing with factor VII. The intrinsic pathway is also referred to as the propagator pathway since this pathway drives fibrin formation after the initial predominance of the extrinsic pathway fades in the coagulation process. Both the extrinsic and intrinsic pathways meet at the common pathway where the end result is the formation of fibrin.

#### 2.11.1.1 The Extrinsic/Initiator/Tissue Factor Pathway

The extrinsic pathway derived its name since an "extrinsic" agent was required to activate the clotting factors. This extravascular factor is known as tissue factor (TF), which is also factor III [20]. Factor III along with factor VII comprises the extrinsic pathway. Tissue factor (TF) is expressed in the vascular smooth muscle, pericytes, and fibroblasts within the vessel wall and in the tissue surrounding the vasculature. TF has been proposed to form a "hemostatic envelope" around blood vessels [20–22]. At the site of injury, tissue factor is exposed which binds circulating factor VII and catalyzes its conversion to activated factor VII (VIIa). Factor VIIa then catalyzes the conversion of factor X to activated factor X in the common pathway. Factor VIIa also activates factor IX [2, 4, 23].

**Extrinsic Factors**
III, VII

#### 2.11.1.2 The Intrinsic/Propagator Pathway

The intrinsic pathway is also referred to as the propagator pathway. The factors that constitute the intrinsic pathway include factors IX, XI, and XII. Factor XII is listed as the first reaction in the pathway. Factor XII is a protein which circulates in plasma. It is activated by contact with collagen in an injured vessel. Activated factor XII (XIIa) catalyzes the activation of factor XI. High-molecular-weight kininogen (HMWK) acts as a cofactor in this conversion and prekallikrein accelerates the reaction. Factor XIa then catalyzes the activation of factor IX (Christmas factor). Factor IXa then activates factor X in the common pathway [2].

**Intrinsic Factors**
IX, XI, XIII

#### 2.11.1.3 Common Pathway

Within the common pathway, three factors undergo proteolysis culminating in the conversion of fibrinogen to fibrin. Factor X becomes activated by products from the extrinsic and intrinsic pathways. Activated factor X (Xa) catalyzes the conversion of factor II (prothrombin) to thrombin. Thrombin then catalyzes the conversion of fibrinogen to fibrin (Fig. 2.1) [3, 10].

**Common Pathway Factors**
I, II, X

Using knowledge of the coagulation reactions, the proposed sequence of events after vessel injury has been described in terms of primary and secondary hemostasis. Primary hemostasis is the reactions leading to formation of the platelet plug. Secondary hemostasis is the formation of fibrin at the platelet plug via the coagulation cascade.

The platelet plug is formed by initial vessel constriction and activation of platelets. Activated platelets then adhere and aggregate to the site of injury via membrane glycoprotein receptors (GP). GPIb/IX/V binds von Willebrand factor (vWF) in the subendothelium. GPVI directly binds exposed collagen. Platelet aggregation then occurs with adjacent platelet GPIa/IIb binding of fibrinogen. The coagulation cascade is then initiated when tissue factor (TF), which is factor III, binds with factor VIIa. These two factors comprise the extrinsic pathway. The complex of FIII/FVIIa catalyzes the conversion of factor X in the common pathway.

### 2.11.2 Cell-Based Model of Hemostasis

The cascade model of coagulation, introduced in 1964, has had a significant impact on understanding of how fibrin is formed. However, researchers and clinicians had known for years this model alone could not readily explain situations encountered clinically. For instance, deficiencies in factor XII do not result in pathologic hemorrhage, whereas deficiencies in factors VIII and IX and hemophilia A and B, respectively, are consistently linked to pathologic hemorrhage [4]. It had also become obvious to researchers that membrane phospholipids were essential for in vivo thrombin and fibrin formation. Accumulation of data led researchers to develop surface-dependent and cell-dependent models of hemostasis that has now become a modern theory of in vivo hemostasis known as the cell-based model of hemostasis [4, 8, 18, 23–26]. Cell-based hemostasis links the enzymatic activation of factors as described above with specific cells accumulating at the site of vascular injury. A brief description of this model is as follows:

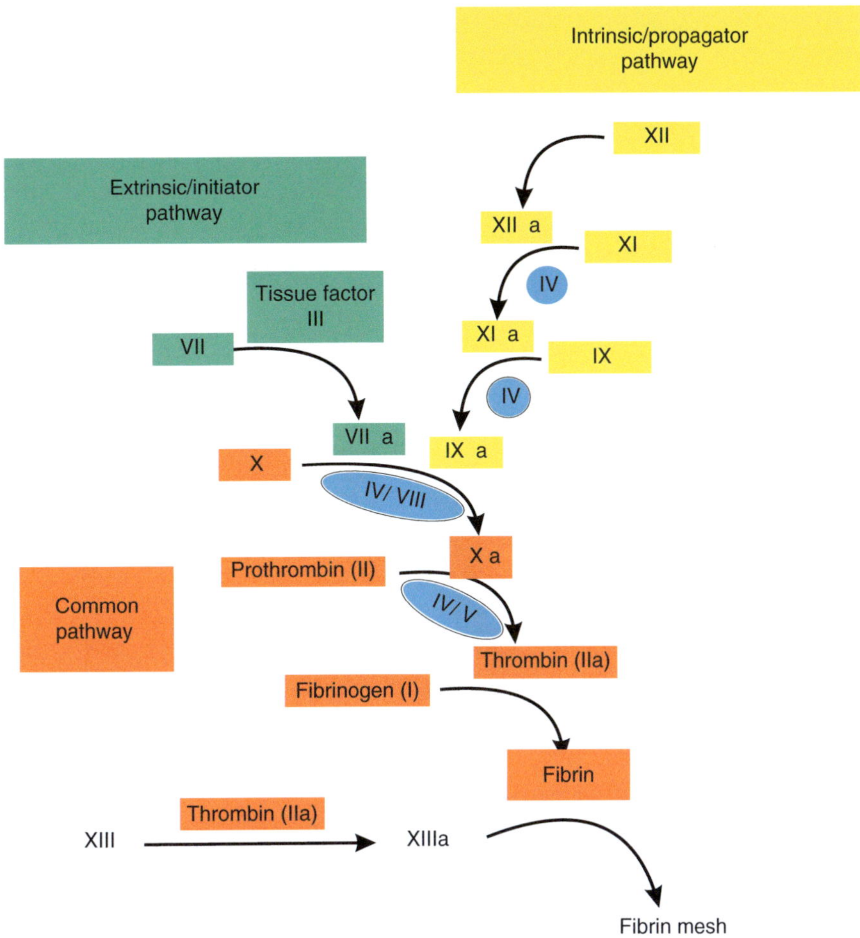


**Fig. 2.1** Coagulation cascade: Biochemical Model

The process of coagulation begins when tissue factor (FIII) is exposed to blood at the site of injury. As discussed above, tissue factor is a transmembrane protein found in certain perivascular cells. Tissue factor functions as a receptor and cofactor for FVII. Factor VII circulates in the blood, and if a disruption of the vessel wall is encountered, FVII will adhere to the TF in the membranes of exposed cells—fibroblasts, etc. Once bound to TF, FVII becomes activated to FVIIa. The TF/FVIIa cell membrane-bound complex then activates factor X and factor IX. Factor Xa reacts with cofactor Va to produce a small amount of thrombin at the TF/FVIIa complex. This thrombin serves several functions: activates platelets and activates factors V, VIII, and XI. These reactions are restricted to the TF-bearing cells since FXa is immediately inactivated by the natural anticoagulants antithrombin (AT) and tissue factor pathway inhibitor (TFPI).

The other factor activated by the TF/FVIIa complex, FIXa, is not inactivated by TFPI and only slowly by AT and, therefore, can diffuse to the surface of the activated platelets that are adhering to the injury site and aggregating by mechanisms previously discussed. Factor IXa binds to platelet receptors. Activated platelets also bind factors Va, VIIIa, and XIa. The platelet-bound activated factors Va, VIIIa, IXa, and XIa are now responsible for further activation of plasma FX leading to a significant amount of thrombin production on the platelet surface. This thrombin is now the catalyst for converting fibrinogen to fibrin and for activating factor XIII which will stabilize the clot [4, 18].

This cell-based model is divided into three overlapping processes: initiation, amplification, and propagation. Initiation refers to the phase when exposed cell membrane tissue factor binds FVII, and the TF/VIIa cell-bound complex activates factor X leading to a small amount of thrombin production. Amplification is when the thrombin produced during initiation activates platelets and factors V, VIII, and XI. These activations set in motion the procoagulant response which will lead to an explosion of thrombin production at the platelet membrane surface considered the propagation phase [4].

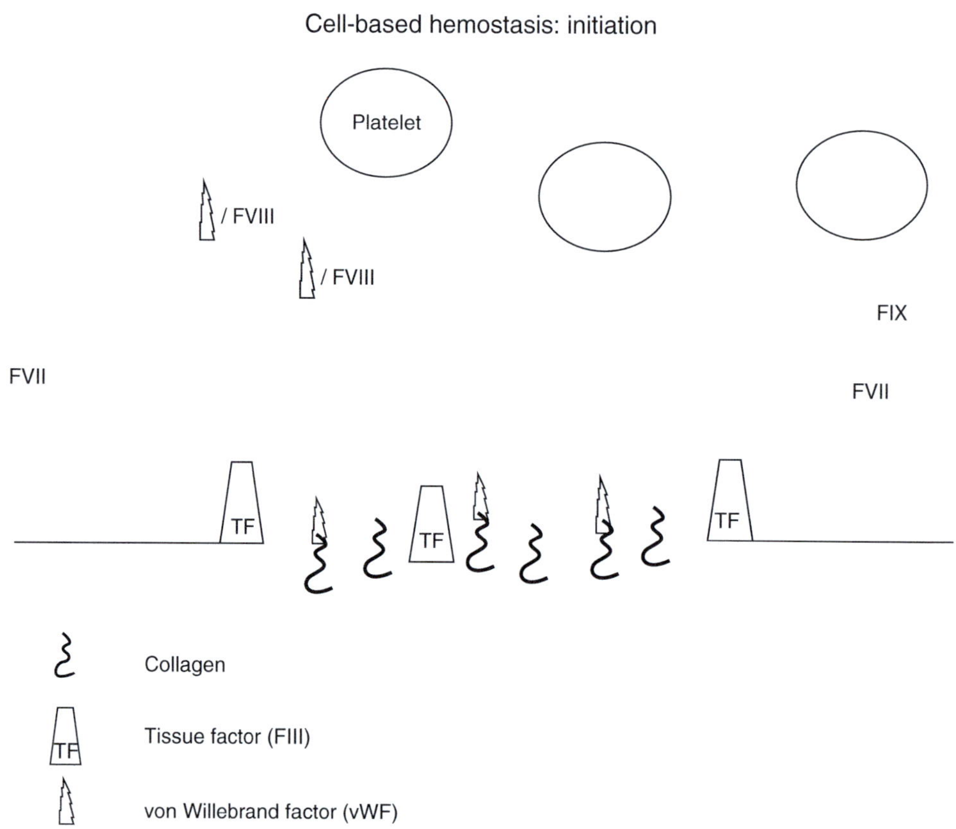

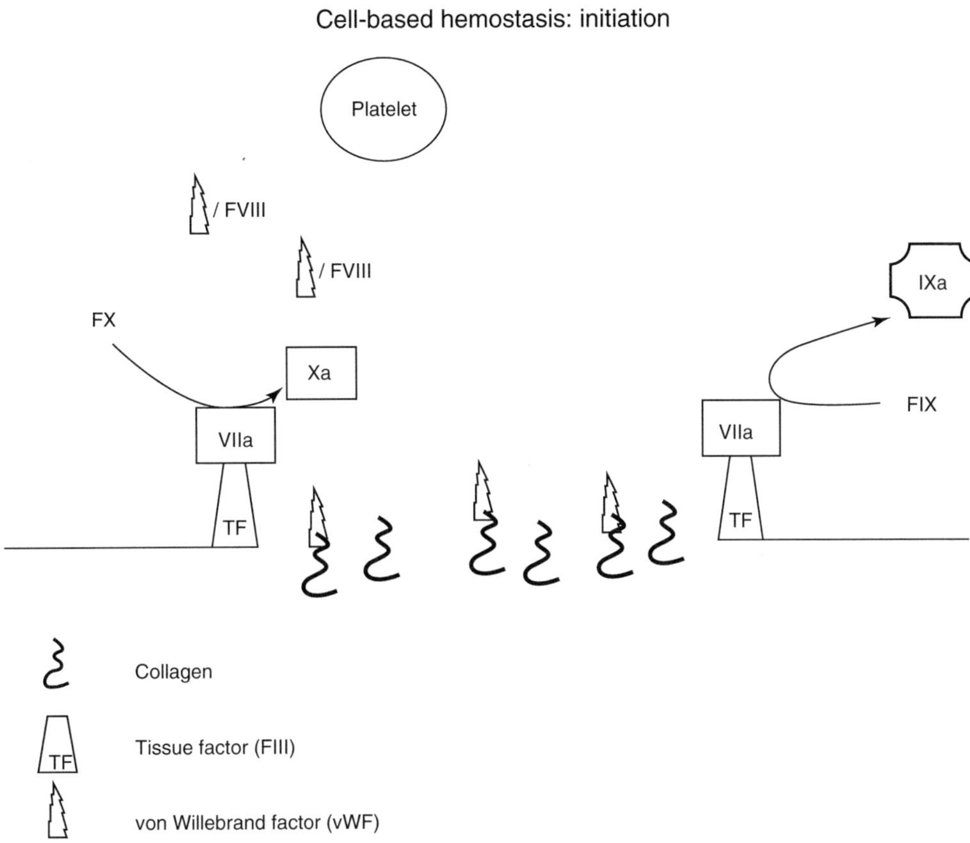
Cell-based hemostasis: initiation
Platelet
/ FVIII
/ FVIII
FX
Xa
VIIa
TF
IXa
FIX
VIIa
TF
Collagen
Tissue factor (FIII)
von Willebrand factor (vWF)

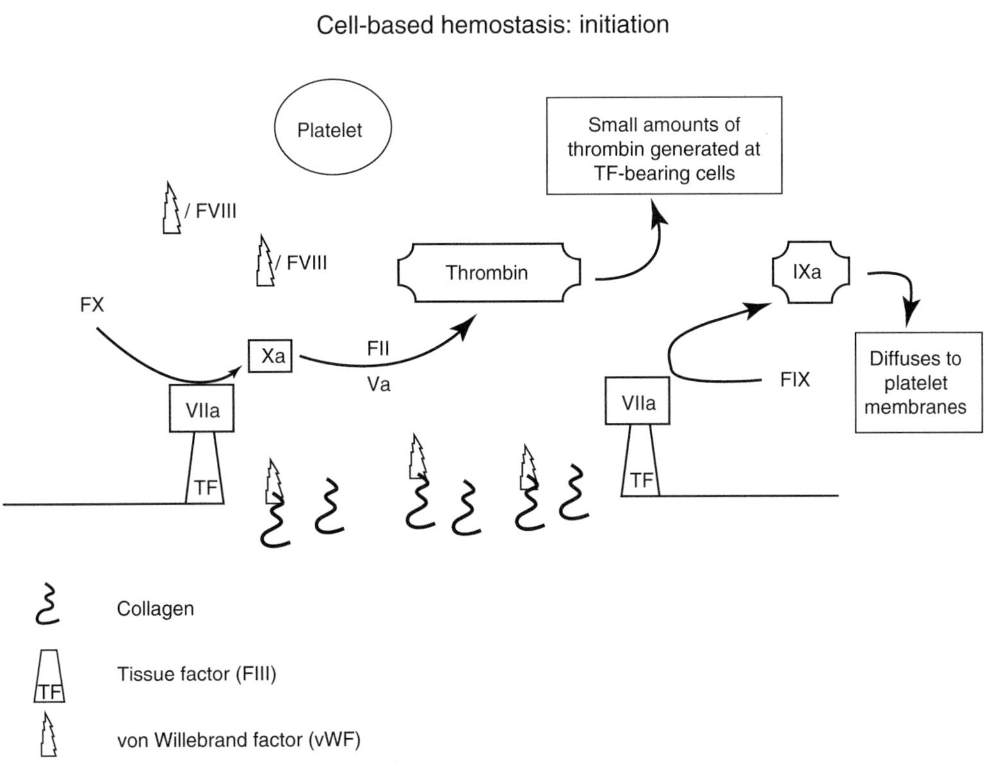
Cell-based hemostasis: initiation
Platelet
Small amounts of thrombin generated at TF-bearing cells
/ FVIII
/ FVIII
Thrombin
IXa
FX
Xa
FII
Va
VIIa
TF
FIX
VIIa
TF
Diffuses to platelet membranes
Collagen
Tissue factor (FIII)
von Willebrand factor (vWF)

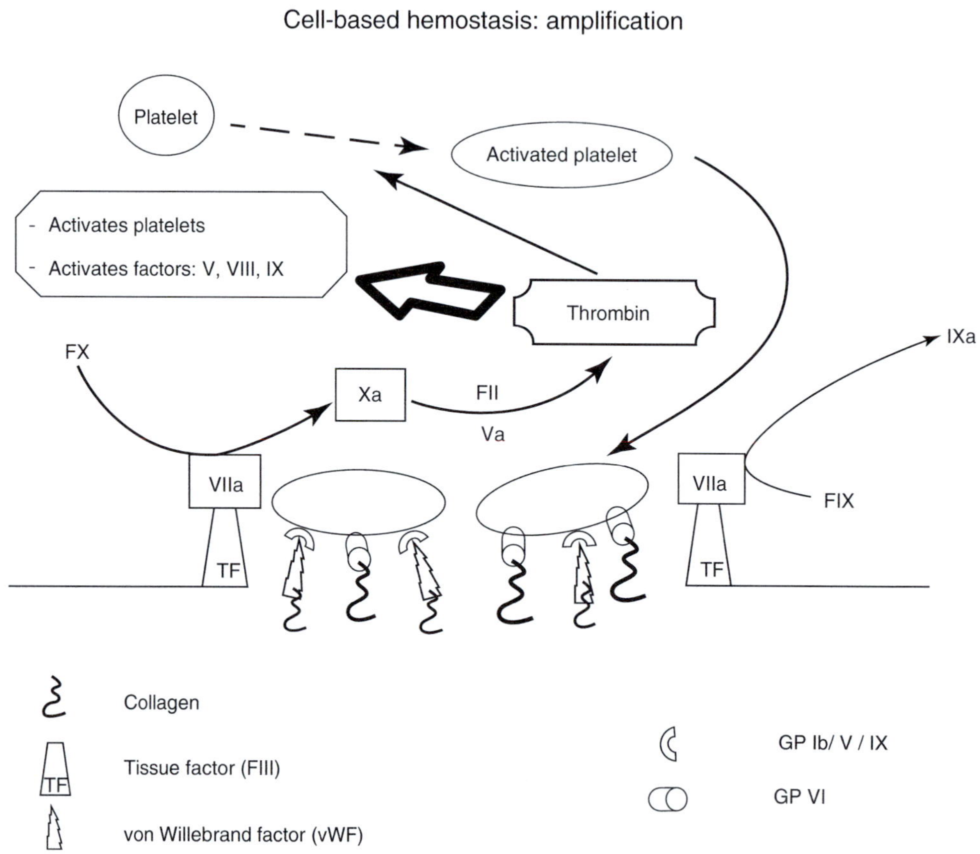
Cell-based hemostasis: amplification
Platelet
Activated platelet
- Activates platelets
- Activates factors: V, VIII, IX
Thrombin
FX
Xa
FII
Va
IXa
VIIa
TF
VIIa
FIX
TF
Collagen
Tissue factor (FIII)
von Willebrand factor (vWF)
GP Ib/ V / IX
GP VI

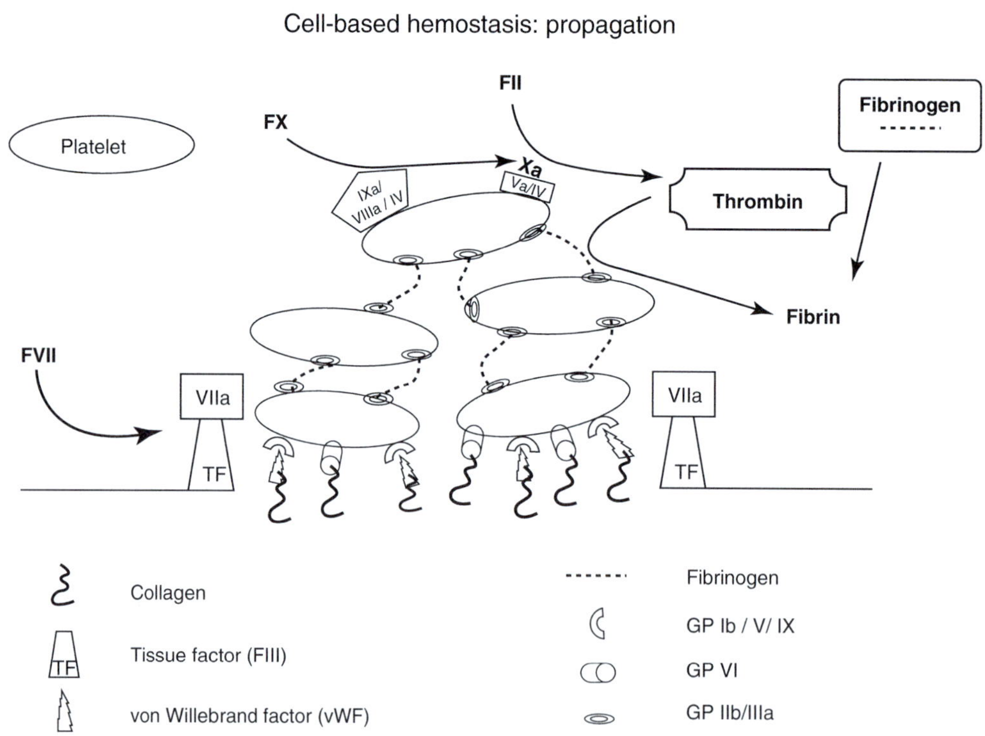
Cell-based hemostasis: propagation
FII
Fibrinogen
FX
Platelet
Xa
IXa/ VIIIa / IV
Va/IV
Thrombin
Fibrin
FVII
VIIa
VIIa
TF
TF
Collagen
Tissue factor (FIII)
von Willebrand factor (vWF)
Fibrinogen
GP Ib / V/ IX
GP VI
GP IIb/IIIa

Diagrams adapted from: Selective Readings in Oral and Maxillofacial Surgery [27].

### 2.11.3 Thrombus

The summation of cellular and enzymatic processes is the formation of the thrombus or clot immediately at the site of disruption of blood vessel integrity. The thrombus thus contains platelets and fibrin. The platelets were anchored to the wound by glycoprotein receptor binding to exposed vWF and collagen at the injury. The platelets aggregate by membrane glycoprotein receptor binding of fibrinogen.

## References


1. Jaques LB. Nomenclature for blood clotting factors. Can Med Assoc J. 1960;82:1327–30.
2. Hall JE. Guyton and hall textbook of medical physiology. 12th ed. Philadelphia: W.B. Saunders Company; 2011.
3. Macik BG. Hemostasis. In: Moylan JA, editor. Surgical critical care. St. Louis: Mosby-Year Book, Inc.; 1994. p. 697–718.
4. Hoffman M, Monroe DM. Coagulation 2006: a modern view of hemostasis. Hematol Oncol Clin North Am. 2007;21(1):1–11.
5. Tanaka KA, Levy JH. Regulation of thrombin activity—pharmacologic and structural aspects. Hematol Oncol Clin North Am. 2007;21(1):33–50.
6. Furie B, Furie BC. Molecular and cellular biology of blood coagulation. N Engl J Med. 1992;326(12):800–6.
7. Mackman N. The many faces of tissue factor. J Thromb Haemost. 2009;7(Suppl 1):136–9.
8. McMichael M. New models of hemostasis. Top Companion Anim Med. 2012;27(2):40–5.
9. Vadivel K, Bajaj SP. Structural biology of factor VIIa/tissue factor initiated coagulation. Front Biosci (Landmark Ed). 2012;17:2476–94.
10. Guyton AC, Hall JE. Textbook of medical physiology. 11th ed. Philadelphia: Elsevier Inc.; 2006.
11. Shuman MA. Endothelial cell structure and function. In: Hoffman R, Benz J, Edward J, Shattil SJ, Furie B, Cohen HJ, Silberstein LE, editors. Hematology basic principles and practice. 2nd ed. New York: Churchill Livingstone Inc.; 1995. p. 1552–65.
12. Yau JW, Teoh H, Verma S. Endothelial cell control of thrombosis. BMC Cardiovasc Disord. 2015;15:130.
13. Sisk AL. Vasoconstrictors in local anesthesia for dentistry. Anesth Prog. 1992;39(6):187–93.
14. Leong M, Phillips LG. Wound healing. In: Townsend CM, Beauchamp RD, Evers BM, Mattox KL, editors. Sabiston textbook of surgery, the biological basis of modern surgical practice. 19th ed. Philadelphia: Elsevier Saunders; 2012. p. 151–77.
15. Chapin JC, Hajjar KA. Fibrinolysis and the control of blood coagulation. Blood Rev. 2015;29(1):17–24.
16. Palta S, Saroa R, Palta A. Overview of the coagulation system. Indian J Anaesth. 2014;58(5):515–23.
17. Davie EW, Ratnoff OD. Waterfall sequence for intrinsic blood clotting. Science. 1964;145(3638): 1310–2.
18. Romney G, Glick M. An updated concept of coagulation with clinical implications. J Am Dent Assoc. 2009;140(5):567–74.
19. Davie EW. A brief historical review of the waterfall/cascade of blood coagulation. J Biol Chem. 2003;278(51):50819–32.
20. Mackman N. The role of tissue factor and factor VIIa in hemostasis. Anesth Analg. 2009;108(5):1447–52.
21. Mackman N, Taubman M. Tissue factor: past, present, and future. Arterioscler Thromb Vasc Biol. 2009;29(12):1986–8.
22. Drake TA, Morrissey JH, Edgington TS. Selective cellular expression of tissue factor in human tissues. Implications for disorders of hemostasis and thrombosis. Am J Pathol. 1989;134(5):1087–97.
23. Mann KG, Krishnaswamy S, Lawson JH. Surface-dependent hemostasis. Semin Hematol. 1992;29(3): 213–26.
24. Hoffman M, Monroe DM 3rd. A cell-based model of hemostasis. Thromb Haemost. 2001;85(6):958–65.
25. Monroe DM, Hoffman M, Roberts HR. Platelets and thrombin generation. Arterioscler Thromb Vasc Biol. 2002;22(9):1381–9.
26. Heemskerk JW, Mattheij NJ, Cosemans JM. Platelet-based coagulation: different populations, different functions. J Thromb Haemost. 2013;11(1):2–16.
27. Szumita RP, Szumita P. Hemostasis: a clinical review of physiology, pathology, pharmacology, and perioperative management. Selected Readings in Oral and Maxillofacial Surgery. 2013;21(3). www.selectedreadingsoms.com.

# Part II

# Pathophysiology and Pharmacotherapy of Hemostasis in Dentistry

# 3 Review of von Willebrand Disease and Perioperative Management in Dentistry

Richard P. Szumita

**Abstract**

von Willebrand disease (vWD) is the most common inherited coagulation disorder. In addition, vWD can also be acquired later in life in patients with no previous history of pathologic bleeding. vWD is the result of either a quantitative deficit or a qualitative defect in von Willebrand factor (vWF). Each patient's disease is classified based on the type of defect in vWF. Dental and surgical management of patients with vWD is based on the severity of their disease, and several systemic and local treatments are available to allow for the hemorrhage control. This chapter will review important aspects of vWF, classification of vWD, and treatment of the dental patient with vWD.

## 3.1 von Willebrand Disease

von Willebrand disease (vWD) results from either a decrease in the quantity of, or a structural defect in, vWF. vWD is classified according to the type of alteration in vWF. When all types are considered, vWD is the most common inherited bleeding disorder. Clinically, there is significant variability in patient presentation and degree of bleeding risk [1–7, 11].

R. P. Szumita
Department of Dentistry/Oral and Maxillofacial Surgery, St. Joseph's University Medical Center, Paterson, NJ, USA

Private Practice, Little Falls, NJ, USA
e-mail: Szumita@northeastoralsurgerycenter.com

## 3.2 von Willebrand Factor (vWF)

The primary structure of von Willebrand factor (vWF) is a large glycosylated protein which is synthesized in endothelial cells and megakaryocytes (platelet precursors) [7, 9, 10]. vWF is found in platelets, endothelial cells, basement membrane of blood vessels, and circulating in plasma. The primary functions of vWF are to promote attachment of platelets to areas of vessel injury and to act as a carrier molecule for circulating factor VIII (FVIII), stabilizing this important factor in plasma [2, 5, 9, 11–13].

Following initial assembly of the large protein structure in the nucleus of endothelial cells and megakaryocytes, vWF undergoes modifications in the endoplasmic reticulum and Golgi apparatus resulting in the formation of multimeric (multiple repeating segments) complexes of varying molecular weights. The size of the mature vWF helps determine its location. Smaller vWF is secreted



R. P. Szumita, P. M. Szumita (eds.), *Hemostasis in Dentistry*, https://doi.org/10.1007/978-3-319-71240-6_3

into circulation, while larger multimers of vWF are stored in α-granules of the platelets or Weibel–Palade bodies of endothelial cells. vWF released into circulation bind with factor VIII (antihemophilic factor) protecting the factor from degradation [5, 7, 9]. vWF stored in endothelial cells is released into both the circulation and the adjacent subendothelium upon stimulation by thrombin, fibrin, or desmopressin (DDAVP). vWF contained in the α-granules of platelets is released upon vessel injury [11, 12].

The multimeric nature of the protein structure of the mature vWF allows it to possess unique binding sites for platelet membrane receptors, collagen, and factor VIII. There are four binding sites on vWF which interact with platelet membrane receptor (GpIb/IX/V) involved in platelet adhesion, platelet membrane receptor (GpIIb/IIIa) integral in platelet aggregation, subendothelial collagen exposed after endothelial damage, and factor VIII [9, 11–13].

von Willebrand factor is an important adhesive protein aiding in platelet adhesion to the injured tissue by binding with collagen and with the platelet membrane receptor, GPIb/IX/V [14, 15].

Exposed collagen in the subendothelium of injured perivascular tissue serves two major functions. First, collagen is a potent platelet activator. Second, collagen serves as a binding site for platelet adhesion via vWF or as direct binding to platelet membrane receptor GPVI [16–18].

## 3.3 Classification of vWD

vWD is primarily an inherited disease, but acquired vWD has also been noted. Acquired forms of the disease are associated with pathologic conditions. Both forms are discussed below.

The most widely known classification system describes the hereditary form of vWD [1]. This system classifies vWD into three general types: 1, 2, and 3. Types 1 and 3 vWD encompass quantitative deficits in vWF. Type 2 vWD includes qualitative defects in vWF. Including all types of vWD, the prevalence is approximately 1–3% in the general population [10].

Type 1 vWD is the most common form of the disease accounting for roughly 70–80% of all cases of vWD. Type 1 is due to a decrease in vWF levels (usually 5–50% of normal). The vWF that is synthesized is structurally and functionally normal [2, 5, 13].

Type 2 vWD is the second most common form of the disease accounting for approximately 10–30% of all cases [1]. Type 2 vWD is a result of a structural (qualitative) abnormality of vWF and is further subdivided into four additional subtypes: 2A, 2B, 2M, and 2 N. Each of the subtypes represents a unique qualitative defect [2, 5, 11].

Type 2A vWD is a result of the absence of high molecular weight multimer forms of vWF (smaller molecule) resulting in decreased binding sites on the protein. This reduces the platelet adhesion and collagen binding [2].

Type 2B vWD results from a mutation in the binding site on vWF with platelet GpIb. This mutation results in an increased affinity for circulating vWF binding to platelets in circulation. This gain-of-function trait leads to platelet clumping and often results in varying degrees of thrombocytopenia [5].

Type 2M vWD is characterized by defective platelet adhesion. This decreased activity is similar to type 2A. However, unlike type 2A, the protein structure of vWF does not lack the multimers making it structurally more "normal." Similar to type 2B, the defect in platelet binding is due to mutations of the platelet binding sites. Unlike type 2B, the mutation results in loss of function [2, 5].

Type 2N vWD is caused by mutations in the binding site for factor VIII (FVIII) resulting in reduced affinity and binding of FVIII. This leads to depressed levels of FVIII and can be confused with hemophilia A [5, 11].

Type 3 vWD is the most severe form of the disease. It is rare with estimated prevalence of 1–3 per million and is characterized by severe quantitative deficiency in vWF in plasma and platelets. Severe mucocutaneous bleeding is seen clinically. In addition, and unlike the other forms of vWD, soft tissue bleeding and bleeding into joints are common [2, 5].

Acquired vWD (AvWD) is a rare form of the disease. This form arises in association with various underlying diseases, including malignancies, autoimmune diseases, and structural cardiac abnormalities (i.e., aortic stenosis) [1, 8, 19]. Patients with AvWD have no prior history of abnormal bleeding and no family history of prolonged bleeding. Bleeding patterns in AvWD is similar to hereditary vWD [8].

**von Willebrand Disease (vWD) Classifications**

*Type 1*: Quantitative (partial) deficit in vWF

*Type 2*: Qualitative defects in vWF

- Type 2A
  - Decreased platelet binding due to lack of normal multimeric form of vWF
- Type 2B
  - Increased affinity for circulating vWF platelet binding; thrombocytopenia present
- Type 2M
  - Decreased platelet binding but with normal multimeric form of vWF
- Type 2N
  - Decreased affinity for factor VIII

*Type 3*: Complete deficiency of vWF

*Acquired vWD*: Arises in associated with certain pathologic diseases; rare.

## 3.4 Clinical Presentation

Diagnosis of vWD is based on three parameters: a history of excessive mucocutaneous bleeding, a family history of excessive bleeding, and laboratory evaluation confirming a quantitative and/or qualitative defect in vWF [5, 11].

Mucocutaneous bleeding includes recurrent gingival bleeding, epistaxis, menorrhagia, prolonged bleeding from lacerations, and easy bruising. Except for type 3 vWD, deep soft tissue bleeding and bleeding into joints are uncommon. Previously undiagnosed vWD have been shown to manifest as prolonged and excessive bleeding following undergoing oral surgical procedures—especially dental extractions [5, 7, 13].

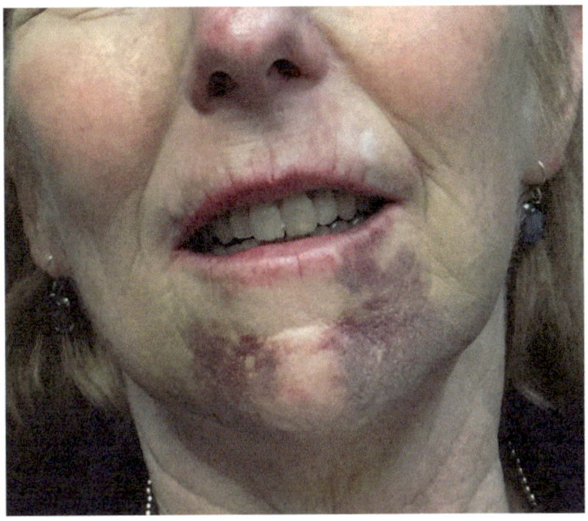

Since types 1, 2A, 2B, and 2M are inherited as an autosomal dominant trait, a family history of bleeding is often elicited during history taking. However, it should be understood that the clinical penetrance of the disease can be variable and a clear family bleeding history is not always present [5, 11].

## 3.5 Management of the Dental Patient with vWD

Dental management of patients with vWD can be divided into two categories. First is the patient without a diagnosis of vWD who presents for dental treatment. The second is management of a patient with a known diagnosis.

Since vWD is the most common inherited bleeding disorder, patients may unknowingly present to the dental office with a yet undiagnosed form of vWD. Especially in younger patients, the removal of teeth (i.e., as part of comprehensive orthodontic treatment) or removal of third molars may be the first significant challenge to their hemostatic system. These oral surgical procedures may uncover their coagulopathy. To minimize this risk, thorough pre-procedural bleeding history should be undertaken. Key questions include a history of frequent and prolonged mucocutaneous bleeding (gingival bleeding and epistaxis), frequent bruising, prolonged bleeding from uncomplicated skin lacerations, and, in females, heavy menses. Any positive response should trigger further questioning of bleeding tendencies and asking about family history of bleeding. If any concern is raised, evaluation with the patient's primary physician and/or a hematologist would be prudent.

In patients who present with a documented diagnosis of vWD, safely delivering dental treatment will be guided by three key elements: reviewing the patient's hematologic history, assessing dental needs and the anticipated procedural risks for bleeding, and communicating and coordinating with the patient's hematologist. The following questions should be included in the patient interview: When was the initial diagnosis of vWD made? Do you know now which type of vWD you have? What types of bleeding have you experienced? How have you controlled bleeding? Have you had dental treatment or surgery since your diagnosis? If so, what treatment was administered to help control bleeding. Have you required hospitalizations for bleeding episodes? Answers to these questions should provide insight to the patient's disease severity, previous effective treatment strategies, and response to treatment.

Next, the dental team is the best suited to assess the risks associated with various dental procedures. The many and various dental and oral surgical procedures are associated with varying degrees of bleeding risk. Recently, a dental bleeding risk assessment and treatment tool (DeBRATT) was devised and studied. Dental procedures were categorized into noninvasive, minimally invasive, moderately invasive, and highly invasive based on tendency to cause bleeding [20]. This tool may prove to be a useful adjunct when communicating with the patient's hematologist.

The last element in the pre-procedural phase is communicating and coordinating with the patient's hematologist. Information to confirm is the type of vWD and severity of disease. The dentist/dental team should relay the anticipated bleeding risk to the hematologist in order to devise appropriate treatment strategies.

Treatment strategies aimed at preventing pathologic bleeding are divided into local and systemic management. The dentist is responsible for deciding upon and implementing the local treatments. The systemic treatments are prescribed and administered by the hematologist.

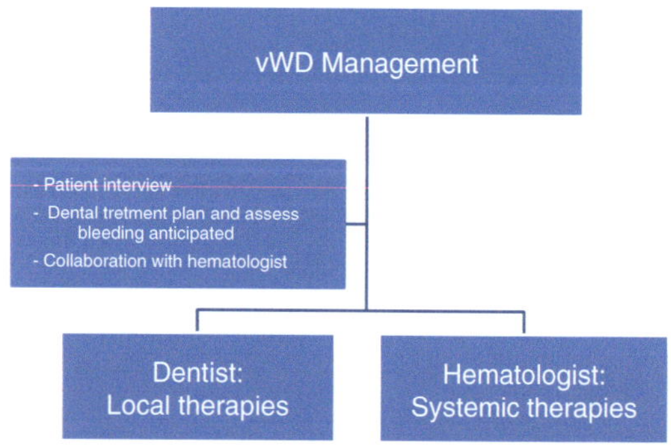


Local treatments are reviewed in detail in Chap. 15. Briefly, precision in performing surgical procedures, careful handling of the soft tissues, and suturing helps limit local bleeding in all patients. Additionally, the application of one or more of the following prohemostatic therapies has also shown to be effective in vWD: hemostatic wound dressings, tissue adhesives, and use of antifibrinolytic oral rinses are the mainstay of the local treatments [4, 7, 21–23]. As in all cases of wound bleeding, careful assessment of the effectiveness of local measures must be performed. Persistent bleeding should not automatically be assumed to be due to failure of systemic therapy. In instances where maximal effective systemic management has been confirmed with the hematologist, careful reevaluation of the source of wound hemorrhage is required. Patient monitoring and proximal control of contributing vessels may also be required [24, 25].

Systemic therapies are prescribed based on the type and severity of vWD and include the use of desmopressin, systemic antifibrinolytics, factor replacement infusions, and transfusions.

Desmopressin (1-deamino-8-arginine vasopressin; DDAVP) is a synthetic analogue of antidiuretic hormone vasopressin. Upon administration, DDAVP transiently increases FVIII and vWF. The mechanism of action has not been fully established, but the release of vWF from endothelial cells is believed to involve DDAVP binding to the transmembrane protein receptor, V2, which signals release of vWF via intracellular cyclic adenosine monophosphate (c-AMP) [1, 5, 13].

DDAVP is used in the management of vWD types 1, 2A, 2M, and 2N. In type 3 vWD, response is likely to be ineffective since most patients do not synthesize vWF. In type 2B, administering DDAVP worsens the thrombocytopenia. In addition, even when indicated, DDAVP does not always produce sufficient clinical response. This is believed to be the result of one of two mechanisms: either by inducing insufficient release of vWF or the half-life of the released vWF is reduced in certain subsets of the disease. Patients with a known diagnosis of vWD often undergo evaluation for the effectiveness of DDAVP therapy [5, 25].

DDAVP is administered via intravenous, subcutaneous, and intranasal routes. Onset of action is immediate and maximizes at 30–60 min. Factor VIII and vWF levels are increased approximately three to fivefold and for approximately 8–12 h. Side effects of use of DDAVP are usually mild and transient. Primary effects include headache, facial flushing, and mild tachycardia. Since DDAVP possesses an antidiuretic effect, fluid restriction for 24 h following administration is often prescribed by the hematologist [4, 5].

The systemic administration of antifibrinolytic agents is also available to the hematologist. Although not specific for treatment of vWD, antifibrinolytics have been shown to be important adjuncts in achieving hemostasis in disease and medication-induced oral bleeding as oral mucosa and saliva contain high levels of plasminogen activators [26]. The available forms of antifibrinolytic agents are aminocaproic acid and tranexamic acid.

Antifibrinolytics are reviewed in Chap. 15. In brief, the mechanism of action of antifibrinolytic agents is the inhibition of the conversion of plasminogen to plasmin by reversibly binding to plasminogen [26]. Plasmin is a proteolytic enzyme that hydrolyzes fibrin [27]. By blocking the effect of plasmin, the forces responsible for dissolving the fibrin are lessened, and the clot is "stabilized." Both aminocaproic acid and tranexamic acid block the conversion of plasminogen to plasmin, thereby stabilizing the forming clot. Aminocaproic acid is supplied as tablets (500 and 1000 mg) and syrup (250 mg/cc) for oral use and an intravenous formulation (5 g/20 cc). Tranexamic acid is supplied as 600 mg tablets and an intravenous formulation of 1000 mg/10 cc [28]. Depending on the dental procedures scheduled to be performed, systemic antifibrinolytics can be administered orally for dental office procedures. In major maxillofacial surgical procedures, the agent can be administered intravenously while in the hospital.

In vWD types 2B and 3, where DDAVP is not indicated, and in cases of failure of DDAVP in the other types of vWD, clotting factor concentrates are available for infusion. Historically, infusion of cryoprecipitate (which contains factors I, VIII, XIII, vWF) had been the main treatment for patients for whom DDAVP was contraindicated or ineffective. The primary drawback with cryoprecipitate is a small risk of transmitting blood-borne infections. Concentrates of factor VIII-vWF, which were initially developed for management of hemophilia A, are now available and recommended for use in vWD. These concentrates are treated to inactivate blood-borne viruses [3, 13]. Factor concentrates are discussed in detail in Chap. 11.

In summary, vWD is primarily an inherited bleeding disorder and is present in approximately 1% of the population. This prevalence essentially guarantees the dental team will encounter and treat patients with this condition. vWD is a complex disease with significant variability in clinical presentations. Patients, especially young patients, may present for dental treatment without having been diagnosed. Careful pretreatment bleeding history should be obtained. A history of unusual and prolonged mucosal bleeding and excessive bruising, especially if unusual bleeding has been noted in a family member, should raise suspicions of possible vWD. In patients with a diagnosis of vWD, the type of disease and the patient's experience with bleeding episodes should be reviewed with the patient and the hematologist. Treatment strategies utilizing local and systemic therapies have proven effective in avoiding excessive bleeding during and following dental and oral and maxillofacial procedures.

## References


1. Mazzeffi MA, Stone ME. Perioperative management of von Willebrand disease: a review for the anesthesiologist. J Clin Anesth. 2011;23(5):418–26.
2. Federici AB. Classification of inherited von Willebrand disease and implications in clinical practice. Thromb Res. 2009;124(Suppl 1):S2–6.
3. Nitu-Whalley IC, Griffioen A, Harrington C, Lee CA. Retrospective review of the management of elective surgery with desmopressin and clotting factor concentrates in patients with von Willebrand disease. Am J Hematol. 2001;66(4):280–4.
4. Israels S, Schwetz N, Boyar R, McNicol A. Bleeding disorders: characterization, dental considerations and management. J Can Dent Assoc. 2006;72(9):827.
5. Lillicrap D. The basic science, diagnosis, and clinical management of von Willebrand disease. Treatment of Hemophilia. Monograph No. 35. 2008:18.
6. Zulfikar B, Koc B, Ak G, et al. Surgery in patients with von Willebrand disease. Blood Coagul Fibrinolysis. 2016;27(7):812–6.
7. Wilde JT, Cook RJ. von Willebrand disease and its management in oral and maxillofacial surgery. Br J Oral Maxillofac Surg. 1998;36(2):112–8.
8. Hanratty JM, Cowan CG. Acquired von Willebrand disease secondary to hypothyroidism: a rare cause for postextraction hemorrhage. Oral Surg Oral Med Oral Pathol Oral Radiol Endod. 2010;110(3):337–40.
9. Wagner DD, Ginsburg D. Structure, biology, and genetics of von Willebrand factor. In: Hoffman R, et al., editors. Hematology: basic principles and practice. 2nd ed. New York: Churchill Livingstone; 1995. p. 1717–25.
10. Murray EW, Lillicrap D. von Willebrand disease: pathogenesis, classification, and management. Transfus Med Rev. 1996;10(2):93–110.
11. Leebeek FW, Eikenboom JC. Von Willebrand's disease. N Engl J Med. 2016;375(21):2067–80.
12. Springer TA. von Willebrand factor, Jedi knight of the bloodstream. Blood. 2014;124(9):1412–25.
13. Mannucci PM. How I treat patients with von Willebrand disease. Blood. 2001;97(7):1915–9.
14. Sumpio BE, Riley JT, Dardik A. Cells in focus: endothelial cell. Int J Biochem Cell Biol. 2002;34(12):1508–12.
15. Andrews RK, Berndt MC. Platelet physiology and thrombosis. Thromb Res. 2004;114(5–6):447–53.
16. Hall JE. Guyton and hall textbook of medical physiology. 12th ed. Philadelphia: W.B. Saunders Company; 2011.
17. Versteeg HH, Heemskerk JW, Levi M, Reitsma PH. New fundamentals in hemostasis. Physiol Rev. 2013;93(1):327–58.
18. Lowenberg EC, Meijers JC, Levi M. Platelet-vessel wall interaction in health and disease. Neth J Med. 2010;68(6):242–51.
19. Lison S, Dietrich W, Spannagl M. Review article: Unexpected bleeding in the operating room: the role of acquired von Willebrand disease. Anesth Analg. 2012;114(1):73–81.
20. Rasaratnam L, Chowdary P, Pollard D, Subel B, Harrington C, Darbar UR. Risk-based management of dental procedures in patients with inherited bleeding disorders: Development of a Dental Bleeding Risk Assessment and Treatment Tool (DeBRATT). Haemophilia. 2017;23(2):247–54.
21. Federici AB, Sacco R, Stabile F, Carpenedo M, Zingaro E, Mannucci PM. Optimising local therapy during oral surgery in patients with von Willebrand disease: effective results from a retrospective analysis of 63 cases. Haemophilia. 2000;6(2):71–7.
22. Bornert F, Clauss F, Gros CI, et al. Hemostatic management in pediatric patients with type I von Willebrand disease undergoing oral surgery: case report and literature review. J Oral Maxillofac Surg. 2011;69(8):2086–91.
23. Malmquist JP. Complications in oral and maxillofacial surgery: management of hemostasis and bleeding disorders in surgical procedures. Oral Maxillofac Surg Clin North Am. 2011;23(3):387–94.
24. Faverani LP, Gaetti-Jardim EC, Ramalho-Ferreira G, Gulinelli JL, Queiroz TP, Garcia Junior IR. Ligature of external carotid artery as an optional technique in a patient with von Willebrand disease. Braz Dent J. 2011;22(5):435–8.
25. Gill JC. Treatment of urgent bleeding in von Willebrand disease. Thromb Res. 2007;120(Suppl 1):S21–5.
26. Mannucci PM. Hemostatic drugs. N Engl J Med. 1998;339(4):245–53.
27. O'Reilly RA. Anticoagulant, antithrombotic, and thrombolytic drugs. In: Gilman AG, Goodman LS, Rall TW, Murad F, editors. Goodman and Gilman's the pharmacological basis of therapeutics. 7th ed. New York: Macmillan Publishing Company; 1985. p. 1338–62.
28. Hamilton R, editor. Tarascon pocket pharmacopoeia. Burlington, MA: Jones & Bartlett Publishing; 2015.

# 4 Review of Hemophilia A and B and Perioperative Management in Dentistry

Pooja Gangwani and Ryan Richards

**Abstract**

Hemophilia A (classic hemophilia) and hemophilia B (Christmas disease) are inherited disorders of coagulation that can produce life-threatening bleeding. Patients with hemophilia will require special management strategies in order to safely undergo dental treatment. Patient management is optimized when the dental professional has a basic understanding of how these diseases affect hemostasis, is familiar with medical/systemic treatment strategies available to the hematologist, and knows the principles of dental/local management of patients with bleeding risks. In order to help with these goals, this chapter reviews the pathophysiology, clinical presentation, patient evaluation, and basics of medical management of hemophilia. These reviews are presented with an emphasis given to the dental management of patients with hemophilia A and B.

Hemophilia A and hemophilia B are X-linked recessive congenital bleeding disorders caused by deficiency of coagulation factor VIII and factor IX, respectively [1–4]. Hemophilia A is more common than hemophilia B, comprising 80–85% of the total hemophilia population [1–3]. Owing to the inheritance pattern, males are more commonly affected than females [1–3]. However, one third of all cases occur due to spontaneous mutation [1–3]. Hemophilia is noted to occur in all ethnic groups, with no racial or geographic predilection [1, 2].

Hemarthroses and bleeding in soft tissues are characteristic features of hemophilia A and B [1–3]. Intracranial, neck, and gastrointestinal bleeding can be life threatening and warrants immediate treatment [1–3]. Factor levels in the plasma correlate to severity of clinical expression [1–4]. Based on factor levels, hemophilia is categorized into three types, namely, mild (5–40%), moderate (1–5%) and severe (<1%). 50–100% is considered as normal range [1–4]. Generally, patients with mild hemophilia do not bleed spontaneously [1–3]. They only bleed when subjected to surgical procedures, dental extractions, or trauma [1–3]. Excessive bleeding is seen in patients with moderate hemophilia in response to minor surgery or trauma [1–3]. Patients with severe hemophilia bleed spontaneously into joints and muscles in addition to massive bleeding after trauma or surgery [1–3]. The purpose of

P. Gangwani (✉) · R. Richards
Oral and Maxillofacial Surgery, St. Joseph's University Medical Center, Paterson, NJ, USA


R. P. Szumita, P. M. Szumita (eds.), *Hemostasis in Dentistry*, https://doi.org/10.1007/978-3-319-71240-6_4

this chapter is to discuss appropriate management of patients with hemophilia in the setting of oral and maxillofacial surgery.

## 4.1 Pathophysiology

Hemophilia A, also referred to as classic hemophilia, is caused by a deficiency in factor VIII. Hemophilia A is the most common hereditary disease associated with life-threatening hemorrhage [12]. Hemophilia B, also known as Christmas disease, is due to a deficiency in factor IX and produces a disorder clinically indistinguishable from hemophilia A [12]. Both hemophilia A and B are X-linked recessive disorders [1, 2, 12]. As a result of the X-linked inheritance pattern, hemophilia A and B are more commonly seen in males than females [2]. Hemophilia A and B are the only hereditary clotting disorders with a X-linked inheritance pattern (Fig. 4.1) [1].

The genes that encode coagulation factors VIII and IX are located on the long arm of the X-chromosome [1]. The genetic mutations lead to a qualitative decrease in protein activity, a quantitative decrease in protein expression, or both [1]. A father who has hemophilia will produce female offspring that are carriers, but none of his male offspring will be affected [2]. A mother who is a carrier will have 50% chance of producing male offspring with hemophilia and a 50% chance of producing female offspring who is a carrier [2].

In order to understand the pathophysiology of hemophilia, a thorough understanding of the primary and secondary mechanisms of hemostasis is essential. The main function of the hemostatic mechanism is to maintain vascular patency while

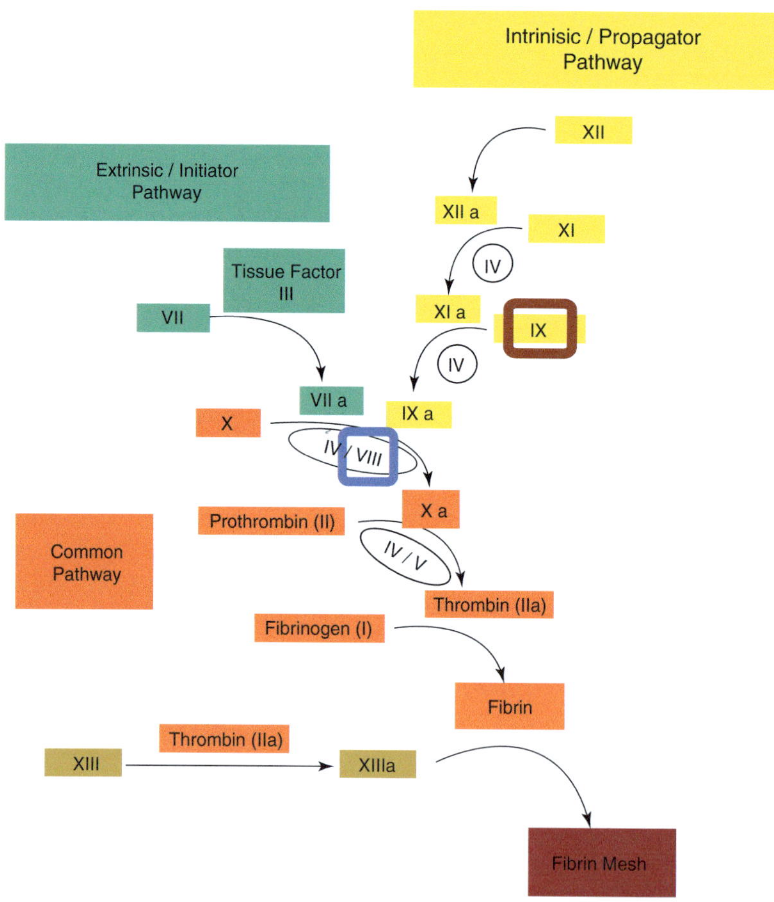


**Fig. 4.1** Factor VIII outlined in blue box; Factor IX outlined in brown box

restoring endothelial continuity when the vasculature is injured [1]. The four principal events in hemostasis are initial vasoconstriction, platelet plug formation, thrombus formation, and eventual fibrous tissue ingrowth into the thrombus [12]. Directly after trauma to a blood vessel, smooth muscle cells within the vascular wall contract, resulting in reduced vessel diameter, are decreasing the blood flow through the injured vessel [12]. When circulating platelets come into contact with collagen fibers exposed through the damaged vascular surface and von Willebrand factor (vWF) that seeps into the tissue, their physical properties change [12]. The activated platelets become adhesive and stick to THE exposed collagen and vWF forming the initial platelet plug [12]. These platelets secrete many factors, including thromboxane $A_2$, which activate adjacent platelets to reinforce the initial platelet plug [12].

The coagulation factors circulate through the vascular system in inactivated forms [1]. Soft tissue trauma causes release of various factors from the vascular wall, activated platelets, and tissue factor. Exposed tissue factor binds activated factor VII forming a tissue factor—factor VII complex [1]. This complex activates factor X and factor IX. Activated factor X converts prothrombin (factor II) to thrombin (activated factor II) [1]. Thrombin activates factor VIII and causes release of activated factor IX [1]. Activated factor VIII and IX along with calcium form the tenase complex, which activates factor X, amplifying the production of thrombin, converting fibrinogen to fibrin leading to fibrin clot formation [1]. Thus, the pathophysiology of hemophilia A and B lies in the reduced quantities of activated factors VIII and IX, reduced tenase complex formation, and dysfunctional clot formation [1].

## 4.2 Laboratory Findings

Proper diagnosis is crucial to management of patients with bleeding disorders. For this purpose, coagulation screening tests and factor assays are employed. Prolongation of activated partial thromboplastin time (PTT) is found in patients with hemophilia [1, 2]. It is increased by 2–3 times higher than normal in severe hemophilia [1, 2], whereas prothrombin time (PT), thrombin time, and bleeding time are noted to be normal [1, 2]. Additional testing such as measurement of factors VIII and IX is performed to confirm and ascertain the level of factor activity [1, 2]. This further helps to classify the disease as mild, moderate, or severe. Positive result of mixing study indicates possibility of presence of inhibitors. In this study, plasma of hemophilia patient is mixed with normal plasma which contains all the clotting factors. The PPT should normalize. Failure to normalize PTT indicates the presence of inhibitors [1–3].

## 4.3 Inhibitors

Development of inhibitors is the most significant complication of hemophilia treatment [1–3, 5]. Inhibitors are specific immunoglobulins (IgG) that are formed against infused factor VIII or IX [1–3]. Infused factors are neutralized by the inhibitors rendering factor VIII or IX ineffective [1–3]. 30% of hemophilia A patients develop inhibitors, whereas incidence in hemophilia B patients is approximately 5% [1–3]. Development of inhibitors is an immune response and it occurs during the first 50 exposures to the factor [1, 5]. Some reports illustrate that inhibitors are formed within the first 20 exposure days [1, 7]. Risk factors include patients with severe disease, family history of inhibitors, and history of blood transfusion prior to factor replacement. Additionally, if patients are exposed to the factor treatment early on in their lifetime, the chance of forming specific antibodies is increased [1, 5, 6]. Some studies have indicated that use of recombinant factor VIII is more likely to cause the development of inhibitors [1]. Bethesda assay is implemented to quantify the inhibitor [1, 3]. Inhibitor titer measurement is expressed as Bethesda units per millimeter [1]. Patients with <5 BU/mL inhibitor titers are considered to have "low titer," whereas patients with ≥5 BU/mL inhibitor titers are considered to have "high titer" [2, 3]. After administration of the factor to a patient with inhibitors, if the titer levels do not increase, the patient is classified as "low responder," and if the titer levels increase, then the patient is classified as "high responder" [2]. Therefore, titer levels and patient's response to the factor play a role in managing hemophilia patients.

## 4.4 Clinical Features

Hemarthroses are a characteristic finding in patients with hemophilia [1, 2]. Knees and elbows are more commonly involved than ankles and shoulders [1, 2]. Wrists and hips are least frequently involved [1, 2]. Symptoms involve swelling, pain, and limited range of motion [1, 2]. Hemarthroses ultimately lead to painful arthropathies and debilitating joint dysfunction [1–3]. Manifestations in patients with severe disease appear in first year of their life, when they begin crawling and walking [1, 3]. Other typical features include easy bruising and bleeding in soft tissues [1–3]. Even though any type of bleeding may occur in patients with hemophilia, recognizing life-threatening bleeds in three areas is imperative: intracranial, iliopsoas, and neck and retropharyngeal space [1–3]. The first area is intracranial hemorrhage (ICH). Majority of deaths in hemophilia patients are attributed ICH [1, 2]. The mortality rate is as high as 20% and most of the patients experience post ICH sequelae [6]. Next in order is bleeding in iliopsoas muscle that can present as pain in the lower abdomen, groin, and/or lower back [1, 3, 7]. There may be altered sensation in the medial aspect of the thigh [3, 7]. Sometimes, loss of patellar reflex secondary to femoral nerve compression is noted [3, 7]. Patients also report painful extension of the hip and weakness of the quadriceps [3, 7]. Large amount of blood is lost in retroperitoneum leading to hypovolemic shock before any symptoms or physical signs appear [1]. Lastly, bleeding in neck and retropharyngeal space can lead to airway embarrassment [1–3].

## 4.5 Medical Management

Factor replacement is required for the treatment of bleeding in patients with hemophilia [1, 2]. They receive factor replacement for the following purposes: prophylactic, treatment of bleeding episodes and perioperatively [1, 2]. Hemophilia prophylaxis is initiated at an early age to reduce the incidence of hemophilic arthropathies [2, 3, 8, 9]. Factor replacement protocol includes episodic treatment, continuous prophylaxis, and intermittent prophylaxis [3, 8]. Episodic treatment is also referred to as on-demand treatment, which comprise of factor replacement at the time of clinically evident bleeding [3, 8]. Continuous prophylaxis consists of primary, secondary, and tertiary prophylaxis [3, 8]. Primary continuous prophylaxis is considered an optimal mode of management before the age of 3 years with or without previous joint bleeds [3, 8, 9]. Secondary continuous prophylaxis prevents progression of joint disease [3, 8, 9]. Treatment is started after two or more bleeding episodes into the joints [3, 8, 9]. Tertiary continuous prophylaxis involves treatment after the joint disease is reported by a physical exam and on plain radiographs of the affected joints [3, 8]. Intermittent prophylaxis, also called as periodic prophylaxis, suggests factor replacement to prevent bleeding for duration not exceeding 45 weeks in a year [3, 8].

## 4.6 Mild Hemophilia A

Majority of patients with mild hemophilia A respond positively to desmopressin 1-deamino-8-D-arginine vasopressin (DDAVP) [1–4, 10]. DDAVP is a synthetic analog of the antidiuretic hormone [1, 10]. The mechanism of action of DDAVP is inadequately understood [1, 10, 11]. It is believed that DDAVP increases levels of von Willebrand factor (VWF), which in turn makes more binding sites for factor VIII available inside the VWF molecules [10, 11]. DDAVP can be administered by various routes, namely, intranasal, intravenous, or subcutaneous [1–3, 10]. The recommended dose for intravenous route: 0.3 μg/kg diluted in 50–100 mL of isotonic saline and infused over 30 min [3, 4, 10], whereas owing to poor absorption intranasally, the recommended dose for intranasal DDAVP is 300 [3, 4, 10]. DDAVP can increase baseline factor VIII levels by three- to fivefold, 30–90 min after its administration [3, 4]. The released factor VIII half-life is about 8–12 h similar to that of the normal circulating protein [2, 4]. Response to DDAVP decreases with repeat administration over a short period of time; this phenomenon is called as tachyphylaxis [1–3]. DDAVP is a synthetic analog of vasopressin [1–3]. It causes water reabsorption from the renal collecting ducts [1–3]. Therefore, excessive water consumption should be avoided to prevent hyponatremia [1–3].

## 4.7 Mild Hemophilia B

Factor IX levels do not increase in the presence of DDAVP; therefore it has no role in the management of hemophilia B [3, 4]. Hence, preoperative administration of factor IX is essential. Factor IX is not an acute phase reactant [4]. Therefore, factor IX levels do not increase in response to surgery or inflammation [4]. Thereupon, postoperative replacement is routinely required to achieve wound healing [4].

## 4.8 Moderate/Severe Hemophilia A and B

A calculated dose of factors VIII and IX is administered 10–20 min prior to the procedure [3, 4]. Administration of 1.0 IU/kg of factors VIII and IX increases the factor levels by 2% and 1%, respectively [2, 3]. Considering the short half-lives, factor VIII is typically administered every 12 h and factor IX every 24 h [2].

## 4.9 Fresh Frozen Plasma (FFP) and Cryoprecipitate

Sometimes, FFP is used to manage coagulation factor deficiencies because it contains all the coagulation factors [3]. One milliliter of FFP is considered equivalent to 1 U of factor activity [3]. Cryoprecipitate contains significant quantities of FVIII, VWF, fibrinogen, and FXIII [3]. A bag of cryoprecipitate may contain 70–80 U of FVIII [3].

## 4.10 Dental Management

As is the case for any new patient encounter, a preoperative evaluation of a patient with hemophilia begins with a through history and physical examination. Components of the history targeted toward hemophilia include family members with history of bleeding problems and history of abnormal bleeding after surgical procedures or trauma [12]. As is the case with many other bleeding disorders, in patients with hemophilia, bleeding after surgery, including oral surgical procedures, is often the first evidence of an underlying coagulopathy [12]. As mentioned earlier, components of the physical exam that may lead the practitioner to suspect an underlying coagulopathy include easy bruising and swelling, pain, and limited range of motion in joints due to hemarthroses.

For patients with known hemophilia, preventive dentistry is of the utmost importance. Frequent dental visits with education on dental hygiene and routine dental prophylaxis are instrumental in minimizing dental caries and periodontal disease [12]. Fluorides, sealants, and diet modifications including carbohydrate restriction should be initiated in childhood and maintained throughout adult life [12]. Early and aggressive dental maintenance can prevent the need for more invasive dental procedures later on.

In patients with known hemophilia requiring more invasive surgical procedures, preoperative consultation with a hematologist is indicated. Often, patients with hemophilia require hospitalization for surgical procedures. The decision to hospitalize the patient is made by thorough communication between the dental practitioner and the hematologist. Factors considered in this decision include the severity of the disease and the nature of the dental procedures. Patients with mild hemophilia and no inhibitors can usually be managed on an outpatient basis without the need for factor replacement [12]. Patient with moderate hemophilia and no inhibitors may require factor replacement for less invasive procedures and will require factor replacement for more invasive oral surgical procedures [12]. Patients with moderate hemophilia can also be treated with DDAVP (desmopressin) and EACA (epsilon-aminocaproic acid) or tranexamic acid [12]. Patients with severe hemophilia will require hospitalization and treatment with factor replacement, DDAVP, EACA, or tranexamic acid [12]. Local measures can also be taken for surgical treatment of patients with hemophilia regardless of severity of disease. Preoperatively, surgical stents can be fabricated to prevent displacement of the clot. Good surgical technique and pressure packings can be useful. Surgical sites can be packed with Gelfoam impregnated with topical thrombin to control postoperative bleeding. Patients should also be seen 24–48 h after surgery to assess postoperative control of bleeding [12].

In conclusion, surgical management of patients with hemophilia can be concerning for both the patient and provider. However, thorough preoperative assessment, coordination with the patient's hematologist, and careful preoperative planning allow safe and effective surgical management of patients with hemophilia.

## References

1. Zimmerman B, Valentino LA. Hemophilia: in review. Pediatr Rev. 2013;34:289–95.
2. Smith JA. Hemophilia: what the oral and maxillofacial surgeon needs to know. Oral Maxillofac Surg Clin North Am. 2016;28:481–9.
3. Srivastava A, Brewer AK, Mauser-Bunschoten EP, Key NS, Kitchen S, Llinas A, Ludlam CA, Mahlangu JN, Mulder K, Poon MC, Street A. Guidelines for the management of hemophilia. Haemophilia. 2013;19:1–47.
4. Mensah PK, Gooding R. Surgery in patients with inherited bleeding disorders. Anesthesia. 2015;70:112–20.
5. Kreuz W, Ettingshausen CE. Inhibitors in patients with haemophilia A. Thromb Res. 2014;134:S22–6.
6. Ljung RCR. Intracranial hemorrhage in hemophilia A and B. Br J Haematol. 2007;140:378–84.
7. Balkan C, Kavakli K, Karapinar D. Iliopsoas haemorrhage in patients with haemophilia: results from one centre. Haemophilia. 2005;11:463–7.
8. Ljung R, Andersson NG. The current status of prophylactic replacement therapy in children and adults with hemophilia. Br J Haematol. 2015;169:777–86.
9. Rodriguez-Merchan EC. Musculoskeletal complications of hemophilia. HSSJ. 2010;6:37–42.
10. Franchini M, Zaffanello M, Lippi G. The use of desmopressin in mild hemophilia A. Blood Coagul Fibrinolysis. 2010;21:615–9.
11. Haberichter SL, Shi Q, Montgomery RR. Regulated release of VWF and FVIII and the biologic implications. Pediatr Blood Cancer. 2006;46:547–53.
12. Little, James W. Dental management of the medically compromised patient, 7th edn. St. Louis, MO; Mosby, 2008.

# Review of Thrombocytopenia and Perioperative Management in Dentistry

5

Hani F. Braidy

**Abstract**
Thrombocytopenia may be caused by a variety of underlying systemic diseases. Mechanisms resulting in low levels of circulating platelets can be categorized into three categories: decrease in platelet production, an increase in platelet sequestration, or peripheral destruction of platelets. Peripheral platelet destruction may be further classified as immune or nonimmune mediated. The management of thrombocytopenia is based on the severity of the underling systemic disorder and clinical extent of the bleeding. A detailed history and physical exam, review of laboratory values, and scope of the anticipated dental procedure will determine the optimal perioperative management of the thrombocytopenic patient.

Platelet disorders generally fall within one of two categories: qualitative, referring to abnormal platelet function, or quantitative, indicating a low platelet count (thrombocytopenia). Both types of conditions can be associated with significant bleeding problems of interest for the clinician. Rarely, an underlying medical condition may produce concomitant qualitative and quantitative platelet disorders such as Bernard-Soulier syndrome. In this chapter, the most common conditions associated with thrombocytopenia and their perioperative management will be reviewed.

## 5.1 Definition of Thrombocytopenia

A normal individual has a platelet count of 150,000–400,000/μL as measured in 95% of the population [1]. By definition, thrombocytopenia is a platelet count of less than 150,000/μL. Thrombocytopenia can be further classified as mild (100,000–150,000/μL), moderate (50,000–99,000/μL), or severe (less than 50,000/μL). According to the 95% confidence interval above, 2.5% of the normal population will have platelet count of less 150,000/μL.

## 5.2 Pathophysiology of Thrombocytopenia

A thorough knowledge of platelet physiology is essential to fully comprehend the various mechanisms leading to thrombocytopenia. The reader is referred to Chap. 2 for an in-depth platelet review. A decreased platelet count can be caused by several mechanisms listed in Table 5.1. In the majority of patients, a single identifiable condition is

H. F. Braidy
Department of Oral and Maxillofacial Surgery, Rutgers University School of Dental Medicine, Newark, NJ, USA


R. P. Szumita, P. M. Szumita (eds.), *Hemostasis in Dentistry*, https://doi.org/10.1007/978-3-319-71240-6_5

**Table 5.1** Pathophysiology of thrombocytopenia

| Pathophysiologic mechanism | Differential diagnosis |
|---|---|
| Decreased production | Nutritional |
| | Congenital |
| | Bone marrow suppression |
| Sequestration | Splenomegaly |
| Increased destruction | Immune mediated |
| | Nonimmune mediated |

often responsible for a low platelet count by means of a distinct mechanism (i.e., primary autoimmune thrombocytopenia causing increased platelet destruction). Rarely, however, the decrease in platelet count may be initiated by multiple simultaneous mechanisms triggered by an illness (i.e. increased platelet destruction and decreased production in HIV-infected individuals [2]).

## 5.3 Decreased Production

The production of platelets can be decreased due to a variety of disease processes such as nutritional deficiencies, congenital conditions, and direct bone marrow damage.

Many nutritional deficiencies are responsible for impaired cell production such as anemia, pancytopenia, and, more rarely, isolated thrombocytopenia. Iron deficiency typically leads to hypochromic and microcytic anemia which may be occasionally associated with thrombocytopenia. Vitamin B12 (cobalamin) and B9 (acid folic, folate) are vital for DNA production and repair as well as for red blood cell maturation. Deficiencies in B12 and folate may trigger a megaloblastic anemia with a concomitant mild thrombocytopenia resulting from decreased platelet production. In the Western hemisphere, the acute and chronic ingestion of alcohol is one of the most common causes for thrombocytopenia. Transient decrease in megakaryocyte production within the bone marrow may be caused by alcohol metabolites such as acetaldehyde. Chronic alcoholism has also been shown to suppress bone marrow, trigger folate deficiency, and cause end-stage liver disease resulting in splenomegaly and increased sequestration of platelets [1].

There is myriad of rare congenital disorders and syndromes exhibiting thrombocytopenia or a defect in platelet function. Some of these disorders present soon after birth due to severe bleeding and bruising such as congenital amegakaryocytic thrombocytopenia, an autosomal recessive disease caused by mutations affecting the thrombopoietin receptor [3]. It has been shown these patients respond favorably to stem cell transplantation. Bernard-Soulier syndrome is also an autosomal recessive disease characterized by giant platelets, thrombocytopenia, and qualitative platelet defects due to decreased or lack of GPIb receptor for von Willebrand factor [3]. Most patients with inherited platelet disorders, however, are discovered later in life as they present with relatively mild cutaneous or mucosal purpura, petechia, and ecchymosis as well as with mild bleeding following minor surgeries such as dental extractions. Upon careful review, patient family history is usually relevant for sporadic bleeding episodes. A few of these inherited platelet disorders are related to autosomal dominant transmission of mutations on the MYH9 gene, which include May-Hegglin anomaly, Sebastian syndrome, Epstein syndrome, and Fechtner syndrome, all characterized by thrombocytopenia, giant platelets, and neutrophil inclusions (Döhle bodies) [4]. Of note for the dentist and the oral maxillofacial surgeon, DiGeorge or velocardiofacial syndrome is a condition associated with craniofacial anomalies including cleft palate and velopharyngeal insufficiency as well as with congenital cardiac malformations and learning disabilities. Mild macrothrombocytopenia can be found in up to 20% of patients which may lead to mild bleeding tendencies [5].

Decreased production of platelets may also be the result of bone marrow suppression by a variety of conditions. In these situations, megakaryocytes are absent or decreased upon review of the bone marrow aspirate. Arrest of megakaryocytopoiesis may be secondary to direct stem cell destruction by cytotoxic drug or replacement of bone marrow by an infiltrative disease process. Multiple drugs are well known to cause bone marrow suppression by direct effect on platelet production. For example, the use of chemotherapeutic drugs in the treatment of Hodgkin's disease typically leads to profound bone marrow suppression and resulting pancytopenia, including severe thrombocytopenia. Gemcitabine and platinum agents such as cisplatin and carboplatin, both of which are used in the treatment of advanced head and neck cancer, for instance, are chemotherapeutic agents notoriously responsible for severe thrombocytopenia. Platelet transfusions are indicated if the platelet count drops to 10,000/μL or if bleeding occurs. Recently, the use of thrombopoietin receptor agonists has shown promise in treating thrombocytopenia-induced chemotherapy by stimulating the production and maturation of megakaryocytes [6]. Although most drug-induced thrombocytopenias are immune in nature, some are known to directly suppress the bone marrow such as thiazide diuretics and tolbutamide [7].

Multiple infiltrative diseases of the bone marrow may cause thrombocytopenia by disrupting megakaryocytopoiesis. Bone marrow malignancies such as leukemia, multiple myeloma, and lymphoma predictably induce a thrombocytopenia accompanied by a pancytopenia. Bone marrow destruction and thrombocytopenia may also occur in the setting of advanced breast or prostate cancer due to their propensity for bone metastasis. Thrombocytopenia is also noted in the setting of myelodysplastic syndromes (MDS) which are a group of diseases affecting the maturation of bone marrow stem cells and result in cytopenias. Patients with MDS may have a history of chemotherapy, radiation, or exposure to toxic agents such as benzene and pesticides. MDS are also associated with a variety of other conditions such as Down's syndrome and aplastic anemia [8].

## 5.4 Sequestration

Approximately 30% of platelets normally reside in the spleen at any given point, where they can be released depending on physiological demands. As the spleen enlarges, the amount of sequestered cells also increases, which decreases the total amount of circulating platelets. Hypersplenism secondary to liver cirrhosis and portal hypertension is the most common cause for pathologic spleen enlargement [1]. The resulting thrombocytopenia is noted to be in the order of 50–100,000μL [9] which may further exacerbate bleeding problems in patients in whom coagulation pathways are already compromised (see Chap. 6). Splenomegaly may also be found in myelofibrosis, a condition whereby normal bone marrow environment is slowly invaded by fibrotic scar tissue due to abnormal proliferation of stem cells and excess release of cytokines. The resulting pancytopenia stimulates splenic extramedullary hematopoiesis and hypersplenism which increases platelet sequestration [10].

## 5.5 Increased Destruction-Immune-Related

An important step in the evaluation of the thrombocytopenic patient where the mechanism of the low platelet count is due to increased destruction is to establish whether increased platelet destruction is of immune or nonimmune origin.

Immune thrombocytopenia (formerly known as immune thrombocytopenic purpura (ITP)), first recognized by Hippocrates, is one of the most frequent causes for thrombocytopenia with an incidence of approximately 4 per 100,000. Harrington and Hollingsworth devised a famous experiment in 1951 that proved critical in understanding the pathophysiology of the disease [1]. Immune destruction of the platelets is thought to be mediated by autoantibodies directed to the glycoproteins receptors, notably GPIIB/IIIA and occasionally GPIB [9]. In idiopathic or primary ITP, which occurs in 80% of patients with immune-mediated thrombocytopenia, no underlying disease can be found. Secondary ITP, which affects 20% of patients with ITP, is seen in patients with history of autoimmune disorders such as systemic lupus erythematosus. In children, ITP is usually of acute onset and preceded by a common viral infection such as varicella zoster, Epstein-Barr, and rubella [11]. It is believed a complex interplay between genetics, cell-mediated immunity, and complement pathway defects is responsible for the production of IgG antibodies against platelets and their subsequent destruction by the reticuloendothelial system, which mostly occurs in the spleen [1]. An acute onset is typically seen in children and often spontaneously resolves without treatment (see Table 5.2). Platelet counts of <20,000/μL are noted and accompanied with mild mucosal bleeding and purpura. Severe bleeding is rare due to upregulation of platelet function and bone marrow production in response to increased destruction. In adults, ITP usually becomes chronic in half of the patients and is often found to be an early manifestation of HIV or hepatitis. Patients with critical symptoms may be first treated with intravenous immunoglobulin (IVIG) or steroids [9]. More advanced lines of therapies in children with recalcitrant symptoms may include splenectomy, rituximab (anti-CD20 monoclonal antibody), and thrombopoietin receptor agonists (such as romiplostim or eltrombopag) [12]. In patients with acute life-threatening hemorrhage, platelet transfusions may be administered but are not expected to increase the platelet count significantly due to the underlying disease process. It is believed the concomitant administration of IVIG and steroid therapies with transfusions may delay the eventual destruction of platelets dispensed [1].

Secondary ITP is, by definition, immune thrombocytopenia in the setting of autoimmune disease such as antiphospholipid syndrome, systemic lupus erythematosus (SLE), rheumatoid arthritis, or Sjögren syndrome. Thrombocytopenia may be found in up to 7–30% of patients with SLE and may even be an initial symptom of the disease [13]. Up to 60% of patients with SLE exhibit antiplatelet antibodies and are associated with severe end-organ disease [14]. In SLE, thrombocytopenia may be caused by a variety of other mechanisms including depressed thrombocytopoiesis, splenomegaly, and bone marrow suppression secondary to immunosuppressants or systemic infections [1]. Clinically, severe hemorrhage is rare and can be managed with platelet transfusions and the concomitant administration of steroids and IVIG.

Lastly, immune-mediated platelet destruction may also be triggered by certain drug reactions (see Table 5.3). Commonly used drugs suspected to activate these rare complex immune responses include heparin, antimalarial agents, platelet inhibitors (aspirin), antibiotics (penicillins, cephalosporins), and analgesics (nonsteroidal anti-inflammatories) [15]. It is thought these drugs elicit an antigenic response once they bind on the platelet protein receptor, namely, GPIIB/IIIA or GPIB. The autoantibodies then target the complex

**Table 5.2** Acute vs chronic immune thrombocytopenic purpura (ITP)

| | Acute | Chronic |
|---|---|---|
| Age of onset | 2–6 years of age | 20–50 years of age |
| Gender predilection | None | Female to male ratio of 3:1 |
| Prior infection | Yes, common | No, unusual |
| Onset of bleeding | Sudden | Gradual |
| Platelet count | <20,000/μL | <20,000/μL |
| Duration | Weeks | Months to years |
| Remission | 90% of patients | Uncommon |
| Seasonal pattern | Winter/spring | None |
| Treatment response rate with steroids | 70% | 30% |
| Treatment response rate with splenectomy | Low | High |

**Table 5.3** Medications commonly associated with thrombocytopenia

| Class of medications | Medications |
|---|---|
| Anti-inflammatory agents | Aspirin, acetaminophen, ibuprofen |
| Cardiovascular agents | Quinidine, amiodarone, propranolol, hydralazine, ACEI, digoxin |
| Antiplatelets | Ticlopidine, abciximab, tirofiban, eptifibatide |
| Antibiotics | Penicillin, ampicillin, trimethoprim-sulfamethoxazole, clindamycin, cephalosporins, ciprofloxacin, macrolides |
| Antihistamines | Ranitidine, famotidine |
| Anticonvulsants | Carbamazepine, phenytoin, diazepam, valproic acid |
| Antiparasitics | Quinine, dapsone |
| Chemotherapeutic drugs | Almost all agents |
| Diuretics | Furosemide, hydrochlorothiazide |
| Others | Corticosteroids, gold salts, fluoxetine, chlorpropamide, allopurinol, heparin |

Abbreviations: *ACE* angiotensin-converting enzyme inhibitor "drug-platelet" through a mechanism called "hapten-dependent antibody" as seen with penicillins or cephalosporins, for example [15]. Other proposed mechanisms include "quinine-type drug" reactions, whereby the presence of the offending medication generates platelet antibodies as seen with quinine (an antimalarial), sulfonamides, and nonsteroidal anti-inflammatory analgesics. Patients usually present with mild ecchymosis and mucosal petechiae which develop following a few days' exposure to the offending medication. The thrombocytopenia promptly resolves as soon as the associated drug is discontinued [15].

Heparin-induced thrombocytopenia (HIT) is a well-known reaction occurring in 1 in 5000 patients [16] and usually presents with decreased platelet count (20,000/μL) in the hospitalized patients requiring anticoagulation for deep vein thrombosis, pulmonary embolism, or coronary artery disease. As opposed to other types of immune-mediated drug thrombocytopenias, HIT predisposes up to 50% of patients to thrombotic events such as vein thrombosis in the legs and pulmonary embolism or, less commonly, stroke and myocardial infarction [16]. In these patients, heparin binds with platelet factor 4 (PF4) which triggers the development of antibodies. These newly formed complexes "antibody-heparin-PF4" subsequently elicit platelet, monocyte, and endothelial activation with aberrant thrombin production, resulting in a consumptive type of thrombocytopenia [16]. Patients with HIT are promptly treated by discontinuing heparin and with the administration of direct thrombin inhibitors such as argatroban and lepirudin [4].

## 5.6 Nonimmune Platelet Destruction

Furthermore, platelets may be peripherally destroyed by a variety of nonimmune-related mechanisms. Disseminated intravascular coagulation (DIC) is a potentially fatal condition in which "the intravascular activation of coagulation is generalized and arising from different causes" [17]. The exuberant activation of coagulation then overwhelms anticoagulant regulator systems in place which are mainly mediated by protein C, antithrombin, and tissue factor pathway inhibitor [18]. As a result, a large amount of fibrin is produced and deposited intravascularly with subsequent thrombosis of small vessels ensuing major organ failure. As platelets and other coagulation factors are depleted by widespread clot formation, hemorrhage ensues and manifests in mucosal, skin, and gastrointestinal tract bleeding. Gram-negative sepsis, incompatible transfusion reactions, brain injury, malignancies, and snakebite venom have all been associated with DIC which carries a mortality risk of up to 50–80% [18]. Treatment of DIC is directed to the management of the underlying associated conditions and the administration of platelet transfusion, cryoprecipitate, and fresh frozen plasma in severe cases associated with hemorrhage. Depending on clinical indications, anticoagulation may be instituted for patients at risk for developing thrombosis or emboli [19].

Another condition associated with a consumptive thrombocytopenia and a prothrombic state is thrombotic thrombocytopenic purpura (TTP). In this rare disease, a metalloprotease (ADAMTS13) responsible for cleaving the large multimeric form of the von Willebrand factor (vWF) is either congenitally missing or decreased due to an autoimmune reaction as seen in systemic lupus erythematosus or HIV [20]. These large multimers aggregate circulating platelets to produce thrombi and trigger vessel occlusion in different organs. Patients with TTP classically exhibit a pentad of fever, thrombocytopenia, hemolytic anemia, renal insufficiency, and neurologic symptoms such as seizures, stroke, coma, or confusion. Hemorrhagic clinical signs include epistaxis, bruising, and hematuria. Due to its rarity, a high degree of suspicion is required to promptly diagnose TTP as any delay in treatment may result in devastating morbidity. If left untreated, mortality approaches 85–100% [4]. TTP is urgently treated with plasma exchange using an automated blood cell separator to exchange the patient plasma for a donor's. Rituximab, an anti-CD20 antibody, has been shown to decrease the frequency of plasma exchanges required and improve remission rates

[20]. Steroids are also routinely administered to decrease the production of ADAMTS13 inhibitor [21]. Severe or life-threatening bleeding in patients with TTP is rare and can be urgently treated with platelet transfusion [22].

In the pregnant patient, nonimmune thrombocytopenia may be caused by preeclampsia, a condition characterized with a new onset hypertension, proteinuria, renal insufficiency, thrombocytopenia, and liver damage. The term eclampsia refers to a preeclamptic patient developing seizures during the peripartum phase. The pathogenesis of preeclampsia is complex and thought to be caused by uteroplacental ischemia [23]. A low platelet count, hypothesized to be the result of increased coagulation activation similar to TTP, can be found in approximately half of preeclamptic women [1]. The thrombocytopenia severity is typically closely associated with the degree of preeclampsia. Additionally, HELLP syndrome can be found in approximately 10–20% of patients with severe preeclampsia. This peripartum complication is characterized by hemolytic anemia, elevated liver enzymes, and low platelet count and closely resembles some of the clinical characteristics and pathophysiology of TTP as well [24]. Bleeding problems are rarely encountered in patient with preeclampsia and HELLP syndrome. In severe cases, delivery of the fetus, corticosteroid therapy, and plasma exchange are considered [25].

## 5.7 Perioperative Management of Thrombocytopenia

### 5.7.1 Detailed History

A thorough history is critical to perform in order to establish a diagnosis and to initiate the appropriate consultation and perioperative management. A history of recurrent epistaxis, severe menorrhagia, spontaneous gingival or gastrointestinal bleeding, and bruises should raise suspicions of a platelet disorder as opposed to a coagulation problem.

Excessive bleeding after surgery or dental extractions is usually the first clinical manifestation of an underlying platelet disorder and should elicit additional testing and consultation with a hematologist. Typically, the postsurgical bleeding associated with thrombocytopenia such as ITP or VwD is immediate and usually mild as the initial "platelet plug" is either absent or ineffective. On the other hand, coagulation disorders such as hemophilia A or B are more often associated with delayed (1–2 days) and often severe bleeding.

A history of new medication exposure such as NSAIDs, Tylenol, penicillin, sulfonamides, heparin, and anticonvulsants, among many others, as well as quinine-containing beverages (such as tonic water), has also been associated with thrombocytopenia.

Alcoholism, malnutrition, and vegetarianism should raise concerns of abnormal production of platelets. A history of severe anemia, end-stage cancers, and myeloproliferative disorders such as lymphoma and leukemia may cause severe bleeding. A report of end-stage liver disease should also elicit the possibility for splenomegaly and platelet sequestration as described earlier in this chapter.

A history of recent acute viral infection in children or chronic infection in adults such as *H. pylori*, hepatitis C, or HIV in a patient with low platelet count is suspicious for immune-mediated thrombocytopenia [26].

A positive family history for bleeding is often found in patients with congenital platelet disorders such as von Willebrand disease, May-Hegglin anomaly, Bernard-Soulier syndrome, or Glanzmann's thrombasthenia.

### 5.7.2 Physical Exam

Dermatologically, thrombocytopenia commonly manifests as bruises, caused by the superficial extravasation of blood within the skin or mucosa, and is more commonly found in dependent areas such as the lower extremities. On the other hand, hemarthrosis and deep muscle bleeding are more commonly associated with coagulation abnormalities (see Table 5.4).

Bruises are typically found to be flat on palpation unless caused by vessel wall inflamma-

**Table 5.4** Physical exam findings in patients with thrombocytopenia and coagulation disorders

| | Thrombocytopenia | Coagulation disorders |
|---|---|---|
| Bleeding site | Skin<br>Mucous membranes<br>(epistaxis, gingiva, GU/GI tracts) | Deep in soft tissue (joints, muscles) |
| Petechia | Yes | No |
| Ecchymosis | Small, superficial | Large, deep |
| Hemarthrosis/muscle bleeding | Extremely rare | Common |
| Hematoma | Rare | Common |
| Bleeding after cuts and scratches | Yes | No |
| Bleeding after surgery or trauma | Immediate<br>Usually mild | Delayed (1–2 days)<br>Often severe |

Abbreviations: *GU* genitourinary, *GI* gastrointestinal

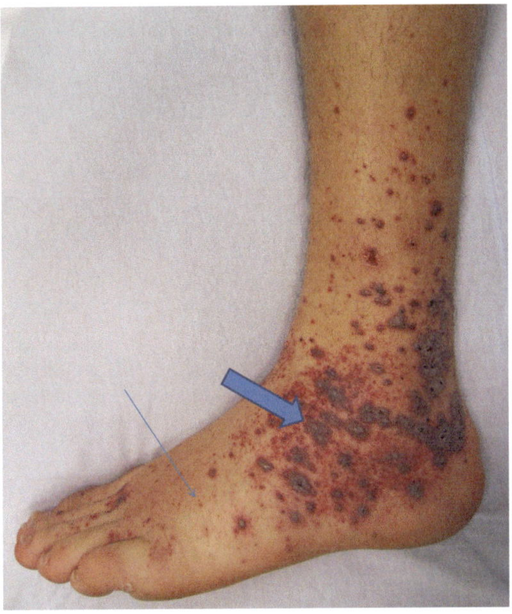

**Fig. 5.1** Petechia (standard arrow) and purpura (block arrow). Image obtained from https://en.wikipedia.org/wiki/Petechia, copyright belongs to James Heilman, MD

tion as seen in patients with Henoch-Schönlein purpura [27] or other vasculitides. In addition, bruises do not blanch under pressure unlike vascular malformations or hemangiomas. Clinically, bruises are further classified according to size. Petechiae are punctate purple hemorrhagic spots less than 3 mm in diameter and are often found in clusters, caused by a ruptured capillary (see Fig. 5.1). Bruises are labeled as purpura (see Fig. 5.1) when measured between 3 and 10 mm and as ecchymosis when found to be larger (>10 mm). In the oral cavity, bruising is referred as "wet purpura" and is clinically associated with increased bleeding severity and morbidity. Other than thrombocytopenia and platelet function defects, many conditions may cause mucocutaneous bruising: physical trauma, vitamin C and K deficiencies, connective tissue diseases, septicemia, and many infectious diseases [28].

In addition to performing a detailed mucocutaneous exam, the clinician must also palpate the liver and the spleen for enlargement. Hepatosplenomegaly may be a sign of liver disease causing platelet sequestration in patient with thrombocytopenia. Additional classic physical signs associated with end-stage liver disease include jaundice, ascites, and spider angiomas. Splenomegaly may also be found in lupus, myelofibrosis, lymphoma, or leukemia [29], all of which are conditions often associated with a low platelet count. Lastly, lymphadenopathy in patients with thrombocytopenia may be associated with an underlying infectious process or malignancy [30].

### 5.7.3 Laboratory Testing

Once a bleeding disorder is suspected upon history and physical exam, thorough testing is undertaken. A first line of bloodwork includes a complete blood count (CBC), a peripheral blood smear (PBS), bleeding time (BT), and coagulation studies such as prothrombin time (PT) and activated partial thromboplastin time (aPTT) (Table 5.5).

**Table 5.5** Main clinical laboratory testing in assessing patients with bleeding tendencies and their interpretation

| Test | Test description | Findings | Causes |
|---|---|---|---|
| CBC | Assessment of red blood cells, white blood cells, and platelet count | Thrombocytopenia | Quantitative platelet defect |
| | | Elevated WBC and concomitant thrombocytopenia | Presence of bacterial or viral infection mediated thrombocytopenia |
| | | Combined anemia and concomitant thrombocytopenia | Bone marrow disorders, infections, nutritional deficiencies |
| Peripheral blood smear | Microscopic morphologic examination of a drop of blood | Clumped platelets | Pseudothrombocytopenia (redraw with non-EDTA coagulant such as sodium citrate or heparin [4]) |
| | | Large or giant platelets | vWd, gray platelet syndrome, MYH9-related diseases, Bernard-Soulier syndrome, and other hereditary thrombocytopenias |
| | | Small platelets | Wiskott-Aldrich syndrome |
| | | Schistocytes (fragmented RBCs) | Intravascular hemolysis seen in TTP, HUS, DIC |
| | | Blasts (immature cells), nucleated RBCs | Myelodysplasia |
| BT | In vivo assessment of platelet function | Elevated | Thrombocytopenia, platelet function defect, connective tissue disease |
| PT and aPTT | Measure of intrinsic and extrinsic pathways of coagulation | Elevated | Warfarin use, vitamin K deficiency, hemophilia, DIC |

Abbreviations: *CBC* complete blood count, *WBC* white blood count, *vWd* von Willebrand disease, *EDTA* ethylenediaminetetraacetic acid, *RBC* red blood cell, *TTP* thrombotic thrombocytopenic purpura, *HUS* hemolytic uremic syndrome, *DIC* disseminated intravascular coagulation, *BT* bleeding time, *PT* prothrombin time, *aPTT* activated partial thromboplastin time

In patients with confirmed thrombocytopenia, the evaluation of the peripheral blood smear is the most critical step to elucidate the etiology for patients with low platelet count (see Fig. 5.2). A concomitant anemia and/or leukopenia should raise the suspicion for myelosuppression which can be ruled out by performing a bone marrow aspiration and biopsy. A bone marrow examination is especially critical in patients more than 60 years of age to rule out myelodysplastic syndrome [31]. Human immunodeficiency virus (HIV) and hepatitis C virus (HCV) tests are also commonly administered as asymptomatic thrombocytopenia is considered to be a marker and early sign for these conditions [32]. Additional testing is mainly indicated when there is suspicion for other underlying systemic diseases such as liver disease (coagulation studies), SLE (antinuclear antibodies), TTP (ADAMTS13 activity), heparin-induced thrombocytopenia (heparin-PF4 antibodies), etc. Consultation with a hematologist or an internist is often required to elucidate the underlying mechanism responsible for the low platelet count.

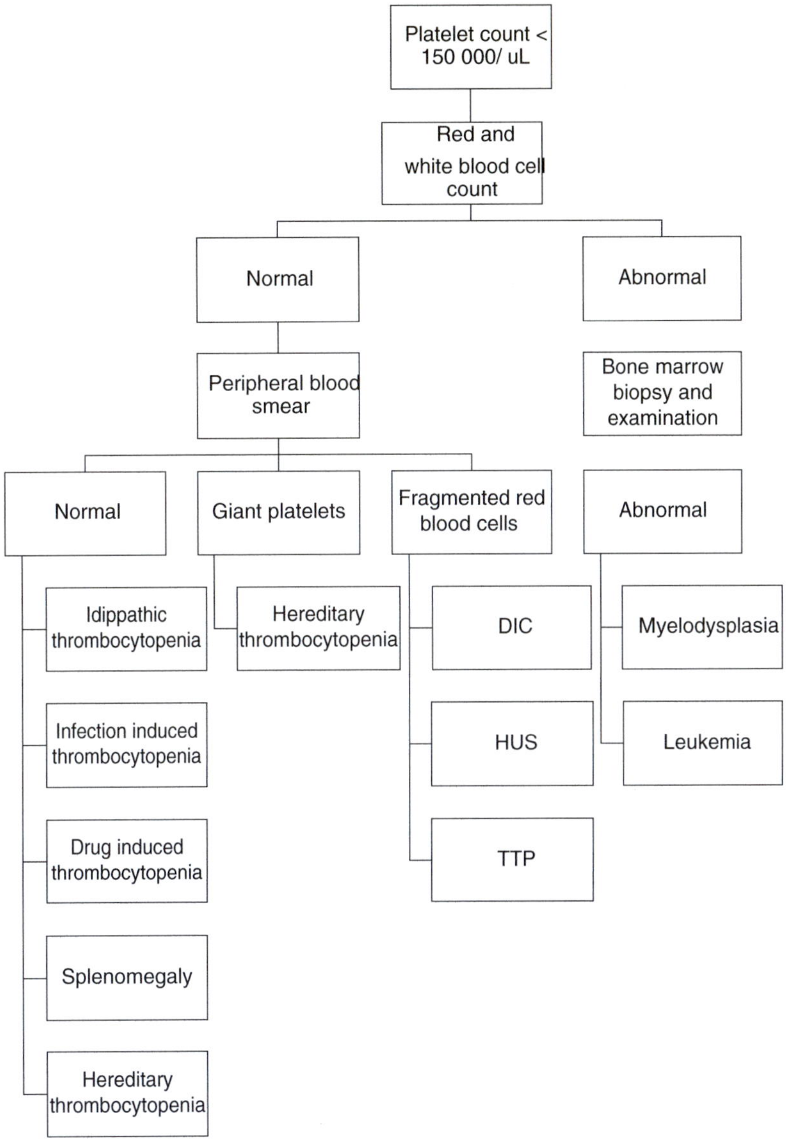


**Fig. 5.2** Diagnostic approach to the patient with thrombocytopenia. Abbreviations: *DIC* disseminated intravascular coagulation, *HUS* hemolytic uremic syndrome, *TTP* thrombotic thrombocytopenic purpura

## 5.8 Management of the Thrombocytopenic Patient

The clinician faces numerous challenges when treating patients at risk for bleeding. A consultation with a hematologist is mandatory to further stratify the risk for hemorrhage and to optimize the thrombocytopenic patient.

The risk for bleeding is not only associated with the type of dental procedure planned but also with the nature of the underlying systemic condition causing the thrombocytopenia as well as the platelet count value. For instance, it is well known the risk for bleeding is amplified in patients with end-stage liver disease due to coagulation pathways disruption in addition to thrombocytopenia. Addressing the deficit in both coagulation factors and platelets is often necessary to optimize cirrhotic patients prior to an invasive procedure. Similarly, patients with Bernard-Soulier syndrome often present with bleeding disproportionate to their level of thrombocytopenia which is due to concomitant platelet adhesion defects. These patients may require a combination of platelet transfusion and factor VIIa [33] to address both quantitative and qualitative platelet defects.

Certain dental procedures, such as extractions, periodontal surgery, placement of endosseous implants, and periapical endodontic surgery, are well known to produce hard or soft tissue bleeding. The administration of inferior alveolar and posterior superior alveolar blocks likewise carries the potential to induce uncontrolled bleeding or hematoma due to the presence of significant local vessels at risk for perforation. Dental procedures associated with a low risk of intraoperative or postoperative bleeding include supraperiosteal injections (buccal infiltrations), supragingival scaling and cleaning, restorative dentistry, fabrication of fixed and removable partial dentures, as well as intracanal endodontic therapy.

Clinically, a platelet count of less than 10,000/μL is classically associated with a risk of spontaneous gastrointestinal or genitourinary tracts bleeding and usually prompts the prophylactic initiation of platelet transfusions depending on the clinical picture [34]. Excluding any concomitant qualitative platelet or coagulation defects, platelet counts of 30,000/μL are considered to be generally safe for local anesthesia administration, including blocks, and for most noninvasive dental procedures [35]. Dental extractions, periodontal surgery, and minor soft tissue surgery are likely to be safe in patients with platelet count above 50,000/μL. Extensive maxillofacial procedures are best performed in patients with counts above 80,000–100,000/μL (see Table 5.6). Below these recommended levels, platelet transfusions are generally recommended to reduce the risk for severe bleeding. Of special concern, procedures performed in the floor of mouth area carry the risk for hematoma formation and resulting airway obstruction. Great care must be taken to avoid injections or extensive flaps in this area.

**Table 5.6** Indications for platelet transfusion based on platelet count threshold and clinical scenario

| Type of indication | Platelet count/μL threshold | Clinical scenario | Dental and OMFS procedures |
|---|---|---|---|
| Therapeutic | Any thrombocytopenic patient[a] | Active bleeding | |
| Prophylactic | 100,000 | Elective neurosurgery, ocular surgery | Extensive maxillofacial surgery (orthognathic surgery, tumor resection, reconstruction, etc.) |
| | 50,000 | General surgery | Invasive dental treatments (dental extractions, periodontal surgery, deep scaling, and root planning, etc.) |
| | 30,000 | | Noninvasive dental treatments (local anesthetics blocks, restorative dentistry, intracanal endodontic treatment, supragingival scaling, etc.) |
| | 20,000–50,000 | Lumbar puncture, central line venous access, endoscopy | |
| | 10,000–20,000 | Bone marrow aspiration of biopsy | |
| | ≤10,000 | Acute leukemia, chronic stable thrombocytopenia, patients undergoing chemotherapy for solid tumors | |

Abbreviations: *OMFS* oral and maxillofacial surgery, *DIC* disseminated intravascular coagulation, *CNS* central nervous system

[a]Platelets are relatively contraindicated in patients with thrombotic thrombocytopenic purpura (TTP), heparin-induced thrombocytopenia (HIT), or immune thrombocytopenia (ITP)

## 5.9 Platelet Transfusion

Platelets may be collected by one of two methods for anticipated transfusions. In the single donor platelet method, also named whole blood-derived platelets or random donor pooled platelets, whole blood is mixed with citrate anticoagulant and centrifuged at low and high speed (double centrifugation). 40–70 cc of the supernatant, which contains approximately $5.0 \times 10^{10}$ platelets, is then labeled as "one unit." One unit of platelet concentrate predictably increases the platelet count only 5000–10,000/μL in the average size adult. Therefore, platelets are typically administered as a package of 6 units (from six random donors), raising baseline platelets 30,000–60,000/μL. This method allows for quick, efficient, and inexpensive collection of platelets for transfusion. On the other hand, the transfusion recipient is exposed to multiple donors, increasing the risk for infection transmission and allergic reactions. The apheresis method allows for platelet collection from a single donor thereby limiting the recipient exposure to antigens. In this technique, whole blood from a random or selected (i.e., family member, HLA-compatible, etc.) donor circulates through a platelet apheresis machine which separates the platelets and plasma from the red blood cells which are ultimately returned to the donor. This method of platelet collections typically yields approximately $3 \times 10^{11}$ platelets suspended in 200 cc of plasma, which is enough to raise the platelet count 30,000–50,000/μL. One unit of apheresed platelets is therefore equivalent to a pool of 4–6 units of random donor platelets. Both pooled and apheresed platelets are collected and stored at room temperature (22 °C, as opposed to 4 °C for red blood cells [34]) under continuous agitation. Refrigeration is known to inactivate platelets and increase macrophage-mediated clearance from the circulation [36]. The typical shelf life for both collection methods is only approximately 5 days following collection due to increased risks for bacterial contamination [37].

Platelets may be "therapeutically" transfused in thrombocytopenic patients who are actively bleeding, with the goal of maintaining a platelet count of at least 50,000/μL until the hemorrhage is controlled. Furthermore, preserving a platelet count of more than 100,000/μL is advocated in patients with central nervous system bleeding or DIC due to increased risks for morbidity [38]. Platelets may also be "prophylactically" transfused to optimize thrombocytopenic patients undergoing elective invasive medical or dental procedures (see Table 5.6). Lastly, a subset of patients with severe chronic thrombocytopenia (less than 10,000 platelets/μL) secondary underlying systemic disease (as discussed previously in this chapter) may benefit from platelet transfusion to prevent spontaneous bleeding.

Prophylactic platelet transfusions in preparation for elective surgical or dental procedures can be administered either as in an inpatient or outpatient setting through a peripheral or central intravenous access. A unit of apheresed platelets or a pack of sixpooled donor units, which is the standard adult dose for prophylactic transfusion, should be infused over 30–60 min, once a day. Patients actively bleeding will typically require repeated transfusions based on the clinical situation. Patient's vital signs including temperature must be monitored during the transfusion process. A platelet count is taken immediately prior to and following the transfusion to confirm the anticipated platelet response. Generally, the platelet count peaks in the first hour following the infusion of platelets, followed by a gradual decrease over the following 3 days [38].

Complications associated with platelet transfusions are generally rare and summarized in Table 5.7. The most common complication associated with platelet transfusion is allergic reactions which manifests as pruritus and urticaria in minor cases or hypotension and anaphylactic shock in the most severe instances. Febrile transfusion reactions are also common and thought to be triggered by various inflammatory mediators released by donors' neutrophils normally found in small quantity within the platelets. The risk for bacterial infection transmission is approximately 1 in 2000 transfusions, 15 times more frequent than for red blood cell administration. This increased risk associated found in platelet transfusion is caused by rapid proliferation of bacteria at room temperature [38]. Inadequate increase in

**Table 5.7** Most common complications associated with platelet transfusion

| Complication | | Incidence |
|---|---|---|
| Alloimmunization and refractoriness to platelet transfusion | | 28–44% |
| Febrile reactions | | 7% |
| Allergic reactions | | 2% |
| Bacterial infection (sepsis) | | 1:75,000 |
| Transfusion-related acute lung injury | | 1:140,000 |
| Viral infection | HIV | 1:2.3 million |
| | Hepatitis B | 1:2.6 million |
| | Hepatitis C | 1:3.3 million |
| | CMV (in leukoreduced platelets) | 1:13.5 million |

Abbreviations: *CMV* cytomegalovirus

platelet count following transfusion may be seen in 28–44% of patients [39]. Refractoriness to platelet transfusion is often caused by a systemic infection, fever, platelet sequestration by the spleen, and certain medications. In addition, autoimmune inactivation of platelets is thought to occur in approximately 20% of patients and is often mediated by antibodies targeting human leukocyte antigens (HLA) expressed by platelets through a process called alloimmunization. Alloimmune inactivation of platelets is reduced by leucocyte reduction and irradiation of the transfused platelets. In patients with history of alloimmunization, the use of HLA-compatible and crossed-matched platelets may improve platelet count response posttransfusion [37].

Platelet transfusions are relatively contraindicated in consumptive thrombocytopenias such as thrombotic thrombocytopenic purpura (TTP) and heparin-induced thrombocytopenia (HIT). In these potentially fatal disorders, patients are at high risk for developing widespread end-organ thrombosis. Transfusing platelets to correct the resulting thrombocytopenia may only "add fuel to the fire" and is only reserved in cases of severe hemorrhage. Platelet transfusions are relatively contraindicated in patients with immune thrombocytopenia (ITP) due to their anticipated autoimmune destruction. Fortunately, patients with ITP are found to be at relatively low risk for bleeding due to highly effective and upregulated residual circulating platelets (typically >30,000/μL). As mentioned earlier in this chapter, ITP is primarily managed with intravenous immunoglobulin (IVIG) or steroids while reserving platelet transfusion for life-threatening hemorrhage.

## 5.10 Additional Considerations in the Management of the Thrombocytopenic Dental Patient

Following the detailed review of the patient's history and physical examination, laboratory values, and hematology consultation, the dentist will need to determine whether to treat the patient in a hospital or office setting. As mentioned previously, procedures at low risk for bleeding in patients with platelet count above 30,000/μL can safely be performed in a dental office. Patients requiring platelet prophylactic transfusions or undergoing invasive procedures such as dental extractions are ideally managed in a hospital outpatient setting which facilitates the coordination of care and gives the dentist greater resources to manage surgical complications. When required, platelet transfusion should occur at the beginning of the day to allow enough processing time for a pre/post platelet count. The surgical procedure would then be promptly initiated after verifying a satisfactory increase in platelet count. Following the procedure, the patient is monitored for at least 1–2 h to confirm persisting hemostasis and dissipation of the epinephrine contained in local anesthetic solutions. Intraoperative or postoperative platelet transfusion may be required depending on platelet response, baseline platelet count, surgical procedure extent, or persisting hemorrhage. It is also advisable to schedule patients at risk for postoperative bleeding at the beginning of the work week which allows flexibility should a complication occur. Communication with the treating hematologist is therefore key to coordinate the treatment phases described above. In a retrospective study of 68 thrombocytopenic patients with a mean platelet count of 44,000/μL, 32 patients required prophylactic transfusions prior to dental extractions. Postoperative bleeding was noted in only five patients in whom local measures and aminocaproic acid rinse were successfully used to control the hemorrhage. According to the authors of the study, extractions in thrombocytopenic patients are relatively safe provided adequate hematological workup and medical optimization [40].

The preoperative construction of a surgical stent is often useful in providing postoperative pressure to the surgical site and carrying local hemostatic agents to the wound. An impression of the arch is taken and plaster is poured to fabricate working models. The cast is then modified (i.e., teeth removed, alveoloplasty simulated, etc.) before a soft vacuum forming mouthguard material is "sucked down" with the vacuum-forming machine (Patterson Dental, St. Paul, MN).

The use of careful surgical technique is imperative when managing patient at risk for postoperative bleeding. Releasing incisions and extensive flaps should be realistically avoided to minimize soft tissue injury. Conservative bony removal and tooth sectioning are advised to reduce hard tissue bleeding. Granulation tissue should be carefully curetted and removed as it may be responsible for postoperative bleeding. If possible, primary closure with sutures should be achieved to help stabilize the clot. It is imperative the dentist or oral maxillofacial surgeon provides their patients with detailed postoperative surgical instructions aimed to reduce the risks for bleeding. These typically include biting on cotton gauzes, maintaining a soft diet, avoiding spitting and rinsing for the first day, etc. Multiple local hemostatic and pharmacological agents are available to the dentist and described in detail in Chap. 15. With proper planning and medical and surgical management, re-bleeding should be uncommon. Should a patient present with postoperative bleeding, local hemostatic measures are promptly re-implemented. Failure to obtain enduring hemostasis should urge the clinician to reconsult the hematologist and obtain a new platelet count and coagulation profile.

## 5.11 Summary

As reviewed in this chapter, thrombocytopenia may be caused by a decrease in platelet production, increased sequestration, or peripheral platelet destruction. A low platelet count may be associated with life-threatening hemorrhage and therefore profoundly affects dental management of these medically compromised patients. Proper preoperative evaluation, laboratory workup, and consultation with the hematologist are critical to establish and sequence the appropriate treatment plan and to reduce the risks for bleeding.

## References


1. JAL RD-K. Thrombocytopenia. In: Williams hematology [Internet]. 9th ed. New York, NY: McGraw-Hill Education; 2016. p. 1993–2035.
2. Scaradavou A. HIV-related thrombocytopenia. Blood Rev. 2002;16(1):73–6. PubMed PMID: 11914001
3. Drachman JG. Inherited thrombocytopenia: when a low platelet count does not mean ITP. Blood. 2004;103(2):390–8. PubMed PMID: 14504084
4. Konkle BA. Disorders of platelets and vessel wall. In: Kasper D, Fauci A, Hauser S, Longo D, Jameson JL, Loscalzo J, editors. Harrison's principles of internal medicine. 19th ed. New York, NY: McGraw-Hill Education; 2015.
5. Nurden AT, Nurden P. Inherited thrombocytopenias. Haematologica. 2007;92(9):1158–64. PubMed PMID: 17768118
6. Kuter DJ. Managing thrombocytopenia associated with cancer chemotherapy. Oncology. 2015;29(4):282–94. PubMed PMID: 25952492.
7. Visentin GP, Liu CY. Drug-induced thrombocytopenia. Hematol Oncol Clin North Am. 2007;21(4):685–96. vi. PubMed PMID: 17666285. Pubmed Central PMCID: 1993236
8. Hasserjian RP. Myelodysplastic syndromes. In: Hematopathology [Internet]. Philadelphia, PA: Elsevier; 2017. p. 793–815.
9. Rinder CATHM. Disorders of hemostasis: bleeding. In: Andreoli and Carpenter's cecil essentials of medicine [Internet]. Philadelphia, PA: Elsevier; 2016. p. 544–63.
10. Manson HGWJIOCLM. Blood disease. In: Davidson's principles and practice of medicine [Internet]. Philadelphia, PA: Elsevier; 2014. p. 989–1056.
11. Rand ML, Wright JF. Virus-associated idiopathic thrombocytopenic purpura. Transfus Sci. 1998;19(3):253–9. PubMed PMID: 10351137
12. Toltl DMACPLJ. Diseases of platelet number: immune thrombocytopenia, neonatal alloimmune thrombocytopenia, and posttransfusion purpura. In:

Hematology: basic principles and practice [Internet]. Philadelphia, PA: Elsevier; 2013. p. 1883–94.
13. Leung WH, Wong KL, Lau CP, Wong CK, Liu HW. Association between antiphospholipid antibodies and cardiac abnormalities in patients with systemic lupus erythematosus. Am J Med. 1990;89(4):411–9. PubMed PMID: Medline: 2121029. English
14. Macchi L, Rispal P, Clofent-Sanchez G, Pellegrin JL, Nurden P, Leng B, et al. Anti-platelet antibodies in patients with systemic lupus erythematosus and the primary antiphospholipid antibody syndrome: their relationship with the observed thrombocytopenia. Br J Haematol. 1997;98(2):336–41. PubMed PMID: Medline: 9266930. English
15. Aster RH, Bougie DW. Drug-induced immune thrombocytopenia. N Engl J Med. 2007;357(6):580–7. PubMed PMID: 17687133
16. Greinacher A. Clinical practice. Heparin-induced thrombocytopenia. N Engl J Med. 2015;373(3):252–61. PubMed PMID: 26176382
17. Taylor FB Jr, Toh CH, Hoots WK, Wada H, Levi M, Scientific Subcommittee on Disseminated Intravascular Coagulation of the International Society on T, et al. Towards definition, clinical and laboratory criteria, and a scoring system for disseminated intravascular coagulation. Thromb Haemost. 2001;86(5):1327–30. PubMed PMID: Medline: 11816725. English
18. Boral BM, Williams DJ, Boral LI. Disseminated intravascular coagulation. Am J Clin Pathol. 2016;146(6):670–80. PubMed PMID: 28013226
19. Andreoli T, Benjamin I, Griggs R, Wing E. Andreoli and Carpenter's cecil essentials of Medicine: Elsevier Health Sciences; 2010. Available from: http://www.r2library.com/Resource/Title/1416061096.
20. Blombery P, Scully M. Management of thrombotic thrombocytopenic purpura: current perspectives. J Blood Med. 2014;5:15–23. PubMed PMID: 24523598. Pubmed Central PMCID: 3921093
21. Balduini CL, Gugliotta L, Luppi M, Laurenti L, Klersy C, Pieresca C, et al. High versus standard dose methylprednisolone in the acute phase of idiopathic thrombotic thrombocytopenic purpura: a randomized study. Ann Hematol. 2010;89(6):591–6. PubMed PMID: 20033409
22. Swisher KK, Terrell DR, Vesely SK, Kremer Hovinga JA, Lammle B, George JN. Clinical outcomes after platelet transfusions in patients with thrombotic thrombocytopenic purpura. Transfusion. 2009;49(5):873–87. PubMed PMID: 19210323
23. Mustafa R, Ahmed S, Gupta A, Venuto RC. A comprehensive review of hypertension in pregnancy. J Pregnancy. 2012;2012:105918. PubMed PMID: 22685661. Pubmed Central PMCID: 3366228
24. Pourrat O, Coudroy R, Pierre F. Differentiation between severe HELLP syndrome and thrombotic microangiopathy, thrombotic thrombocytopenic purpura and other imitators. Eur J Obstet Gynecol Reprod Biol. 2015;189:68–72. PubMed PMID: Medline: 25879992. English
25. Erkurt MA, Berber I, Berktas HB, Kuku I, Kaya E, Koroglu M, et al. A life-saving therapy in class I HELLP syndrome: therapeutic plasma exchange. Transfus Apher Sci. 2015;52(2):194–8. PubMed PMID: 25595543
26. Johnsen J. Pathogenesis in immune thrombocytopenia: new insights. Hematology Am Soc Hematol Educ Program. 2012;2012:306–12. PubMed PMID: 23233597
27. Saulsbury FT. Clinical update: Henoch-Schonlein purpura. Lancet. 2007;369(9566):976–8. PubMed PMID: 17382810
28. Khair K, Liesner R. Bruising and bleeding in infants and children—a practical approach. Br J Haematol. 2006;133(3):221–31. PubMed PMID: 16643424
29. O'Reilly RA. Splenomegaly in 2,505 patients in a large university medical center from 1913 to 1995. 1913 to 1962: 2,056 patients. West J Med. 1998;169(2):78–87. PubMed PMID: 9735688. Pubmed Central PMCID: 1305176
30. George JN. Approach to the adult with unexplained thrombocytopenia. In: Post T, editor. UpToDate, UpToDate. Waltham, MA; 2017.
31. Stasi R. How to approach thrombocytopenia. Hematology Am Soc Hematol Educ Program. 2012;2012:191–7. PubMed PMID: Medline: 23233580. English
32. Neunert C, Lim W, Crowther M, Cohen A, Solberg L Jr, Crowther MA, et al. The American Society of Hematology 2011 evidence-based practice guideline for immune thrombocytopenia. Blood. 2011;117(16):4190–207. PubMed PMID: Medline: 21325604. English
33. Israels S, Schwetz N, Boyar R, McNicol A. Bleeding disorders: characterization, dental considerations and management. Journal. 2006;72(9):827. PubMed PMID: 17109803
34. Slichter SJ. Evidence-based platelet transfusion guidelines. Hematology Am Soc Hematol Educ Program. 2007:172–8. PubMed PMID: 18024626
35. British Committee for Standards in Haematology General Haematology Task F. Guidelines for the investigation and management of idiopathic thrombocytopenic purpura in adults, children and in pregnancy. Br J Haematol. 2003;120(4):574–96. PubMed PMID: 12588344
36. Rumjantseva V, Hoffmeister KM. Novel and unexpected clearance mechanisms for cold platelets. Transfus Apher Sci. 2010;42(1):63–70. PubMed PMID: 19932055. Pubmed Central PMCID: 4303245
37. Thiagarajan P, Afshar-Kharghan V. Platelet transfusion therapy. Hematol Oncol Clin North Am. 2013;27(3):629–43. PubMed PMID: 23714315
38. Yuan S. Clinical and laboratory aspects of platelet transfusion therapy. In: UpToDate [Internet], UpToDate. Waltham, MA; 2016.
39. Goldfinger D. Refractoriness to platelet transfusion therapy. In: UpToDate [Internet]. Waltham, MA: UpToDate; 2016.
40. Fillmore WJ, Leavitt BD, Arce K. Dental extraction in the thrombocytopenic patient is safe and complications are easily managed. J Oral Maxillofac Surg. 2013;71(10):1647–52. PubMed PMID: 23932116

# Review of Liver Disease and Perioperative Management in Dentistry

6

Hillel Ephros and Ilya L. Garibyan

**Abstract**

The liver has numerous essential functions, and multifactorial liver disease presents many challenges for the delivery of medical and dental care. Dental professionals who treat patients in various stages of the disease must be aware of the associated disturbances in hemostasis and the increased likelihood of bleeding postoperatively and during dental and oral surgical procedures. Thus, managing liver disease patients in the dental office or a hospital requires an understanding of the disease's progression, an ability to interpret laboratory tests, and proper preparation to manage hemostatic complications.

H. Ephros (✉)
Department of Dentistry/Oral and Maxillofacial Surgery, St. Joseph's University Medical Center, Paterson, NJ, USA
e-mail: ephrosh@sjhmc.org

I. L. Garibyan
Oral and Maxillofacial Surgery Resident, St. Joseph's University Medical Center, Paterson, NJ, USA

## 6.1 Liver Disease: A Brief Review of Types, Etiologies, Pathophysiology, Signs, and Symptoms

In the United States, an estimated 5.5 million people have chronic liver disease; it claims the lives of approximately 25,000 Americans each year. Additionally, more than 300,000 people are hospitalized annually due to cirrhosis [1]. Among the most common causes of liver disease in the United States are alcohol abuse, chronic hepatitis B or C, and fatty liver disease (Table 6.1) [1]. During acute stages of liver disease, hepatocellular damage occurs, but the liver retains normal function after withdrawal of the causative agent or treatment of the underlying cause. However, after years of continuous injury, the process may become irreversible and fibrous scarring is noted, resulting in impaired liver function. At this stage, the disease progresses to a chronic state, and normal hepatic architecture is replaced with interconnecting bands of fibrous tissue. Normal liver function is altered due to inadequate blood flow and ongoing damage to hepatocytes [2]. This may lead to portal hypertension, ascites, splenomegaly, and esophageal varices. Ultimately, this process results in cirrhosis, hepatocellular necrosis, and hepatic failure, and the patient will require a liver transplant.



R. P. Szumita, P. M. Szumita (eds.), *Hemostasis in Dentistry*, https://doi.org/10.1007/978-3-319-71240-6_6

**Table 6.1** Etiology of chronic liver disease in the United States

| Etiology | Approximate frequency in the United States (%) |
|---|---|
| Hepatitis C | 25 |
| Alcoholic liver disease | 20 |
| Chronic hepatitis C and alcoholic liver disease | 15 |
| Hepatitis B | 15 |
| Cirrhosis of unknown etiology | 15 |
| All other causes | 10 |

Adapted from Firriolo et al. [1]

**Table 6.2** Rebalancing hemostatic mechanisms in liver disease

| Phase | Promoting bleeding | Promoting thrombosis |
|---|---|---|
| Primary hemostasis | • Thrombocytopenia<br>• Platelet function defects<br>• Enhanced inhibition of platelet function | • Elevated VWF<br>• Decreased inactivation of VWF |
| Secondary hemostasis | • Decreased levels of coagulation factors II, V, VII, IX, X and XI<br>• Quantitative and qualitative fibrinogen abnormalities | • Decreased levels of various anticoagulants<br>• Elevated factor VIII |
| Fibrinolysis | • Low levels of alpha 2 anti-plasmin, factor XIII and thrombin-activated fibrinolysis inhibitor (TAFI) | • Decreased plasminogen |

Adapted from http://www.iltseducation.com/documents/Mallett_ILTScoag.pdf

## 6.2 Disturbances in Hemostasis Associated with Liver Disease

The liver plays a central role in coagulation in both primary and secondary hemostasis. It produces 11 of the 13 coagulation factors involved in the coagulation cascade and plays a role in clearing these products from circulation. This process has been described in great detail elsewhere in this book. Furthermore, the liver produces thrombopoietin, which regulates the production of platelets from megakaryocytes and serves as a storehouse for vitamin K, which is essential to the activation of coagulation factors II, VII, IX, and X [3]. Therefore, patients with end-stage liver disease may have a decreased platelet count and reduced production of coagulation factors, all of which may lead to disturbances in hemostasis.

Thrombocytopenia may add to the complexity of these disturbances. A decreased platelet count may be secondary to alcoholic marrow suppression or caused by decreased hepatic synthesis of thrombopoietin. Platelet number and function are also affected by portal hypertension through altered endothelial function and increased sequestration associated with splenomegaly. However, platelet procoagulant activity is generally preserved in patients with cirrhosis [4]. This is attributed to an elevated von Willebrand factor (VWF), which enhances platelet adhesion and counteracts the defects from thrombocytopenia and platelet dysfunction [5].

Patients with cirrhosis frequently acquire a disorder of hemostasis secondary to their disease but are susceptible to both bleeding complications and thrombotic disease. These patients can have elevated levels of VWF and factor VIII as well as decreased levels of anticoagulants such as protein C and antithrombin [6, 7].

An improved understanding of hemostatic mechanisms and the pathogenesis of liver disease has led to the concept of "rebalanced hemostasis" (Table 6.2), in which hemostatic changes that promote bleeding can be counterbalanced by hemostatic changes that promote thrombosis. Consequently, many liver disease patients currently undergo surgery without any blood product transfusion. The hemostatic balance in these patients, however, can be unstable, and occurrences of both bleeding and thrombotic complications during surgery may occur [6].

## 6.3 Pretreatment Evaluation of the Liver Disease Patient: The History and Physical Examination, Blood and Other Testing

Prior to initiating any procedures, the clinician must obtain a thorough history, conduct a physical exam, order pertinent laboratory tests, and consult the patient's physician. The bleeding risk in the patient with liver disease should be assessed through these means. Risk stratification may be documented by using classifications such as the Child-Pugh and Model for End-Stage Liver Disease (MELD) score (Table 6.3).

Clinical examination of the oral cavity and surrounding regions may reveal evidence of liver dysfunction with the presence of petechiae, jaundiced mucosal tissues, gingival bleeding, parotid enlargement, generalized mucosal erythema, and icteric mucosal changes. Also, glossitis may be seen in patients with alcoholic hepatitis [8] and alcohol-related nutritional deficiencies (see Figs. 6.1 and 6.2). The remainder of the complete physical exam is also likely to yield findings associated with the underlying condition. However, physical examination alone is not ade-

**Table 6.3** Modified Child-Pugh classifications

| Parameter | 1 | 2 | 3 |
|---|---|---|---|
| Ascites | None | Slight | Moderate—severe |
| Encephalopathy | None | Slight—moderate | Moderate—severe |
| Bilirubin (mg/dl) | <2.0 | 2–3 | >3.0 |
| Albumin (mg/L) | >3.5 | 2.8–3.5 | <2.8 |
| PT seconds increase over control | 1–3 | 4–6 | >6.0 |

| Key | |
|---|---|
| Total score | Child-Pugh class |
| 5–6 | A |
| 7–9 | B |
| 10–15 | C |

Adapted from Firriolo et al. [1]

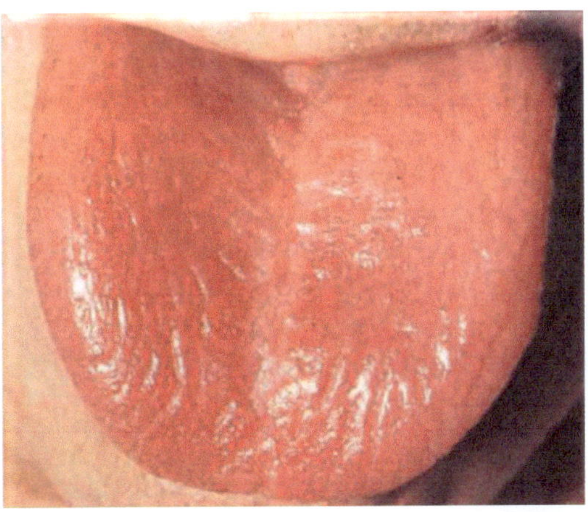

**Fig. 6.1** Tongue of chronic alcoholic

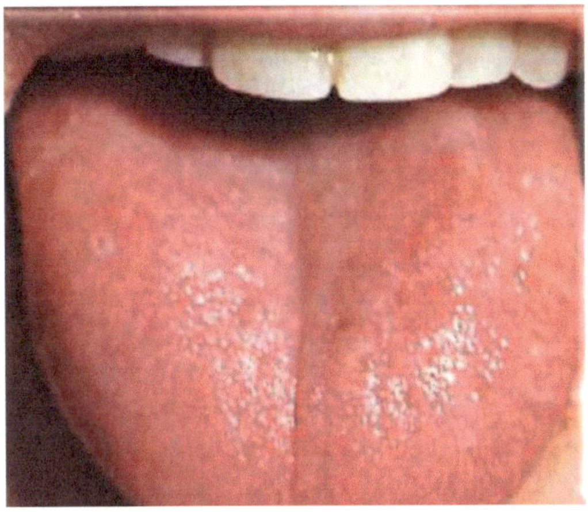

**Fig. 6.2** Glossitis from nutritional deficiencies

quate to assess the stage of liver disease and the risk of bleeding. As such, the history, with a particular focus on previous surgery and bleeding episodes, physical findings, and pertinent laboratory test results are all important elements in the database that serves as the basis for collaborative management of these patients with their primary care physicians and specialists as indicated.

The dentist should be aware of the Child-Pugh classification scheme and the MELD score for liver disease patients and their use in preoperative assessment. The Child-Pugh classification is commonly used and helps to determine long-term prognosis based on disease progression [9]. The classification assesses ascites, encephalopathy, bilirubin, albumin, and prothrombin time (PT). Although there is no direct correlation between Child-Pugh class and hemostasis, a patient with higher Child-Pugh score is likely to have an increased bleeding risk.

MELD score, which is used to determine the extent of the coagulopathy or the severity of liver failure, is currently being used to prioritize candidates for liver transplant. It is based on a patient's serum bilirubin, creatinine international normalized ratio (INR) and, as of 2016, serum sodium level. However, this score does not predict which of these patients will require perioperative transfusion [6].

Liver function laboratory tests help to assess liver disease status. However, there is no definitive laboratory test that determines the degree of hepatic failure, and these tests are limited in their ability to predict bleeding risk [10]. Laboratory tests commonly used in patients with potentially impaired hemostasis include platelet count, prothrombin time (PT), activated partial thromboplastin time (aPTT), and INR. If any of these tests are abnormal in patients with known liver disease, consultation with the patient's physician is required. It is critical that the treating clinician understand the relative value of INR in liver disease as compared with its utility in determining the therapeutic range of anticoagulation. For individuals with normal hemostatic mechanisms who are prescribed medications to achieve therapeutic anticoagulation, INR is an appropriate tool and is predictive of bleeding risk. Much has been written in the dental and oral surgical literature supporting the safety of minor surgical procedures with INR values up to 3.5 or even higher in that population. It must be clear that in patients with liver disease, the same surgical procedures should not be undertaken if there are significant elevations in INR. This laboratory value is not correlated with bleeding risk in a linear fashion as it is with individuals using warfarin. Moreover, even small elevations in INR may be associated with potentially catastrophic bleeding in the presence of liver disease. Abnormal results may contribute to the risk stratification process and to the development of a plan for perioperative management that may include administration of fresh frozen plasma (FFP) and/or blood products.

The PT and aPTT are commonly used laboratory tests for patients with cirrhosis even though these tests are known to be poor predictors of bleeding. PT test results will be elevated with decreased hepatic synthesis of coagulation factor VII with cirrhosis that affect more than 50% of the liver. Therefore, small elevations in PT, which will be reported as INR, represent a significant liver damage and should alert the clinician for possible complications during procedure. However, as indicated above, there is no direct correlation between increased bleeding during oral surgery procedures and abnormal PT [9].

Patients with chronic liver disease will often present with anemia that may be normocytic. It may also be microcytic and hypochromic, usually as a result of blood loss from the gastrointestinal tract, or macrocytic, a function of alcoholism and nutritional deficiency. Anemia in this population may also be related to suppression of erythropoiesis or to hemolysis secondary to hypersplenism [1]. Thrombocytopenia is not uncommon and should alert the clinician to an increased bleeding risk, but it does not provide information regarding platelet function. Qualitative issues may be present with normal numbers of platelets. If the platelet count falls below 40,000/mm$^3$, the procedure should be withheld, and the patient will require preoperative blood products to correct thrombocytopenia prior to any procedure [9].

It is important to note that conventional laboratory testing does not adequately reflect the "rebalanced hemostasis" of liver disease [6]. These values do measure specific changes that may promote bleeding and thrombosis but may not capture the bigger picture as it occurs in vivo [2]. However, due to their availability and the persistence of long-standing practices in medicine, they are widely used to estimate bleeding risk in patients with liver disease.

In light of the limitations of standard laboratory tests, there are new global coagulation assays that mimic the in vivo environment and reflect the effects of procoagulants, anticoagulants, and platelets. One such test is the thrombin generation assay. This test measures thrombin by using tissue factor to initiate coagulation in the presence of platelets [11]. Thromboelastography (TEG) is another test that can provide continuous tracing of all the hemostatic functions that lead to clot formation. This test takes into account primary hemostasis, coagulation, and fibrinolysis. Both tests may more completely and accurately represent what occurs in vivo, but further clinical trials are needed to determine their predictive value with respect to bleeding risks and thrombosis in patients with cirrhosis [5, 12].

## 6.4 Dental and Oral Surgical Management of the Adult Patient with Liver Disease

Dental providers are often asked to evaluate and treat patients at various stages of liver disease. This may include assessment of the remaining dentition and restorations as well as interventions from minimally invasive to significant surgical procedures. Clinicians should carefully evaluate the history, including previous bleeding, as well as physical findings to help determine whether the patient can be treated in the dental office or the hospital. Communication and collaboration with the patient's physician are necessary to optimize outcomes and enhance patient safety. As previously discussed, routine laboratory tests are important but may not be statistically significant in predicting bleeding risks [13].

The dentist should be aware of episodes of preoperative, intraoperative, and postoperative bleeding while treating liver disease patients. Morimoto et al. [14] and Thomson et al. [15] report isolated cases of severe hemorrhagic complications occurring during extraction of teeth of patients with liver diseases [16].

If oral surgical procedures are required, special attention should be paid to minimizing trauma. For more invasive procedures, an infusion of fresh frozen plasma or blood products should be considered [16]. DePaola [17] reported that 8 of 39 of the patients undergoing dental extractions in one series were given preoperative fresh plasma and coagulation-promoting medication. Nevertheless, three of the eight patients still experienced hemorrhagic complications [7].

Therefore, the hospital setting is appropriate for conducting oral surgical procedures or any dental procedures with the potential to cause bleeding on a patient with end-stage liver disease. The dental office is not an ideal site for management of serious bleeding, and in this population with the likelihood of significant comorbidities, bleeding may not be the only issue to arise.

## 6.5 Perioperative Issues and their Management

### 6.5.1 The Preoperative Period

The critical issues addressed during the preoperative assessment relate to patient safety. Can the procedure be done in a dental office, and if so, what modifications might be required? If not, referral to a hospital dental service and collaboration with the patient's primary care physician and appropriate specialists are recommended. Risk stratification is based on the type of the procedure as well as the current status of the patient's liver disease. According to Ward et al. [13], patients requiring more than ten dental extractions are at high risk of experiencing prolonged postoperative bleeding, suggesting the need for a higher level of management and hospital admission for observation. Guidelines are useful; however, risk stratification is best served by a careful assessment of each patient and his/her surgical needs.

Risk stratification requires a complete history and physical examination as well as pertinent laboratory tests and consultation with the patient's physician. While being mindful of the limitations of laboratory testing, particularly in this population, test results do contribute to the process of evaluating the relative bleeding risk and the need for preoperative administration of FFP and blood products.

Rose and Kay [18] suggested that patients will need transfusion with FFP for INR of 3.0 or greater and platelet transfusion for counts less than 50,000/mm$^3$. In more recent studies, simple dental extractions were performed in patients with INR values of 2.5 and platelet counts of 30,000/mm$^3$. In one series, blood transfusions were not needed, and postoperative bleeding was controlled with local hemostatic measures [19]. In a 2017 publication by Cocero et al., 1183 extractions in 318 patients in various stages of liver disease were analyzed. The authors concluded that patients with platelet counts greater than 40,000/mm$^3$ and INR values lower than 2.5 are considered low risk. The authors of both of these studies concluded that INR of 2.5 or greater is a better predictor of bleeding risk than platelet count [13, 20].

### 6.5.2 Intraoperative Management

During the procedure, the clinician must be prepared to control bleeding. Hemostasis can be achieved with local measures such as pressure, sutures, surgical splint with periodontal packing, oxidized cellulose, absorbable gelatin, local anesthesia, fibrin glue, and cyanoacrylate spray. If local

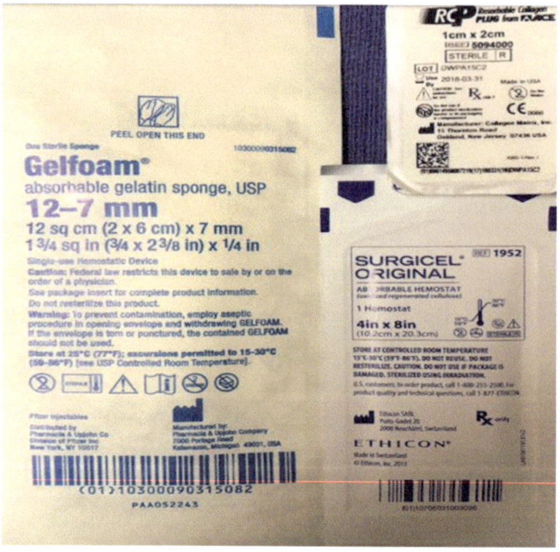


Fig. 6.3 Local hemostatic measures

measures are unsuccessful, the patient may require transfusions of FFP, platelets, cryoprecipitate, and vitamin K injections [13, 21, 22] (see Fig. 6.3). On rare occasion, uncontrollable bleeding may occur during surgical removal of teeth. In such an event, in addition to the measures noted above, the procedure should be abandoned, and the patient may require transfusions of packed cells [7].

### 6.5.3 The Postoperative Period

The patient is still at an increased risk for bleeding in the postoperative period and requires a period of observation and close follow-up after discharge from the clinician's direct care. Reports of secondary bleeding after dental extractions have been published, and in one series, these were successfully treated by local measures [16].

Instructions routinely provided after dental extractions should be modified, if indicated, to reflect the special needs of patients in this population. For pain management, a consideration should be given to postoperative medications and their chance to increase postoperative bleeding. The use of aspirin and nonsteroidal anti-inflammatory drugs in patients with chronic liver disease should be avoided. Both medications have antiplatelet effects and have increased chance of reaching toxic levels due to higher bioavailability in patients with cirrhosis [23]. Acetaminophen containing analgesics are also generally avoided in the liver disease population.

## 6.6 Pediatric Patients

There is not a great deal of data on the impact of liver disease on hemostasis in children. Decisions based upon extrapolation from adult studies may not be fully informed given age-related physiologic differences and the nature of hepatic pathology in the pediatric population. Diseases affecting the liver, including inborn errors of metabolism, may have profound effects on hemostasis, some of which are more marked in pediatric patients. Invasive dental or oral and maxillofacial procedures on such patients require collaborative management with the appropriate pediatric specialists in a setting that best supports the safety and comfort of the child [24].

## 6.7 Liver Transplant Patients

Patients awaiting liver transplant may be referred to dental professionals for evaluation of non-restorable teeth and eradication of active oral disease. Those patients with extensive periodontal disease and carious teeth may require full mouth extraction and the fabrication of dentures. This has been suggested to minimize posttransplant morbidity and mortality associated with infection in patients who are immunosuppressed [16]. These patients, some of whom are Child stage C, may be at an increased risk for bleeding due to chronic liver disease and cirrhosis. In one small series, 7 of 16 patients awaiting liver transplant (43.8%) developed hemorrhagic complications in the course of preoperative dental treatment [7]. Even with aggressive preoperative preparation and perioperative management, patients in this population who require multiple extractions are at a significant risk of postoperative bleeding [13].

During the first 3 months following liver transplant, only emergency dental care should be provided. Some authors advocate antibiotic prophylaxis; however, there is a lack of evidence supporting this recommendation. If invasive treatment is necessary, the patient should be admitted to the hospital and treated collaboratively with the transplant team and the patient's primary physician. Following the initial recovery period, nearly normal liver function may be restored. The coagulation profile and blood chemistry values may be close to normal, though they should always be checked before dental treatment. Platelet levels, however, may remain depressed [7].

Special attention should be given to patients with acute rejection posttransplant as these patients are treated with increased immunosuppression. As such, all dental procedures should be postponed, and only emergency care should be rendered, and these patients should be treated to correct coagulation factor abnormalities and low platelet levels prior to any procedure in order to avoid increased bleeding.

**Conclusion**

Patients with liver disease present a number of challenges to the dental team. Multiple insults to the hemostatic mechanism may result in bleeding that is significant enough to complicate the procedure and/or the postoperative course. Less frequently, serious bleeding may be encountered, requiring aggressive management. Preoperative assessment and careful planning are essential and involve far more than simple guidelines based on laboratory test results. While such guidelines may be useful in the treatment of other patients with coagulopathies and bleeding disorders, patients with liver disease must be evaluated comprehensively, risk stratified thoughtfully, and managed with great care in the appropriate setting.

## References


1. John Firriolo F. Dental management of patients with end-stage liver disease. Dent Clin N Am. 2006;50:563–90.
2. Golla K, Epstein JB, Cabay RJ. Ill liver disease: current perspectives on medical and dental management. Oral Surg Oral Med Oral Pathol Oral Radiol Endod. 2004;98:516–21.
3. Feldman M, Friedman LS, Sleisenger MH. Sleisenger and Fordtran's gastrointestinal and liver disease. 7th ed. Philadelphia, PA: Saunders; 2002. p. 1216–20.
4. Tripodi A, Primignani M, Chantarangkul V, et al. Thrombin generation in patients with cirrhosis: the role of platelets. Hepatology. 2006;44(2):440–5.
5. Roberts LN, Patel RK, Arya R. Haemostasis and thrombosis in liver disease. Br J Haematol. 2010;148:507–21.
6. Lisman T, Porte RJ. Rebalanced hemostasis in patients with liver disease: evidence and clinical consequences. Blood. 2010;116:878–85.
7. Haghighi AG, Finder RG, Bennett JD. Systemic disease and bleeding disorders for the oral and maxillofacial surgeon. Oral Maxillofac Surg Clin North Am. 2016;28:461–71.
8. Novacek G, Plachetzky U, Pötzi R, et al. Dental and periodontal disease in patients with cirrhosis—role of etiology of liver disease. J Hepatol. 1995;22:576.
9. Lockhart PB, Gibson J, Pond SH, Leitch J. Dental management considerations for the patient with an acquired coagulopathy. Part 1: Coagulopathies from systemic disease. Br Dent J. 2003;195:439–45.
10. Neuschwander-Tetri BA. Common blood tests for liver disease: which ones are the most useful? Postgrad Med. 1995;98:49–63.
11. Tripodi A. Tests of coagulation in liver disease. Clin Liver Dis. 2009;13:55.
12. Mallett SV, Chowdary P, Burroughs AK. Clinical utility of viscoelastic tests of coagulation in patients with liver disease. Liver Int. 2013;33:961–74.
13. Ward BB, Weideman EM. Long-term postoperative bleeding after dentoalveolar surgery in the pretransplant liver failure patient. J Oral Maxillofac Surg. 2006;64:1469–74.
14. Morimoto A, Morimoto Y, Maki K, Nishida I, Kawahara H, Kimura M. Dental treatment of a prospective recipient of a liver transplant: a case report. Pediatr Dent. 1998;23:75–8.
15. Thomson PJ, Langton SG. Persistent haemorrhage following dental extractions in patients with liver disease: two cautionary tales. Br Dent J. 1996;180:141–4.
16. Niederhagen B, Wolff M, Appel T, et al. Location and sanitation of dental foci in liver transplantation. Transpl Int. 2003;16:173.
17. DePaola LG. Managing the care of patients infected with bloodborne diseases. J Am Dent Assoc. 2003;134:350–8.
18. Rose L, Kay D. Internal medicine for dentistry. St. Louis: Mosby; 1983. p. 425–6.
19. Perdigão JPV. Postoperative bleeding after dental extraction in liver pretransplant patients. J Oral Maxillofac Surg. 2012;70:e177–84.
20. Cocero N, Bezzi M, Martini S, Carossa S. Oral surgical treatment of patients with chronic liver disease: assessments of bleeding and its relationship with thrombocytopenia and blood coagulation parameters. J Oral Maxillofac Surg. 2017;75(1):28–34.

21. Berthier AM, Guillygomarc'h A, Messner M, et al. Use of re- combinant factor VIIa to treat persistent bleeding following dental extractions in two cirrhotic patients. Vox Sang. 2002;82:119.
22. Thomson PJ, Langton SG. Persistent hemorrhage following dental extractions in patients with liver disease: two cautionary tales. Br Dent J. 1996;180:141.
23. Douglas LR, Douglass JB, Sieck JO, Smith PJ. Oral management of the patient with end-stage liver disease and the liver transplant patient. Oral Surg Oral Med Oral Pathol Oral Radiol Endod. 1998;86:55–6.
24. Magnusson M, et al. A conceptual and practical approach to haemostasis in paediatric liver disease. Arch Dis Child. 2016;101:854–9.

# Malignancy and Hemostasis

7

Matthew Idle, Scott Claiborne, Ketan Patel, and Deepak Kademani

**Abstract**

The presence of cancer may predispose the patient to a hypercoagulable state. Approximately 15% of all patients with a malignancy may be affected by some form of thromboembolic disease. Trousseau's syndrome relates to this predisposition to both arterial and venous coagulation in this cohort of patients. This well-documented state affects the local tumor site as well as causes these systemic effects. The additional burden on the patient of potential immobility, chemotherapy, surgery, indwelling lines, and nutritional deficit make thromboembolic disease more prevalent. It must also be borne in mind that malignant disease may also result in a greater bleeding tendency due to dysfunction with components of the coagulation cascade. Additionally, many patients may be on anticoagulant therapy, and bone marrow disorders such as leukemia may cause thrombo-hemorrhagic complications.

The oral surgical management of cancer patients in regard to hemostasis is a complex interplay of history, physical findings, laboratory values, and provider preference. There is limited high-quality information available regarding the specific oral surgery population, and therefore the best recommendations are extrapolated from available studies and guidelines in the medical and surgical literature. The ultimate decision is at the discretion of the treating provider to ensure procedures are executed appropriately, and there is a plan for monitoring in the postoperative period. Certainly the patient and treatment factors which place patients at greater risk for bleeding should be evaluated together in consultation with the patient's oncologist prior to surgery. Once the risk of bleeding is established, laboratory testing guides consideration of preoperative transfusion, further medical management, or alteration of the surgical plan to reduce risk of bleeding intraoperatively. Scheduling surgery to accommodate for the expected bone marrow recovery following the drop in the patient's blood counts is also a helpful measure. Reducing the extent of

M. Idle · S. Claiborne
Oral/Head and Neck Oncologic and Reconstructive Surgery, North Memorial Health Hospital, Minneapolis, MN, USA

K. Patel
Department of Oral and Maxillofacial Surgery, North Memorial Health Hospital, Minneapolis, MN, USA

D. Kademani (✉)
Oral/Head and Neck Oncologic and Reconstructive Surgery, North Memorial Health Hospital, Minneapolis, MN, USA

Department of Oral and Maxillofacial Surgery, North Memorial Health Hospital, Minneapolis, MN, USA

Department of Surgery, North Memorial Health Hospital, Minneapolis, MN, USA
e-mail: Deepak.Kademani@NorthMemorial.com



R. P. Szumita, P. M. Szumita (eds.), *Hemostasis in Dentistry*, https://doi.org/10.1007/978-3-319-71240-6_7

surgery and dividing treatment into multiple visits can decrease the stress on the patient's hemostatic mechanisms. Careful attention to surgical technique to minimize tissue trauma and blood loss is essential, and local hemostatic measures discussed elsewhere are helpful adjuncts.

## 7.1 Introduction

The presence of cancer may predispose the patient to a hypercoagulable state. Approximately 15% of all patients with a malignancy may be affected by some form of thromboembolic disease [1]. Trousseau's syndrome relates to this predisposition to both arterial and venous coagulation in this cohort of patients [2]. This well documented state affects the local tumor site as well as causing these systemic effects [3]. The additional burden on the patient of potential immobility, chemotherapy, surgery, indwelling lines, and nutritional deficit make thromboembolic disease more prevalent [4]. It must also be borne in mind that malignant disease may also result in a greater bleeding tendency due to dysfunction with components of the coagulation cascade. Additionally, many patients may be on anticoagulant therapy, and bone marrow disorders such as leukemia may cause thrombohemorrhagic complications [5].

This chapter seeks to cover all aspects of acquired coagulation disorders related to malignancy and how these may impact on the management of oral disease. The aim is to gain an appreciation of the cancer patient presenting with a tendency toward clotting or hemorrhage and thus have an algorithm in mind for their dental treatment so as to minimize potential complications that may arise.

## 7.2 Hypercoagulability

Thromboembolic manifestations are the most frequent complication of patients with a malignancy [6]. These are most commonly venous thromboembolism (VTE) in the form of either deep vein thrombosis or pulmonary embolism [7]. Malignancy will have effects on all features of Virchow's triad [8]. It is known that abnormalities in the hematological clotting screen may be abnormal with malignancy even if there is no evidence of clinical manifestations [9]. A solid-state tumor has the ability to leak fibrin into the local environment and also has effects systemically. This along with fibrinolysis is more predominant in patients with metastatic disease thereby increasing the preponderance for hypercoagulability [10].

Recently interesting developments have shown a strong correlation between platelets and cancer-related thrombosis [11]. A subset of platelets called COAT (collagen and thrombin) have a high level of factor V bound to the surface and are related to thromboembolic events [12, 13]. High factor VIII levels and low protein C levels also had a predictive value for thrombosis in patients with malignancy [14].

## 7.3 Tumor Effects

The presence of a tumor may have several local effects, as procoagulant molecules are evident of the surface of cancer cells [15]. In addition, as the tumor shed cells, this initiates a blood-borne phase of the clotting cascade. These metastatic cells encourage thrombus formation surrounding them containing both fibrin and platelets [16, 17]. It was originally postulated that for tumors to spread via a hematogenous route, then activation of the coagulation cascade was necessary [18]. This has subsequently been proven in animal models to be the case [16, 17].

Tissue factor (TF) seems to play a central role in tumor-related coagulation [7]. TF is needed for activation of clotting factors in plasma. It forms a complex with factors VII and VIIa that then initiate the coagulation protease cascade [19]. TF expression is increased not only by cancer cells but also by the tissue surrounding the tumor [20, 21]. The subsequent thromboembolic events caused then result in hypoxia and the expression of vascular endothelial growth factor (VEGF) resulting in angiogenesis and cancer growth [22].

There is a measurable aspect to this as shown by a study that demonstrated increased venous thromboembolism in patients with high tumor expression of TF [23]. In mouse models that focused specifically on colorectal cancers, activation of the oncogene, k-ras, and inactivation of the tumor suppressor protein, p53, caused increased TF expression [24]. Many studies show that TF is critical to overall survival. Its expression is related to increased angiogenesis, poorer histological differentiation, and a higher rate of blood-borne metastasis leading to a less favorable outcome. The processes by which TF causes tumor progression have been proposed by Langer and Bokemeyer to be either coagulation-dependent or coagulation-independent mechanisms [7]. With regard to the mechanisms that are dependent, the production of thrombin with the subsequent conversion of fibrinogen to fibrin causes the activation of platelets and the formations of an extracellular matrix that leads to tumorigenesis. The independent mechanism functions via TF and factor IIa complexes signaled through protease-activated receptors. This process causes enhanced cell proliferation with invasion and angiogenesis that is associated with tumor progression and decreased survival. It is the TF in the cytoplasm that purportedly causes the upregulation of VEGF and subsequent angiogenesis [25]. The current thinking is that TF present in the bloodstream is more likely to be the cause of VTE in cancer patients than TF produced from the primary tumor. It is via this pathway that it can have a direct effect on hypercoagulability. A retrospective analysis showed that the incidence of VTE was 35% in patients who demonstrated TF-positive microparticles as opposed to 0% without evidence of these microparticles [26]. These microparticles are usually introduced into the circulation directly from the cancer cells and can thus exert their effect. Correlation has been demonstrated between levels of these TF-related microparticles and D-dimer that has emerged once again as a valuable measure of coagulability [27]. Several other studies have demonstrated that the surgical removal in patients who had localized tumors resulted in a corresponding rapid decrease in the TF-related microparticles [7]. The mechanism by which TF promotes metastases is also linked closely with it promotion of hemostasis. With regard to lung metastases, it has been directly proven that the formation of a fibrin-platelet clot around tumor cells enables both spreading and protection from natural killer cell-mediated cytotoxicity [28]. In mouse models disruption of this TF-initiated cascade effectively suppressed lung metastases [29]. However, this has not been demonstrated effectively in clinical models due to concerns regarding the risks of bleeding associated with anti-TF treatment. Outside of lung metastasis, the inhibition of Trousseau's syndrome by blocking TF has been investigated in experimental and preclinical studies by either the downregulation of TF or the destruction of TF-expressing tumor cells. Overall, the TF-related link between hypercoagulability and cancer spread has also not been convincingly proven, and further work is currently ongoing. Several other molecules have also been described to have a procoagulant effect in malignancy.

Cancer procoagulant, fibrinolytic molecules and cytokines (e.g., TNF-α and IL-1β) that are released by tumor cells have also been shown to have thrombotic effects [30].

The proinflammatory cytokine tumor necrosis factor alpha orchestrates complex multicellular processes through a wide variety of changes that it induces in cell functions. TNF-alpha is produced by tumor cells constitutively and in turn induces the expression of tissue factor by the vascular endothelial cells [31, 32].

Cancer procoagulant (CP) is another such procoagulant. CP is a cysteine protease which is a substrate for factor X in the coagulation cascade. CP can activate factor X independently and cleaves its heavy chain site at a different location compared to other known factor X activators [30, 33, 34]. CP has been detected in several extracts of tumor cells [30, 35, 36]. CP has been shown to be elevated up to 85% of cancer patients [30, 37].

Platelets also play a major role in the tumor microenvironment. They play a crucial role in promoting tumor growth and metastasis. In solid tumors, many studies have shown that platelets play a major role in protecting tumor cells from natural killer (NK) cell-mediated lysis [38, 39]. Furthermore, platelet-coated tumor cells were physically shielded from lysis by NK cells, and this protection is not a result of passive agglutination but required platelet activation. Upon aggregation by tumor cells or physiological factors, platelets mobilize to their surface membrane glucocorticoid-induced TNF-related ligand (GITRL). This leads to the platelet-coated tumor cell are protected, from NK lytic activity and also interferon-gamma secretion due to the interaction of the GITRL interaction with its receptor GITR on the NK cells. Soluble factors are also secreted by these platelets which inhibit NK antitumor activity. Therefore, platelets not only protect tumor cells from NK-mediated lysis within the circulation but also potentially within the tumor microenvironment via signaling by secreting soluble factors [40, 41].

In hematological malignancies, platelets on the contrary are inhibited from aggregation. Platelets derived from acute and chronic myeloid leukemia (AML and CML) patients tend to have impaired platelet responsiveness to physiological responses. In addition, they may have platelet storage deficiency and, commonly in AML, disease- and treatment-induced thrombocytopenia [42–45].

Tumors may have an additional physical effect causing thrombosis by disturbing bloodflow. This can be via direct pressure causing alteration in flow or injury to the intima of the vessels [1]. This is particularly notable in renal cell carcinoma that is strongly associated with inferior vena cava thrombosis [46]. This has been shown to be the case in 4–10% of renal tumors [47].

## 7.4 Chemotherapy

The treatment of malignant disease with chemotherapy is associated with an increase in the risk of developing VTE by up to six times that of the control group [48, 49]. Most patients who develop VTE do so in the outpatient setting [50]. A significant amount of research was done in the field of breast cancer, and it was shown that both tamoxifen and chemotherapy increased the risk of VTE [51, 52]. Cisplatin-based chemotherapy demonstrated the prevalence of VTE to be 17% compared to 7% for any chemotherapy [53, 54]. It is postulated that this is independently related to endothelial injury, hypomagnesemia, and raised levels of von Willebrand factor [55, 56]. Overall, the acknowledgment is that the polypharmacy of chemotherapy can increase the risk of VTE. The use of anticoagulants, to reduce thromboembolic events in patients undergoing chemotherapy for malignancy, will also impact on the management by the dentist. This will be discussed later in this chapter.

## 7.5 Medical Devices

The management of patients with malignancy, particularly those undergoing chemotherapy, will usually necessitate the placement of a central venous catheter (CVC). This will facilitate the administration of drugs and sampling blood for hematology and chemistry. It is acknowledged that the presence of this device will increase the risk of DVT particularly in the upper limb on the same side and also consequently PE [57]. The injury to the vessel wall that occurs upon its placement may contribute to an increased rate of thrombotic event [58]. This has been documented to occur in 2/3 of patients with cancer. Catheters placed in the left subclavian vein appear to have an increased risk compared to those on the right [59]. Several other variables exist that can affect the development of a DVT related to CVCs including the material used to construct the catheter and the fluid infused through it. The use of total parenteral nutrition is more likely to cause a DVT than a crystalloid solution [60]. It has also been proposed that increasing the number of lumens of the CVC may increase DVT rates. Finally, catheters that contain the use of polyvinyl chloride are more thrombogenic than those containing polyurethane [61].

## 7.6 Surgery

The management of oncology patients for outpatient dental or oral surgical procedures begins with a multifactorial medical and dental assessment. The proposed procedure and its complexity should be considered in relation to the patient's overall health status and expected prognosis in consultation with the patient's oncologist. With modern advances in cancer treatment, patients are often managed with chronic chemotherapy or immunotherapy even in the face of metastatic disease and have a much longer life expectancy than in the past. Dental providers are therefore tasked with managing this new subset of complex patients.

Oncology patients require careful attention to the history and physical examination in preparation for invasive procedures. Important features of the history should be identification of the type of cancer, its stage, the proposed or current treatment regimen, and current medications. Treatment approaches may include a combination of surgery, radiotherapy, chemotherapy, or immunotherapy. The management may also differ based on prognosis and whether the intent is curative or palliative therapy. Knowledge of the care provided is essential in determining the duration and magnitude of impact on hemostasis, immune response, and wound healing prior to undergoing surgical procedures.

The medical treatment of cancer often results in hemodynamic changes which place the patient at increased risk of intraoperative or postoperative hemorrhage, and this is a key component to assessing the patient's candidacy for surgery. Consultation with the patient's oncologist will provide additional details and provide the dental provider a risk assessment regarding the care of patient. In general, the most ideal approach is to provide dental examinations and management of dental pathology prior to initiation of radiation or oncologic treatment. In the event that this is not the case, the dentist must be prepared to be involved in treatment of patients with pre-existing cancer diagnoses and ongoing treatment.

Medical history taking is the most important component of evaluating hemostatic function [62]. At the consultation appointment, all patients should be questioned regarding any pre-existing bleeding disorders, easy or frequent bruising, prolonged bleeding with minor trauma or prior surgery, or episodes of spontaneous bleeding. Melena or hematochezia, hematuria, menorrhagia, epistaxis, and bleeding from mucous membranes are signs of derangement of hemostasis. Examination of the patient should not only be focused on the oral cavity but on the patient as a whole. Evidence of prior bleeding may be seen on a routine physical examination and include petechiae, ecchymosis, or hematomas. Pallor of the conjunctiva and cutaneous ecchymosis may indicate significant anemia. Jaundice, icteric sclera, and abdominal fullness could signify liver dysfunction related to chemotherapy toxicity or previous disease. While a full physical examination is not the responsibility of the dentist, careful attention may prompt further investigation by history or laboratory studies.

Hemostatic derangements are commonly found on laboratory testing in cancer patients, related to severity of disease and duration of both illness and treatment. One study of 40 patients with solid tumors found 80% had two or more abnormal hemostatic tests; another showed an even higher proportion at 92% [63]. A significant portion of the patients had elevated D-dimer levels, which signified a hypercoagulable state, as previously discussed. However, thrombocytopenia was noted in 12.5% and coagulopathy signified by prolonged PT/PTT in 40%, indicating risk of bleeding. Along with the prolonged PT/PTT, there was also a significant difference between the normal control group's platelet count and the cancer patients [64]. Both of these findings are indicative of the abnormal hemostasis and supportive of the need for laboratory studies in patients with known malignancy.

The presurgical laboratory workup of patients with malignancy focuses on the hematological and immune system abnormalities commonly seen either as a result of treatment or from the cancer itself. Cancer infiltration of the bone marrow may be seen in primary lesions such as lymphoma or from metastatic spread from virtually all cancers. Breast, prostate, and lung are the most common cancers associated with bone marrow invasion [65]. Once the bone marrow is 80% saturated with cancer cells, the production of myeloid and lymphoid cell lines are significantly inhibited, leading to reduction in circulating red blood cells (anemia), platelets (thrombocytopenia), and white blood cells (leukopenia) [66]. Bone marrow suppression is also a common side effect of many chemotherapeutic drugs and results in similar cytopenias. Radiation may induce some bone marrow suppression by encompassing those sites during treatment; however, it is less commonly seen than with patients receiving chemotherapy [67]. Platelet function abnormalities have also been reported with malignancy, due to the myeloproliferative process, but these are challenging to diagnose. Bleeding time testing is notoriously unreliable and it has limited usefulness [68]. A platelet function test is expensive and seldom warranted as a baseline evaluation. A key factor in evaluating these patients is the timing of any previous chemotherapy or planned cycles. The effect of treatment on the bone marrow is a cyclic process which follows a generally predictable pattern in which the platelet count begins to fall approximately day 7 following treatment, reaches the low-point at day 14, and returns back to baseline levels between days 28 and 35 [69].

As indicated above, cancer patients are more likely to have a coexisting coagulopathy in addition to the myelosuppressive effects of chemotherapy and radiation. The causes are varied. Malnutrition can lead to vitamin K deficiency and therefore inadequate production of active coagulation factors [70]. Hepatotoxicity of chemotherapeutic drugs (methotrexate, fludarabine, azacytidine) can cause abnormal hepatic synthetic function of clotting factors, although the effects are usually transient [71]. Disseminated intravascular coagulation (DIC) may be found in approximately 7% of cancer patients, with either the hypercoagulable form (clotting) or the hypocoagulable form which induces bleeding from lysis of fibrin clots. Circulating heparin-like anticoagulants are produced in occasional patients afflicted with multiple myeloma [72]. Coagulopathy can be identified by elevated prothrombin time (PT) and standardized INR results as well as prolonged partial thromboplastin time (PTT). In general, the INR should be within the range of 2–3 for elective dental procedures in an outpatient setting. Patients with coexisting coagulopathy, thrombocytopenia, or anemia are a challenge even for the most routine of oral surgeries. These patients may benefit from a hospital setting where easy access to blood products is available in the case of significant bleeding. Vitamin K or fresh frozen plasma may sometimes be required to transfuse active clotting factors to correct hemorrhage in patients with underlying coagulopathy [73].

Thrombocytopenia is usually identified on a complete blood count by reduction in the platelet count below the normal level of 150,000–400,000. The causes are generally decreased production by myelosuppression, increased destruction by drug-related effects, and sequestration by splenomegaly. Chemotherapy causes approximately 2/3 of all thrombocytopenia in cancer patients [74]. Values below 100,000 often require reduction in chemotherapy dosing [75]. Severe platelet deficiency of less than 50,000 occurs in 20–25% of those receiving chemotherapy, according to 2 major studies of 4956 patients [76, 77]. Despite this high frequency of significant thrombocytopenia, spontaneous bleeding is a less frequent complication, occurring in only 9% of treatment cycles [78]. The highest risk has long been thought to occur when platelet counts drop below 20,000, which was established in the 1960s in a study of patients with acute leukemia [79]. This has been the standard threshold for platelet transfusion in patients who are otherwise asymptomatic and not undergoing surgical procedures in the hopes of reducing spontaneous hemorrhage [80].

Subsequent authors have challenged the absolute use of the platelet count as the only variable to determine risk. The study by Ducher found 84% of significant bleeding events began when the platelet count was between 20,000 and 50,000, with a population of 1274 patients. This is evidence of significant variability from patient to patient regarding bleeding at specific platelet counts, which is important when considering the threshold for transfusion or the safety of even minor surgery procedures. A more recent study by Friedman found that platelet count was not correlated at all with episodes of bleeding, and the most significant factor was a history of prior bleeding events [81]. A retrospective study by Slichter supports the previous conclusions and found importance not in the platelet count, but in a history of bleeding within 5 days [82]. Another study indicated a prior history of bleeding, presence of bone marrow metastasis, and highly myelosuppressive chemotherapy were all associated with hemorrhage [83]. Certain chemotherapeutic drugs are known to have higher incidence of myelosuppression. Cisplatin, methotrexate, fluorouracil, vincristine, cyclophosphamide, doxorubicin, and etoposide are medications causing thrombocytopenia severe enough to warrant delay in radiation therapy [84]. Elting in 2002 identified cisplatin, carboplatin, lomustine, carmustine, dacarbazine, and mitomycin C as agents considered extremely toxic to bone marrow which were more associated with bleeding [85]. Many other agents have intermediate risk.

All of these factors in addition to the laboratory values should be considered when assessing oncologic patients and their risk stratification in preparation for oral surgical procedures. The studies cited above all dealt with asymptomatic patients who were not undergoing surgical procedures. The risk of uncontrolled hemorrhage is likely higher during surgery as increased stress is placed on the coagulation process. Current guidelines from the American, British, and Canadian systems for surgery (excluding neurosurgery) reflect this concern and consider preoperative transfusion indicated to maintain a platelet count >50,000 [86–88]. Thrombocytopenic patients have been found to be safe for routine dental extractions, in a single study with some limitations. Fillmore in 2013 studied 68 patients with a platelet count under 100,000 and found 7.4% had postoperative hemorrhage, which responded to local measures [89]. The study concluded that neither the transfusions nor hemostatic measures had any outcome on bleeding risk, although the authors indicated the use of local measures remains the judgment of the treating dentist. This study is of limited sample size and did not seek to stratify the results based on severity of thrombocytopenia; therefore the results are of limited value. The authors did seem to reflect the recommendations by others that oral surgical procedures are safe above the 50,000 platelet level. More substantial research is indicated for the safety of oral surgical procedures in this patient population.

Anemia is defined as decreased red blood cell mass, amount of hemoglobin, or volume of RBCs based on standardized numbers set by gender [90]. Normal hemoglobin values are between 12–16 g/dL for women and 14–18 g/dL for men [91]. The World Health Organization classifies anemia as mild (10 mg/dL to the lower limit of normal), moderate (8–9.9 g/dL), severe (6.5–7.9 g/dL), and life-threatening (<6.5 g/dL). While anemia does not cause intraoperative bleeding, significant bleeding may worsen pre-existing anemia, increasing postoperative morbidity, and it is therefore important to note in the operative management of oncology patients. One study identified 63% of patients with cancer diagnosis presented with anemia, which increased with advancing cancer stage [92]. Anemia may result from many different mechanisms in cancer patients. Patients with gastrointestinal lumen cancers or genitourinary cancers may lose blood through direct bleeding from the neoplasm itself. Those with bone marrow invasion or metastasis lack ability to produce active red blood cells. The inflammatory products of cancers (IL-1, IL-6, TNF-α) can also restrict survival of red blood cell precursors, leading to anemia [93]. Hemolysis of existing RBCs may be the result of autoimmune processes or drug related [94]. Malnutrition is a common cofactor in cancer which reduces iron stores and therefore leads to anemia [95]. However, the most common cause of anemia in cancer patients by far is treatment with chemotherapy or radiation, inducing a suppression of red cell production.

A routine complete blood count includes both hemoglobin and hematocrit values, will promptly identify anemia, and should be included in basic preoperative laboratory testing for these patients as mentioned previously because it will also screen for thrombocytopenia. The management of cancer-associated anemia is complex but in general utilizes iron supplementation, erythropoietic-stimulating agents (ESAs), and blood transfusions [96]. In placebo-controlled trials of ESAs, 2–3 weeks was required before a significant difference was found between the epoetin and placebo groups [97, 98]. Therefore, transfusion is the recommended option when rapid correction of hemoglobin levels is required [95]. This could be for emergent surgeries or more severe or symptomatic anemia. In general, stable patients with hemoglobin levels of 7–8 do not require red blood cell transfusion unless major bleeding is expected [99]. Patients with mild to moderate anemia are usually able to be managed as outpatient surgeries, while symptomatic or severe anemia may require blood transfusion prior to surgical procedures or warrant completion of those procedures in a hospital setting. Identifying anemia during preoperative evaluation, optimizing hemoglobin levels, and minimizing blood loss during surgery are key components to the management of cancer patients undergoing oral surgery, who often require simultaneous management of thrombocytopenia or anticoagulation.

In summary, the oral surgical management of cancer patients in regard to hemostasis is a complex interplay of history, physical findings, laboratory values, and provider preference. There is limited high-quality information available regarding the specific oral surgery population, and therefore the best recommendations are extrapolated from available studies and guidelines in the medical and surgical literature. The ultimate decision is at the discretion of the treating provider to ensure procedures are executed appropriately, and there is a plan for monitoring in the postoperative period. Certainly the patient and treatment factors which place patients at greater risk for bleeding should be evaluated together in consultation with the patient's oncologist prior to surgery. Once the risk of bleeding is established, laboratory testing guides consideration of preoperative transfusion, further medical management, or alteration of the surgical plan to reduce risk of bleeding intraoperatively. Scheduling surgery to accommodate for the expected bone marrow recovery following the drop in the patient's blood counts is also a helpful measure. Reducing the extent of surgery and dividing treatment into multiple visits can decrease the stress on the patient's hemostatic mechanisms. Careful attention to surgical technique to minimize tissue trauma and blood loss is essential, and local hemostatic measures discussed elsewhere are helpful adjuncts [100].

## References


1. Letai A, Kuter DJ. Cancer, coagulation and anticoagulation. Oncologist. 1999;4:443–9.
2. Varki A. Trousseau's syndrome: multiple definitions and multiple mechanisms. Blood. 2007;110(6):1723–9.
3. Nagy JA, Brown LF, Senger DR, et al. Pathogenesis of tumor stroma generation: a critical role for leaky blood vessels and fibrin deposition. Biochim Biophys Acta. 1989;948(3):305–26.
4. Khorana AA, Connolly GC. Assessing risk of venous thromboembolism in the patient with cancer. J Clin Oncol. 2009;27(29):4839–47.
5. Jain A, Gupta N, Singh T, et al. A study of haemostatic parameters in patients of chronic myeloid leukaemia. J Clin Diagn Res. 2016;10(7):OC19–23.
6. Zhu YW, Feng TB, Zhou XJ, et al. Routine hemostasis and hemogram parameters: valuable assessments for coagulation disorder and chemotherapy in cancer patients. Chin Med J. 2016;129(15):1772–7.
7. Langer F, Bokemeyer C. Crosstalk between cancer and haemostasis. Hamostaseologie. 2012;32:95–104.
8. Lip GY, Chin BS, Blann AD. Cancer and the prothrombotic state. Lancet Oncol. 2002;3:27–34.
9. Falanga A, Marchetti M, Vignoli A. Coagulation and cancer: biological and clinical aspects. J Thromb Haemost. 2013;11(2):223–33.
10. Falanga A, Marchetti M, Vignoli A, et al. Clotting mechanisms and cancer: implications in thrombus formation and tumor progression. Clin Adv Hematol Oncol. 2003;1:673–8.
11. Riedl J, Pabinger I, Ay C. Platelets in cancer and thrombosis. Hamostaseologie. 2015;34:54–62.
12. Tafur AJ, Dale G, Cherry M, et al. Prospective evaluation of protein C and factor VIII in prediction of cancer-associated thrombosis. Thromb Res. 2015;136(6):1120–5.
13. Alberio L, Safa O, Clemetson KJ, et al. Surface expression and functional characterization of alpha-granule factor V in human platelets: effects of ionophore A23187, thrombin, collagen, and convulxin. Blood. 2000;95:1694–702.
14. Vormittag R, Simanek R, Ay C, et al. High factor VIII levels independently predict venous thromboembolism in cancer patients: the cancer and thrombosis study. Arterioscler Thromb Vasc Biol. 2009;29:2176–81.
15. Donati MB. Cancer and thrombosis: from phlegmasia alba dolens to transgenic mice. Thromb Haemost. 1995;74:278–81.
16. Ruf W, Mueller BM. Thrombin generation and the pathogenesis of cancer. Semin Thromb Hemost. 2006;32(Suppl 1):61–8.
17. Palumbo JS. Mechanisms linking tumor cell-associated procoagulant function to tumor dissemination. Semin Thromb Hemost. 2008;34:154–60.
18. Falanga A. Biological and clinical aspects of anticancer effects of antithrombotics. Pathophysiol Haemost Thromb. 2003/2004;33:389–92.

19. Mackman N. The role of tissue factor and factor VIIa in haemostasis. Anesth Analg. 2009;108(5):1447–52.
20. Ohta S, Wada H, Nakazaki T, et al. Expression of tissue factor is associated with clinical features and angiogenesis in prostate cancer. Anticancer Res. 2002;22:2991–6.
21. Garnier D, Milsom C, Magnus N, et al. Role of the tissue factor pathway in the biology of tumor initiating cells. Thromb Res. 2010;125(Suppl 2):S44–50.
22. Rong Y, Durden DL, Van Meir EG, et al. 'Pseudopalisading' necrosis in glioblastoma: a familiar morphologic feature that links vascular pathology, hypoxia, and angiogenesis. J Neuropathol Exp Neurol. 2006;65:529–39.
23. Khorana AA, Ahrendt SA, Ryan CK, et al. Tissue factor expression, angiogenesis, and thrombosis in pancreatic cancer. Clin Cancer Res. 2007;13:2870–5.
24. Yu JL, May L, Lhotak V, et al. Oncogenic events regulate tissue factor expression in colorectal cancer cells: implications for tumor progression and angiogenesis. Blood. 2005;105:1734–41.
25. Abe K, Shoji M, Chen J, et al. Regulation of vascular endothelial growth factor production and angiogenesis by the cytoplasmic tail of tissue factor. Proc Natl Acad Sci USA. 1999;96:8663–8.
26. Zwicker JI, Liebman HA, Neuberg D, et al. Tumor derived tissue factor-bearing microparticles are associated with venous thromboembolic events in malignancy. Clin Cancer Res. 2009;15:6830–40.
27. Del Conde I, Bharwani LD, Dietzen DJ, et al. Microvesicle-associated tissue factor and Trousseau's syndrome. J Thromb Haemost. 2007;5:70–4.
28. Im JH, Fu W, Wang H, et al. Coagulation facilitates tumor cell spreading in the pulmonary vasculature during early metastatic colony formation. Cancer Res. 2004;64:8613–9.
29. Amirkhosravi A, Mousa SA, Amaya M, et al. Assessment of anti-metastatic effects of anticoagulant and antiplatelet agents using animal models of experimental lung metastasis. Methods Mol Biol. 2010;663:241–59.
30. Caine GJ, Stonelake PS, Lip GYH, et al. The hypercoagulable state of malignancy: pathogenesis and current debate. Neoplasia. 2002;4(6):465–73.
31. Nemerson Y. The tissue factor pathway of blood coagulation. Semin Hematol. 1992;29(3):170–6.
32. Semeraro N, Colucci M. Tissue factor in health and disease. Thromb Haemost. 1997;78(1):759–64.
33. Gordon SG, Mourad AM. The site of activation of factor X by cancer procoagulant. Blood Coagul Fibrinolysis. 1991;2(6):735–9.
34. Mielicki WP, Gordon SG. Three-stage chromogenic assay for the analysis of activation properties of factor X by cancer procoagulant. Blood Coagul Fibrinolysis. 1993;4(3):441–6.
35. Falanga A, Gordon SG. Isolation and characterization of cancer procoagulant: a cysteine proteinase from malignant tissue. Biochemistry. 1985;24(20):5558–67.
36. Donati MB, Gambacorti-Passerini C, Casali B, et al. Cancer procoagulant in human tumor cells: evidence from melanoma patients. Cancer Res. 1986;46(12 Pt 1):6471–4.
37. Gordon SG, Cross BA. An enzyme-linked immunosorbent assay for cancer procoagulant and its potential as a new tumor marker. Cancer Res. 1990;50(19):6229–34.
38. Nieswandt B, Hafner M, Echtenacher B, et al. Lysis of tumor cells by natural killer cells in mice is impeded by platelets. Cancer Res. 1999;59(6):1295–300.
39. Palumbo JS, Talmage KE, Massari JV, et al. Platelets and fibrin(ogen) increase metastatic potential by impeding natural killer cell-mediated elimination of tumor cells. Blood. 2005;105(1):178–85.
40. Placke T, Örgel M, Schaller M, et al. Platelet-derived MHC class I confers a pseudonormal phenotype to cancer cells that subverts the antitumor reactivity of natural killer immune cells. Cancer Res. 2012;72(2):440–8.
41. Placke T, Salih HR, Kopp HG. GITR ligand provided by thrombopoietic cells inhibits NK cell antitumor activity. J Immunol. 2012;189(1):154–60.
42. Mehta P, Lawson D, Ward MB, et al. Effect of human tumor cells on platelet aggregation: potential relevance to pattern of metastasis. Cancer Res. 1986;46(10):5061–3.
43. Fäldt R, Ankerst J, Zoucas E. Inhibition of platelet aggregation by myeloid leukaemic cells demonstrated in vitro. Br J Haematol. 1987;66(4):529–34.
44. Pulte D, Furman RR, Broekman MJ, et al. CD39 expression on T lymphocytes correlates with severity of disease in patients with chronic lymphocytic leukemia. Clin Lymphoma Myeloma Leuk. 2011;11(4):367–72.
45. Jaime-Pérez JC, Cantú-Rodríguez OG, Herrera-Garza JL, et al. Platelet aggregation in children with acute lymphoblastic leukemia during induction of remission therapy. Arch Med Res. 2004;35(2):141–4.
46. Nouh MA, Inui M, Kakehi Y. Renal cell carcinoma with IVC thrombi; current concepts and future perspectives. Clin Med Oncol. 2008;2:247–56.
47. Mootha RK, Butler R, Laucirica R, et al. Renal cell carcinoma with infra renal vena caval tumor thrombus. Urology. 1999;54:561–5.
48. Heit JA, Silverstein MD, Mohr DN, et al. Risk factors for deep vein thrombosis and pulmonary embolism: a population-based case-control study. Arch Intern Med. 2000;160:809–15.
49. Blom JW, Vanderschoot JP, Oostindier MJ, et al. Incidence of venous thrombosis in a large cohort of 66,329 cancer patients: results of a record linkage study. J Thromb Haemost. 2006;4:529–35.
50. Khorana AA. Cancer and coagulation. Am J Hematol. 2012;87:S82–7.
51. Fisher B, Constantino J, Redmond C, et al. A randomized clinical trial evaluating tamoxifen in the treatment of patients with node negative breast cancer who have estrogen-receptor positive tumors. N Engl J Med. 1989;320:479–84.

52. Pritchard KI, Paterson AHG, Paul NA, et al. Increased thromboembolic complications with concurrent tamoxifen and chemotherapy in a randomised trial of adjuvant therapy for women with breast cancer. J Clin Oncol. 1996;14:2731–7.
53. Moore RA, Adel N, Riedel E, et al. High incidence of thromboembolic events in patients treated with Cisplatin-based chemotherapy: a large retrospective analysis. J Clin Oncol. 2011;29(25):3466–73.
54. Otten H-MMB, Mathijssen J, ten Cate H, et al. Symptomatic venous thromboembolism in cancer patients treated with chemotherapy: an underestimated phenomenon. Arch Intern Med. 2004;164(2):190–4.
55. Dursun B, He Z, Somerset H, et al. Caspases and calpain are independent mediators of Cisplatin-induced endothelial cell necrosis. Am J Physiol Renal Physiol. 2006;291(3):F578–87.
56. Togna GI, Togna AR, Franconi M, et al. Cisplatin triggers platelet activation. Thromb Res. 2000;99(5):503–9.
57. Bona R. Thrombotic complications of central venous catheters in cancer patients. Semin Thromb Haemost. 1999;25:147–55.
58. Falanga A, Marchetti M. Anticancer treatment and thrombosis. Thromb Res. 2012;129(3):353–9.
59. DeCicco M, Matovic M, Balesterri L, et al. Central venous thrombosis: an early and frequent complication in cancer patients bearing long-term silastic catheter. A prospective study. Thromb Res. 1997;86:101–13.
60. Koksoy C, Kuzu A, Erden I, et al. The risk factors in central venous catheter-related thrombosis. Aust N Z J Surg. 1995;65:796–8.
61. Monreal M, Raventos A, Lerma R, et al. Pulmonary embolism in patients with upper extremity DVT associated to venous central lines—a prospective study. Thromb Haemost. 1994;72:548–50.
62. Houry S, Georgeac C, Hay JM, et al. A prospective multicenter evaluation of preoperative hemostatic screening tests. Am J Surg. 1995;170:19–23.
63. Sun NC, McAfee WM, Hum GJ, et al. Haemostatic abnormalities in malignancy: a prospective study in one hundred eight patients. Am J Clin Pathol. 1979;71:10–6.
64. Mohammed M, Mansoor M, Taher M. Hemostatic derangements in patients with solid malignant tumors. J Pak Med Stud. 2013;3(1):1–9.
65. Agarwal AM, Prchal JT. Anemia associated with marrow infiltration (chapter 44). In: Lichtman MA, Kipps TJ, Seligsohn U, editors. Williams hematology. 8th ed. New York, NY: McGraw-Hill; 2010.
66. Kuter DJ. Managing thrombocytopenia associated with cancer chemotherapy. Oncology. 2015;29(4):282–94.
67. Pedersen-Bjergaard J. Radiotherapy and chemotherapy-induced myelodysplasia and acute myeloid leukemia: a review. Leuk Res. 1992;16:61.
68. Glassman AB. Hemostatic abnormalities associated with cancer and its therapy. Ann Clin Lab Sci. 1997;27(6):391–5.
69. Shimazaki C, Inabi T, Uchiyama H, et al. Serum thrombopoietin levels in patients undergoing autologous peripheral blood stem cell transplantation. Bone Marrow Transplant. 1997;19:771–5.
70. Manzullo EF, Sahai SK, Weed HG. Preoperative evaluation and management of patients with cancer. In: Post TW, editor. UpToDate. Waltham, MA: UpToDate; 2014.
71. Thatishetty AV, Agresti N, O'Brien CB. Chemotherapy-induced hepatotoxicity. Clin Liver Dis. 2013;17(4):671–86.
72. Glaspy JA. Disturbances in hemostasis in patients with B-cell malignancies. Semin Thromb Hemostat. 1992;18:440–8.
73. Fellin F. Perioperative evaluation of patients with hematologic disorders (chapter 6). In: Merli GJ, Weitz HH, editors. Medical management of the surgical patient. 3rd ed. Philadelphia, PA: Elsevier; 2008.
74. Wu Y, Aravind S, Ranganathan G, et al. Anemia and thrombocytopenia in patients undergoing chemotherapy for solid tumors: a description study of a large outpatient oncology practice database, 2000–2007. Clin Ther. 2009;31(Pt 2):2416–32.
75. Cairo MS. Dose reductions and delays: limitations of myelosuppressive chemotherapy. Oncology. 2000;9(Suppl 8):21–31.
76. Dutcher JP, Schiffer CA, Aisner J, et al. Incidence of thrombocytopenia and serious hemorrhage among patients with solid tumors. Cancer. 1984;53:557–62.
77. Elting L, Rubenstein E, Loewy J, et al. Incidence and outcomes of chemotherapy-induced thrombocytopenia in patients with solid tumors. Support Care Cancer. 1996;4:238.
78. Piatek C, Akhtari M. Thrombocytopenia: optimizing approaches in cancer patients. Oncology. 2015;29(4):297–8.
79. Gaydos LA, Freireich EJ, Mantel N. The quantitative relation between platelet count and hemorrhage in patients with acute leukemia. N Engl J Med. 1962;266:905–9.
80. Pisciotto PT, Benson K, Hume H, et al. Prophylactic versus therapeutic platelet transfusion practices in hematology and/or oncology patients. Transfusion. 1995;35:498–502.
81. Friedmann AM, Sengul H, Lehmann H, et al. Do basic laboratory tests or clinical observations predict bleeding in thrombocytopenic oncology patients? A reevaluation of prophylactic platelet transfusions. Transfus Med Rev. 2002;16(1):34–45.
82. Slichter SJ. Relationship between platelet count and bleeding risk in thrombocytopenic patients. Transfus Med Rev. 2004 Jul;18(3):153–67.
83. Elting L, Martin C, Cantor S, et al. A clinical prediction rule to guide the use of prophylactic platelet growth factors and platelet transfusions. Proc Am Soc Clin Oncol. 1998;421a:17.
84. MacManus M, Lamborn K, Khan W, et al. Radiotherapy-associated neutropenia and thrombocytopenia: analysis of risk factors and development of a predictive model. Blood. 1997;89:2303–10.

85. Elting L, Martin C, Kurtin D, et al. The bleeding risk index: a clinical prediction rule to guide the prophylactic use of platelet transfusions in patients with lymphoma or solid tumors. Cancer. 2002;94:3252–62.
86. Kaufman RM, Djulbegovic B, Gernsheimer T, et al. Platelet transfusion: a clinical practice guideline from the American Association of Blood Banks. Ann Intern Med. 2015;162(3):205–13.
87. Padhi S, Kemmis-Betty S, Rajesh S, et al. Blood transfusion: summary of NICE guidance. BMJ. 2015;351:h5832.
88. Lin Y, Foltz LM. Proposed guidelines for platelet transfusion. BCMJ. 2005;47(5):245–8.
89. Fillmore WJ, Leavitt BD, Arce K. Dental extraction in the thrombocytopenic patient is safe and complications are easily managed. J Oral Maxillofac Surg. 2013;71(10):1647–52.
90. Napolitano L. Perioperative anemia. Surg Clin North Am. 2005;85:1215–27.
91. Rodgers GM, Becker PS, Bennett CL, et al. Cancer and chemotherapy induced anemia. J Natl Compr Canc Netw. 2008;6:536.
92. Maccio A, Madeddu C, Gramignano G, et al. The role of inflammation, iron, and nutritional status in cancer-related anemia: results of a large, prospective, observational study. Haematologica. 2015;100:124.
93. Weiss G, Goodnough LT. Anemia of chronic disease. N Engl J Med. 2005;352:1011–23.
94. Engelfriet CP, Overbeeke MA, von dem Borne AE. Autoimmune hemolytic anemia. Semin Hematol. 1992;29:3.
95. Neoh K, Stanworth S, Pasricha SR, et al. Estimating prevalence of functional iron deficiency anaemia in advanced cancer. Support Care Cancer. 2017;25(4):1209–14.
96. Gilreath JA, Stenehjem DD, Rodgers GM. Diagnosis and treatment of cancer related anemia. Am J Hematol. 2014;89:203–12.
97. Cascinu S, Fedeli A, Del Ferro E, et al. Recombinant human erythropoietin treatment in cisplatin associated anemia: a randomized, double blind trial with placebo. J Clin Oncol. 1994;12:1058.
98. Abels R. Erythropoietin for anemia in cancer patients. Eur J Cancer. 1993;29A(Suppl 2):S2.
99. Hébert PC, Wells G, et al. A multicenter, randomized, controlled clinical trial of transfusion requirements in critical care. N Engl J Med. 1999;340(6):409–17. Erratum in: N Engl J Med. 1999;340(13):1056.
100. Henderson JM, Bergman S, Salama A, et al. Management of the oral and maxillofacial surgery patient with thrombocytopenia. J Oral Maxillofac Surg. 2001;59(4):421–7.

# 8 Stratifying Thromboembolic Risk: Why Is Your Patient on Antithrombotic Medications?

Benjamin Hohlfelder

**Abstract**

Utilization of antithrombotic medications is extremely prevalent and may be indicated for a variety of disease states. Additionally, innovation and advancements in pharmacotherapy have increased the number of antithrombotic medications available to prescribers, the combinations of medications utilized, and durations of usage with these therapies. Understanding why patients are on certain antithrombotic therapies and the risks of discontinuing these therapies is a vital component of preparation for dental procedures patients may undergo. This chapter will highlight the most common indications for antithrombotic therapy, suggested medications for each disease state, along with recommended intensity and duration of treatment.

Thromboembolic disease represents a significant cause of morbidity and mortality [1]. Anticoagulant and antiplatelet therapy are the mainstay of therapy in the treatment and prevention of thromboembolic disease [1]. The use of oral antithrombotic medications is extremely prevalent in the United States and globally. A survey of adults aged 45–75 in the United States showed that over half of people in this age group used aspirin [2], and approximately six million patients utilize anticoagulant medications in the United States annually [3]. With an aging patient population, increased awareness of the risks of thromboembolic disease, and improved therapies in the management of thromboembolic disease, this number can only be expected to rise in the coming years [2, 3].

Antithrombotic therapy is frequently indicated for disease states that can lead to arterial and venous thromboembolism [1]. This chapter will highlight many of the common indications for antithrombotic therapy, the common agents utilized for treatment or prevention of these disease states, and the durations of treatment with these agents (Table 8.1). The indications highlighted are not an exhaustive list of reasons for patients to be utilizing these medications, but encompass a majority of patients requiring antithrombotic therapy.

## 8.1 Atrial Fibrillation

Atrial fibrillation represents the most common indication for chronic anticoagulation therapy. It was estimated that in 2010, approximately 33.5 million people worldwide were living with atrial fibrillation [4]. The atrial arrhythmia occurs when there is rapid firing of electrical signals

B. Hohlfelder
Cleveland Clinic, Cleveland, OH, USA
e-mail: hohlfeb@ccf.org





R. P. Szumita, P. M. Szumita (eds.), *Hemostasis in Dentistry*, https://doi.org/10.1007/978-3-319-71240-6_8

**Table 8.1** Indications for antithrombotic therapy and general recommendation for antithrombotic therapy

| Indication for antithrombotic therapy | General recommendations for antithrombotic therapy |
|---|---|
| Atrial fibrillation | Assess $CHADS_2$-VASc Score:<br>• For patients with $CHADS_2$-VASc Score < 2, aspirin monotherapy<br>• For patients with $CHADS_2$-VASc Score ≥ 2, lifelong anticoagulation with warfarin (goal INR 2.0–3.0) or DOAC |
| Venous thromboembolism (VTE) | Anticoagulation with warfarin (goal INR 2.0–3.0) or DOAC<br>Duration of therapy:<br>• Provoked VTE: 3–6 months<br>• Idiopathic VTE: 6–12 months<br>• Recurrent VTE: at least 6 months, with consideration for lifelong therapy |
| Prosthetic heart valves | Valve repair procedures: aspirin monotherapy<br>Bioprosthetic valve replacement:<br>• Aortic or pulmonary valve-aspirin monotherapy<br>• Mitral or tricuspid valve-warfarin (goal INR 2.0–3.0) for 3 months followed by aspirin monotherapy; or aspirin monotherapy<br>Mechanical valve replacement:<br>• Aortic or pulmonary valve-warfarin (goal INR 2.0–3.0) for lifelong therapy (exception – may consider goal INR 1.5–2.0 for OnX valve aortic valve replacement)<br>• Mitral or tricuspid valve-warfarin (goal INR 2.5–3.5) for lifelong therapy |
| Hypercoagulable states | No specific recommendations for hypercoagulable states. If thromboembolic disease develops in the setting of a hypercoagulable state, it may influence duration and intensity of antithrombotic therapy |
| Primary prevention of cardiovascular disease (CVD) | Aspirin monotherapy recommended for:<br>• Age ≥ 50 years old (ACCP guidelines)<br>• Risk of CVD > 10% over a 10-year period (AHA guidelines)<br>• Patients with diabetes and an intermediate risk of CVD (5–10% risk over a 10-year period) (AHA guidelines)<br>• Chronic kidney disease, (GFR < 45 mL/min but not severe kidney disease) (AHA guidelines) |
| Coronary artery disease (CAD) | Stable ischemic heart disease:<br>• Aspirin monotherapy or DAPT<br>CABG:<br>• Aspirin monotherapy<br>Percutaneous coronary Intervention with stenting<br>• Bare metal stent-DAPT for at least 1 month followed by aspirin monotherapy<br>• Drug-eluting stent-DAPT for at least 3–6 months (12 months preferred) followed by aspirin monotherapy<br>• Continue DAPT for as long as tolerable/acceptable from a risk of bleeding perspective |
| Ischemic stroke | Cardioembolic stroke:<br>• Warfarin (goal INR 2.0–3.0) or DOAC depending on etiology of cardioembolism<br>Non-cardioembolic stroke:<br>• Aspirin monotherapy<br>• Aspirin/extended-release dipyridamole (Aggrenox®)<br>• Clopidogrel |

*DOAC* direct oral anticoagulant, *ACCP* American College of Chest Physicians, *AHA* American Heart Association, *DAPT* dual antiplatelet therapy

triggered by the pulmonary veins [5–7]. Several additional mechanisms may contribute to the development and persistence of atrial fibrillation, including autonomic tone, atrial remodeling and fibrosis, the presence of reentrance pathways, and inflammatory oxidative stress [7, 8]. The end result is an arrhythmia that produces an RR interval with no distinct pattern, which is frequently referred to as an irregularly irregular cardiac rhythm [8–11].

There are several risk factors for the development of atrial fibrillation [9, 10, 12]. Age is the most commonly recognized risk factor, with the risk of developing AF increasing significantly in patients over age 60 [13]. Other risk factors for developing AF include hypertension, diabetes mellitus, coronary artery disease and those with a history of myocardial infarction, structural or valvular heart disease, or heart failure [10, 12, 13]. In some cases, there may be a familial or genetic component to the risk of AF [14, 15]. Recent studies have identified that up to 30% of patients with AF have a familial history of the disease [14, 15]. The KCNE2, KCNJ2, and KCNQ1 genes have been implicated in disrupting electrical signals within the myocardium but have only been identified in a few instances [14, 15]. The familial risk of AF may be more related to the familial risk of developing several of the cardiovascular and endocrine disorders that are also risk factors for development of AF.

The most feared and common complication of AF is thromboembolic disease, most notably ischemic stroke [16]. Compared to patients without AF, patients with the dysrhythmia are at a fivefold higher risk of stroke. Thrombus formation can occur in AF through several proposed mechanisms [10, 11]. As the atrium fibrillates, blood stasis may allow for clot to form. The presence of a left atrial appendage may also provide an additional area for stasis. Atrial endothelial dysfunction has also been observed in patients with AF. Changes in atrial endothelium can lead to a proinflammatory state and a subsequent hypercoagulable state. Upregulation in plasminogen activator inhibitor-1 and downregulation of thrombin factor pathway inhibitor have been observed. Ultimately, in the absence of antithrombotic therapies, patients with AF have an annual stroke risk between 1.9% and 18.2% depending on the presence of other risk factors [17, 18].

Just as there are many risk factors for the development of AF, several factors influence the risk of thromboembolic disease in patients with AF [17, 18]. Notable risk factors include age, diabetes mellitus, history of stroke or transient ischemic attack (TIA), and hypertension. The use of a clinical scoring tool can help to stratify patients who are in need of chronic anticoagulant therapy. The CHADS2 score (Fig. 8.1) was developed using data from the

| Risk Factor | Points Assigned |
|---|---|
| Congestive Heart Failure | 1 |
| Hypertension | 1 |
| Age ≥ 75 | 1 |
| Diabetes Mellitus | 1 |
| History of Stroke | 2 |

| CHADS$_2$ Score | Annual Stroke Risk |
|---|---|
| 0 | 1.9% |
| 1 | 2.8% |
| 2 | 4.0% |
| 3 | 5.9% |
| 4 | 8.5% |
| 5 | 12.5% |
| 6 | 18.9% |

**Fig. 8.1** CHADS2 Risk Scoring Tool. The CHADS2 Risk Scoring Tool can help clinicians evaluate a patient with atrial fibrillation's annual stroke risk. While guidelines now recommend the use of CHADS2-VASc over CHADS2, previous recommendations suggested that patients with a CHADS2 score of 2 or higher should be chronically anticoagulated. Patients with a CHADS2 score of 0 or 1 could be managed with aspirin alone

| Risk Factor | Points Assigned |
|---|---|
| Congestive Heart Failure | 1 |
| Hypertension | 1 |
| Age ≥ 75 | 2 |
| Diabetes Mellitus | 1 |
| History of Stroke | 2 |
| Vascular Disease (PAD, MI, etc.) | 1 |
| Age 65-74 | 1 |
| Sex Category | 1 |
| PAD, peripheral artery disease<br>MI, myocardial infarction | |

| $CHADS_2$ Score | Annual Stroke Risk |
|---|---|
| 0 | 0% |
| 1 | 1.3% |
| 2 | 2.2% |
| 3 | 3.2% |
| 4 | 4.0% |
| 5 | 6.7% |
| 6 | 9.8% |
| 7 | 9.6% |
| 8 | 12.5% |
| 9 | 15.2% |

**Fig. 8.2** CHADS2-VASc Risk Scoring Tool. The CHADS2-VASc Risk Scoring Tool can help clinicians evaluate a patient with atrial fibrillation's annual stroke risk. Guideline recommendations suggest that patients with a CHADS2-VASc score of 2 or higher should be chronically anticoagulated, when the risk of bleeding does not outweigh benefits of anticoagulation. Patients with a CHADS2-VASc score of 0 or 1 may be managed with aspirin alone

National Registry for AF and has been utilized to estimate the yearly stroke risk [19]. Previous guidelines have recommended that patients with a CHADS2 score ≥ 2 should be chronically anticoagulated, while patients with a CHADS2 score < 2 could be treated with aspirin alone. More recently, the CHADS2-VASc (Fig. 8.2) provided an updated risk scoring tool that incorporated additional risk factors for stroke in AF [18]. Guidelines recommend that patients with a CHADS2-VASc score ≥ 2 should be chronically anticoagulated [20]. Patients with a CHADS2-VASc score of 0 or 1 may be adequately protected with aspirin.

Risk scoring tools have also been established to help guide clinicians as to their patients' risk of bleeding while on anticoagulation [21]. The HAS-BLED score (Fig. 8.3) was developed using data from the Euro Heart Survey on AF and can be used to predict a patient's annual risk of major bleeding on anticoagulation [22]. Risk factors identified in the HAS-BLED score include hypertension, abnormal renal or hepatic function, age, and bleeding history. It is important to note that some of the variables in HAS-BLED refer to patients who are currently utilizing anticoagulant therapy and cannot accurately predict a patient's bleeding risk prior to initiation of anticoagulation. Similarly, a comparison of a patient's CHADS2-VASc and HAS-BLED score to determine the net clinical benefit of anticoagulation has not been validated [23]. A HAS-BLED score ≥ 3 will indicate that a patient is at a higher risk of bleeding. However, a HAS-BLED score ≥ 3 does not necessitate cessation of anticoagulation [22]. Rather, these risk stratification tools simply provide clinicians with additional resources when weighing the risks and benefits of anticoagulation.

Oral anticoagulation is the mainstay of therapy for stroke prevention in AF. For decades, warfarin has been the primary agent used for this indication. Compared with placebo, warfarin has been shown to reduce the risk of thromboembo-

| Risk Factor | Points Assigned |
|---|---|
| Hypertension (uncontrolled; systolic > 160 mm Hg) | 1 |
| Abnormal renal function (dialysis; transplant; SCr> 2.25) | 1 |
| Abnormal hepatic function (cirrhosis; bilirubin or ALT/AST > 2x ULN) | 1 |
| Stroke (prior history of stroke) | 1 |
| Bleeding history (prior major bleeding or disposition to bleed) | 1 |
| Labile INRs (Unstable/high INR; time in therapeutic range <60%) | 1 |
| Elderly (Age > 65) | 1 |
| Drugs (Alcohol use > 8 drinks/week; | 1 |
| NSAID/antiplatelet use) | 1 |

**Fig. 8.3** HAS-BLED Risk Scoring Tool. The HAS-BLED risk scoring tool to evaluate a patient's risk of bleeding while on warfarin. To fully evaluate the HAS-BLED score, patients must already be on warfarin. A HAS-BLED score ≥ 3 indicates that a patient is at a higher risk of bleeding. However, an elevated HAS-BLED score does not necessarily indicate a need to stop anticoagulation therapy, rather that a clinician should undertake an assessment of the risks and benefits of therapy

lism by two thirds [24]. The ACTIVE-W trial group sought to determine if antiplatelet therapy was sufficient to prevent stroke in AF. However, in comparison with the combination of aspirin and clopidogrel, warfarin was shown to be superior for the prevention of vascular events, with no difference in major bleeding between the two groups [25].

Recently, however, a novel group of oral anticoagulants were developed for stroke prevention in patients with AF. Dabigatran, rivaroxaban, apixaban, and edoxaban have all been approved for use in the United States by the FDA since 2010. They are often referred to by several names: novel oral anticoagulants or non-vitamin K oral anticoagulants (NOACs), target-specific oral anticoagulants (TSOACs), or direct oral anticoagulants (DOACs). Each of these medications was compared to warfarin for stroke prevention in AF in the RELY [26], ROCKET-AF [27], ARISTOTLE [28], and ENGAGE-AF [29] trials, respectively. All four medications were shown to be at least non-inferior to warfarin for stroke prevention in AF, as well as major bleeding associated with therapy. Since their approval, the use of these agents has increased significantly and now is used in approximately 50% of patients on chronic anticoagulation for stroke prevention in AF [30, 31].

## 8.2 Venous Thromboembolism

Venous thromboembolism (VTE) is a disease state that encompasses both deep vein thrombosis (DVT) and pulmonary embolism (PE) [32]. It represents a significant cause of morbidity and mortality and was highlighted by the United States Surgeon General as one of the most common causes of preventable disease in the hospital setting [33]. An estimated 350,000–600,000 people are diagnosed with VTE each year in the United States, with as many as 100,000 VTE-related deaths annually [33]. Additionally, many patients living with VTE suffer from chronic complications of the disease state such as the post-thrombotic syndrome and chronic thromboembolic pulmonary hypertension [32, 34, 35].

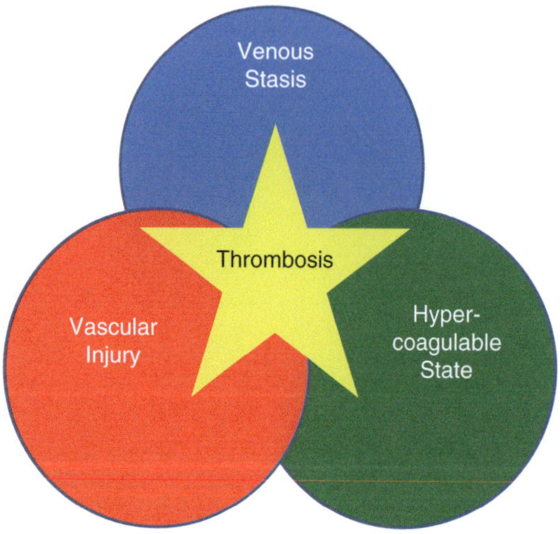


**Fig. 8.4** Virchow's Triad. Virchow's Triad has historically been used to represent the common risk factors for development of venous thromboembolism (VTE). Within each area of the triad, there are several conditions or disease states that may contribute to the risk of VTE. Patients with risk factors in multiple or all aspects of the triad may be at a higher risk for development of VTE

The classic causes for VTE are highlighted in Virchow's triad (Fig. 8.4), which includes the three most common mechanisms for development of VTE [32, 36]. Venous stasis can be caused by several disease states, and a decrease in blood flow rate allows for an increased likelihood of coagulation. Inherited or acquired thrombophilia (will be discussed in a future section) is often diagnosed in the setting of a new VTE event. Lastly, vascular or endothelial injury may significantly increase a patient's risk of developing VTE. This may occur as a direct manipulation of the vasculature, such as during a surgical procedure [37], or as a result of indirect damage to the endothelium, such as in diabetes mellitus [38].

The management of VTE can involve both enteral and parenteral anticoagulants. For chronic management of VTE, oral anticoagulants are generally preferred, while injectable agents such as the low molecular weight heparins (LMWH) or fondaparinux may be utilized in certain clinical situations [39]. As with atrial fibrillation, warfarin has been the mainstay of oral therapy for treatment of VTE [39]. The DOACs have also undergone clinical trials to determine their efficacy in the treatment of VTE. Dabigatran, rivaroxaban, apixaban, and edoxaban were compared with warfarin in the treatment of VTE in the RE-COVER [40], EINSTEIN-VTE [41, 42], AMPLIFY [43], and Hokusai-VTE [44] trials, respectively. Compared with warfarin, each of the DOACs demonstrated non-inferior efficacy and safety [40–44]. Therapy with apixaban and edoxaban was also associated with a decreased rate of major and clinically relevant nonmajor bleeding when compared with warfarin [43, 44].

As previously described, patients with active malignancy are at an increased risk of developing VTE [45, 46]. For this subset of patients, warfarin therapy may present many challenges, including but not limited to decreased oral intake and changes in diet, nausea and vomiting, drug interactions with chemotherapeutic and supportive care agents, and changes in hepatic function [45, 46]. The CLOT trial compared therapy with the LMWH dalteparin to therapy with warfarin for treatment of VTE [47]. Compared with warfarin, dalteparin significantly reduced the rate of recurrent VTE without an increase in major bleeding. As a result, the National Comprehensive Cancer Network Guidelines for Cancer-Associated VTE Disease issued a Category 1 recommendation that LMWH monotherapy is the preferred treatment option for the first 6 months in patients with advanced or metastatic cancer [48]. Currently, the DOACs are undergoing clinical investigation to assess their safety and efficacy in this patient population[49].

The appropriate duration of therapy for treatment of VTE remains a clinical controversy [32]. When determining a patient's duration of treatment, several factors must be considered. First, it is important to consider the cause of VTE. VTE that occurs after a patient undergoes major surgery, has had a long-distance travel experience, or occurs during pregnancy, active malignancy or a period of prolonged immobility is considered to be provoked. VTE that occur without a provoking factor are classified as idiopathic [32].

Patients with provoked VTE can generally be treated for a shorter duration of therapy, assuming the provoking factor has been removed or is no longer present in the patient. Idiopathic VTE should be treated for a longer duration. The American College of Chest Physicians (ACCP) guidelines recommend anticoagulation for 3 months in patients with provoked VTE. For patients with idiopathic VTE, a duration of therapy of 6–12 months is suggested [50]. In both scenarios, the patient's risk of bleeding should be weighed with risk of thrombosis when determining the duration of therapy. Patients who develop recurrent VTE will generally warrant prolonged or lifelong anticoagulation, if tolerated from a bleeding risk standpoint [50–52].

## 8.3 Prosthetic Heart Valves

Valvular heart disease is an extremely common condition, especially in patients of advanced age. Patients may undergo surgical or percutaneous cardiac procedures to repair or replace damaged heart valves when the disease is severe, causes physical limitations, or in the setting of mild-moderate disease when undergoing other cardiac procedures [53]. In the United States, over 100,000 procedures take place annually to repair or replace heart valves, and that number is expected to rise with improvements in procedural technology, further options for percutaneous valve replacement, and an aging population [54, 55].

The heart contains four heart valves: the tricuspid and pulmonary valves on the right side of the heart and the mitral and aortic valves on the left side of the heart. Because the left heart performs more work than the right heart, and pumps against significantly higher afterload, the mitral and aortic valves are most commonly impacted in valvular heart disease [53, 54]. The tricuspid and pulmonary valves are generally spared in valvular heart disease. Exceptions to this include cases of pulmonary hypertension, which increases right heart afterload, or endocarditis or rheumatic disease, where infectious processes may cause direct valvular damage [56].

Valvular heart disease presents as two primary etiologies: stenosis and regurgitation [57]. Stenotic valves do not open appropriately. In many cases, calcification of the valve that increases with age occludes the opening and decreases blood flow through the valve. In other cases, the valve leaflets may thicken or stiffen and decrease the open size of the valve. Disease states such as hypertension may worsen this type of valvular disease [56]. Lastly, patients may be born with congenital heart disorders, such as a bicuspid valve, that increase the likelihood of stenosis.

Regurgitation represents the other major subset of valvular heart disease. Valvular regurgitation is defined as an inappropriate closing of valve leaflets that allows for retrograde blood flow [58]. Patients with valvular regurgitation often present with similar symptoms to patients with heart failure, as the retrograde blood flow inhibits cardiac output. Risk factors and causes of valvular regurgitation include hypertension, heart failure, congenital heart diseases, myocardial infarction, rheumatic heart disease, or endocarditis [58, 59].

The choice of antithrombotic agent in a patient undergoing cardiac surgery for valve repair or replacement is often complex [56, 60, 61]. For most patients undergoing valve repair, aspirin is sufficient for antithrombotic prophylaxis. For valve replacement procedures, the need for anticoagulation versus antiplatelet therapy may be dependent on the type of material used for the replacement valve. Bioprosthetic valves may be crafted using porcine or bovine tissue [62]. Mechanical valves are produced from synthetic materials. While mechanical heart valves generally have a longer lifespan than bioprosthetic valves, mechanical valves are more thrombogenic than bioprosthetic valves [62, 63]. Patients who have a mechanical valve implanted will require lifelong anticoagulation in most scenarios [63].

The valve being replaced also impacts the need or degree of antithrombotic therapy. Due to differences in hemodynamics and blood flow across the valves, the tricuspid valve and mitral valve carry a significantly higher risk of thrombosis compared to their pulmonary and aortic counterparts [64]. While antiplatelet therapy is usually sufficient for bioprosthetic aortic valve replacements, anticoagulation may be needed after replacement of mitral or tricuspid valves, even with a bioprosthesis [56, 60, 61].

Lastly, for patients receiving mechanical heart valves, the type of mechanical valve implanted may play a role in the degree to which patients are anticoagulated. Older mechanical valves, such as the caged ball and monoleaflet valves, are less similar physiologically to the native heart valve and are more thrombogenic [63]. Newer valve technology more closely replicates the native heart valve and may require a lower degree of anticoagulation. The newest mechanical heart valve, the On-X valve, has been approved by the FDA for use with a lower INR target (1.5–2.0) when used in the aortic position [65].

As with other indications for anticoagulation, warfarin has been the mainstay of therapy for decades among patients undergoing valve replacement surgery requiring anticoagulant therapy. The duration of anticoagulation and the intensity of anticoagulation, as determined by the goal INR range, are dependent on the valve material and position [56, 60, 61].

With the development of the DOACs, there is hope that these medications can be used for this indication as well. While the majority of studies with these agents have been in patients with nonvalvular atrial fibrillation [26–29], one trial compared dabigatran with warfarin for patients undergoing mechanical aortic or mitral valve replacement [66]. However, dabigatran was associated with an increase in both thromboembolic and bleeding outcomes, and the trial was terminated prematurely. To this point, DOACs are not recommended for use in patients with valvular heart disease or those who have undergone valve replacement procedures [56, 60, 61].

## 8.4 Hypercoagulable States

Hypercoagulable states are a group of inherited or acquired conditions that place patients at a higher risk of thromboembolism [67]. Among the general population, hypercoagulable states are generally uncommon [67]. However, it is becoming increasingly recognized that among patients with thromboembolic disease, hypercoagulable states more commonly play a role [32, 68]. As many as 70% of patients who present with idiopathic VTE may have a form of hypercoagulability upon workup [32, 67, 69]. Hypercoagulable states most frequently manifest in VTE events but may also cause arterial thrombosis [32, 68].

Hypercoagulable states are generally classified as inherited or acquired. Inherited hypercoagulable states are primarily genetic [70, 71] and include protein C and S deficiencies [72], factor V Leiden [71], prothrombin gene mutation, and antithrombin deficiency [73]. In the general population, the incidence of these conditions ranges from less than 1% up to 10%. Examples of acquired hypercoagulable states include antiphospholipid or anticardiolipin antibody syndromes [74], malignancy, myeloproliferative disease [69], and heparin-induced thrombocytopenia [75]. Each hypercoagulable state leads to an increased risk of thromboembolism through a different yet related mechanism. The presence of one of these conditions will lead to activation of the coagulation system or a dysregulation of the body's natural anticoagulant or fibrinolytic systems.

In the absence of a strong family history of one of these hypercoagulable states, a high percentage of hypercoagulable states are diagnosed in the presence of a new thromboembolic event [32]. By itself, the presence of a hypercoagulable state may not indicate a need for anticoagulation [76, 77]. Some hypercoagulable states such as factor V Leiden or hyperhomocysteinemia may only confer a 2–4 times greater likelihood of developing VTE over the course of a patient's life [78].

Hypercoagulable states play a more significant role when determining the duration of anticoagulation after a patient's thromboembolic event. For some lower-risk hypercoagulable states, there is no data to suggest extended duration anticoagulation after a single thromboembolic event [76]. For higher-risk conditions such as antithrombin deficiency or antiphospholipid or anticardiolipin antibody syndromes, guideline recommendations suggest at least 1 year of anticoagulation and up to lifelong anticoagulation

[76]. Ultimately, a patient's duration of anticoagulation should be carefully assessed based on the individual patient's risk of thromboembolism and bleeding complications.

## 8.5 Prevention of Cardiovascular Disease

Cardiovascular diseases (CVD), most notably coronary artery disease and stroke, represent a significant cause of morbidity and mortality [79]. CVD is the most common cause of death in the United States annually, with over 600,000 deaths each year [79, 80]. As such, there is significant interest in the prevention of such CVD.

Several large-scale registries and analyses have helped clearly define those at risk for developing CVD. One of the most notable, the Framingham Heart Study, is an ongoing registry of residents of Framingham, Massachusetts [82]. The study began in 1948 and has spanned three generations of patients. From this study and others, well-recognized risk factors for CVD and strategies to prevent CVD have been identified. Additionally, risk scoring tools, including the Framingham Risk Score, have been developed to better predict and categorize a patient's risk [82–84].

Risk factors for CVD can be classified as modifiable risk factors and non-modifiable risk factors [79, 80]. Hypertension is well recognized as one of the most common risk factors, particularly for the development of stroke. Other modifiable risk factors for CVD include hyperlipidemia, obesity and physical inactivity, a diet high in saturated fats, use of tobacco products, type 2 diabetes, and use of certain medications such as hormonal replacement therapy [81–84]. The most notable non-modifiable risk factors include age, with the risk of stroke doubling with each decade after age 55, gender, with males being at a higher risk, and familial history of CVD [79–84].

In addition to treatment or changes in modifiable risk factors, antithrombotic therapy may be employed to aid in the prevention of CVD. Aspirin is the most frequently utilized antithrombotic agent for this indication. In fact, in the most recent guidelines for primary and secondary prevention of cardiovascular disease, the American College of Chest Physicians recommends the use of low-dose aspirin (75–100 mg) in patients greater than 50 years old, with a level of evidence of Grade IIB [85]. These guidelines do comment that the benefits are relatively minimal and must be weighed with the risk of aspirin adverse effects, including the risk of gastrointestinal bleeding [85, 86].

Other guidelines suggest the use of a risk scoring tool, or assessment of patient risk factors, to determine the need for antithrombotic therapy. The American Heart Association guidelines recommend the use of aspirin for primary prevention in several scenarios: patients with a risk of CVD > 10% over a 10-year period, as determined by a risk scoring tool; patients with diabetes with an intermediate risk of CVD, defined as a 5–10% risk over a 10-year period; or patients with chronic kidney disease, defined as an estimated glomerular filtration rate < 45 mL/min, but does not apply to patients with severe chronic kidney disease (KDIGO Stage 4 or 5) [87].

## 8.6 Coronary Artery Disease

Coronary artery disease (CAD) is one of the most common manifestations of CVD. Nearly 400,000 Americans die of CAD annually, representing the majority of deaths due to CVD [79, 80]. Additionally, nearly 750,000 patients annually will have a myocardial infarction (MI), including over 200,000 in patients who have previously had MI [79, 80]. The risk factors for developing CAD mirror the risk factors for CVD. The most notable risk factors include hypertension, hyperlipidemia, diabetes, obesity, and a familial history of CAD [81–84].

Classification of CAD may be made based on the acuity of the presenting disease, the number and location of coronary arteries impacted by CAD, and interventions taken in the treatment of CAD [88]. Initial deposits of cholesterol and plaque formation in the coronary arteries are generally defined as stable CAD. Stable CAD can be stratified by the percent occlusion of the coronary artery and the number of vessels impacted. Patients who experience chest pain associated with their stable CAD are classified as chronic stable angina [89].

As disease progression occurs, there may be destabilization of plaque formation in the coronary. Plaque destabilization and ultimately rupture may initiate a cascade of sequelae that can ultimately lead to a complete occlusion of the coronary arteries and death. These events are referred to as acute coronary syndromes (ACS) [89, 90]. Disruption of a coronary plaque that leads to partial thrombosis of the coronary artery may be defined as unstable angina (UA) or non-ST segment elevation MI (NSTEMI). These two syndromes differ, as NSTEMI is severe enough to cause myocardial injury and the release of cardiac enzymes and biomarkers [91]. ACS events that progress and occlude the entire coronary artery will present with hallmark ST segment elevations and are defined as ST segment elevation MI (STEMI) [91].

Antiplatelet therapy will be the backbone of chronic management for patients with CAD. For patients with stable CAD not undergoing any coronary intervention, low-dose aspirin should be utilized in the absence of any contraindications [91, 92]. The use of dual antiplatelet therapy (DAPT) has been evaluated for patients with chronic stable CAD. The CHARISMA trial enrolled over 15,000 patients with stable CAD to receive DAPT with clopidogrel and aspirin versus aspirin alone [93]. While no difference in stroke or MI was observed between the two groups, patients with a history of MI had a decrease in the rate stroke or MI, but at the cost of an increased risk of bleeding. As a result, the 2012 ACCF/AHA/ACP/AATS/PCNA/SCAI/STS guidelines recommend DAPT over aspirin alone in high-risk patients with a level of evidence of Grade IIB [92]. They do note that the potential benefits of therapy should be weighed with the increased cost and bleeding risk associated with DAPT.

For patients with ACS, or those with severe stable CAD, revascularization of the coronary arteries is the hallmark of therapy. This can be done through several modalities, including coronary artery bypass graft surgery (CABG), coronary angioplasty and percutaneous coronary intervention (PCI) with stenting, and pharmacologic thrombolysis in the setting of STEMI [92]. The choice of antithrombotic therapy is dependent on the revascularization strategy undertaken and the type of stent placed during PCI. In the case of CABG, aspirin monotherapy is recommended for prevention of graft occlusion. Doses of aspirin may range from 81 to 325 mg daily, although the guidelines note that higher doses (325 mg daily) may be considered to prevent aspirin resistance [94].

The use of clopidogrel post-CABG has been investigated, most commonly in combination with aspirin. In the CURE trial, over 12,000 patients with ACS without ST segment elevations were randomized to receive aspirin or aspirin plus clopidogrel [95]. In a subgroup analysis of patients undergoing CABG, the DAPT group had a reduction in the primary composite outcome of CV death, nonfatal MI, or stroke. However, the majority of the benefit received from DAPT occurred prior to patients undergoing CABG [96]. A subsequent trial, the CASCADE trial, demonstrated no difference in graft patency between aspirin (162 mg daily) and DAPT with clopidogrel plus aspirin [97].

The newer P2Y12 inhibitors prasugrel and ticagrelor have also been studied post-CABG, but primarily as a component of DAPT in comparison with DAPT with clopidogrel. In the TRITON-TIMI-38 trial, patients receiving prasugrel plus aspirin were found to have a lower rate of death after CABG when compared to the clopidogrel plus aspirin group [98]. This benefit, however, came at the cost of a higher rate of blood loss post-CABG. In the PLATO trial, ticagrelor plus aspirin was compared with clopidogrel plus aspirin [99]. Among patients undergoing CABG, there was a nonsignificant reduction in the primary endpoint with ticagrelor, without an increase in post-CABG bleeding. In each of the trials above, DAPT was continued for 1 year after the index event. For now, aspirin monotherapy remains the recommended antiplatelet therapy post-CABG [94].

For patients undergoing PCI, the choice of antiplatelet therapy is dependent on the type of intervention employed. There are two primary types of coronary stents used by interventionalists during PCI. The bare metal stent (BMS) was the first type of stent developed for angioplasty of the coronary arteries [100]. Subsequent developments in stenting technology led to the invention of drug-eluting stents (DES). There are multiple generations of DES [101]. Early generations of DES were coated with sirolimus or paclitaxel. Second-generation DES are coated with zotarolimus or everolimus. The newest technologies focus on the use of bioabsorbable materials in the stent material. With each subsequent generation of stent, there may be a decrease in stent thrombosis and need for coronary revascularization [101].

All patients undergoing PCI will require lifelong antiplatelet therapy, if they are able to tolerate [102]. As with other CAD indications, aspirin is the mainstay of therapy. Generally, low-dose aspirin is recommended for the remainder of a patient's life, as long as there are no contraindications or adverse events associated with aspirin therapy. DAPT also plays an important role, particularly in the initial period following stent placement [102]. The P2Y12 inhibitors clopidogrel, prasugrel, and ticagrelor have all been studied extensively after PCI and coronary angiography.

Clopidogrel, the first P2Y12 inhibitor, helped to establish the need for DAPT after stent placement [103]. The CURE trial, mentioned above, compared DAPT with clopidogrel and aspirin to aspirin alone [95]. Cardiovascular events were significantly reduced in the entire cohort by 21% at 30 days. An increased benefit was observed in the PCI subgroup of the CURE trial, with a 30% reduction in cardiovascular events at 30 days. Several subsequent trials, CLARITY [104], CREDO [105], and CURRENT-OASIS 7 [106], have showed benefits with clopidogrel when added to aspirin and helped to solidify the use of DAPT after PCI as a Grade IA recommendation [102].

Prasugrel has been studied as a part of DAPT, primarily in comparison with DAPT with clopidogrel. In the TRITON-TIMI-38 trial mentioned previously, DAPT with prasugrel was compared with DAPT with clopidogrel in over 13,000 patients [98]. Nearly 100% patients included in the trial underwent PCI, with 99% undergoing angiography and 94% receiving at least one stent. Overall, prasugrel therapy was associated with a 20% reduction in the primary composite endpoint. However, the efficacy benefit was balanced with a significant increase in major bleeding, including a significant increase in life-threatening bleeding and fatal bleeding.

Ticagrelor has been evaluated in a similar fashion to prasugrel. The PLATO trial, described above, compared DAPT with ticagrelor with DAPT with clopidogrel in over 18,000 patients [99]. Over 80% of patients underwent coronary angiography, with over 60% receiving PCI as a part of their therapy. As with prasugrel, there was a significant decrease in the primary composite endpoint with ticagrelor when compared with clopidogrel. However, there was not a significant increase in bleeding associated with DAPT with ticagrelor. There was an increased rate of intracranial hemorrhage with ticagrelor, but fatal bleeding was actually more frequent among the clopidogrel group. Because of this risk-benefit profile, the most recent guideline updates from the ACC/AHA suggest it is reasonable to favor the use of ticagrelor over clopidogrel for DAPT after PCI (Grade IIA) [102].

The minimal duration of DAPT is highly dependent on the type of stent utilized and the speed with which that stent endothelializes. BMS are associated with a higher rate of early stent thrombosis when compared with DES [107]. However, in the absence of a drug-eluting coating, endothelialization occurs at a more rapid rate. In comparison, DES have significantly delayed or even absent endothelialization [108, 109].

Endothelialization is crucial in the prevention of in-stent thrombus formation. This allows for a shorter duration of DAPT with BMS [100]. Current guideline recommendations suggest a minimum of 1 month of DAPT with BMS, with most clinicians favoring a course of at least 3 months of DAPT. For DES, a minimum of 6 months of DAPT is recommended, with most clinicians opting for 12 months of DAPT [102]. In all scenarios, a longer duration of DAPT has been shown to prevent subsequent events, with the trade-off of increased bleeding risk [110]. For patients at high risk or who have experienced recurrent events, many clinicians opt for extended or even lifelong DAPT, when the risk of bleeding and cost associated with therapy is acceptable to the patient.

## 8.7 Ischemic Stroke

Another feared manifestation of CVD is ischemic stroke [111]. Ischemic stroke is responsible for over 100,000 deaths annually in the United States and represents one of the highest economic burdens to the health-care system [112]. Nearly 800,000 people experience a stroke each year, with approximately 75% of these as first time strokes. Risk factors for stroke similarly mirror those for CVD, with hypertension, female gender, and ethnicity playing significant roles [111, 113].

There are several etiologies to ischemic stroke, with significant differences in pathophysiology. The TOAST classification system defines five types of ischemic stroke: large artery atherosclerosis, cardioembolic, small-vessel occlusion, stroke of other determined etiologies, and stroke of undetermined etiology [114]. Stroke of undetermined etiology may also be referred to as cryptogenic stroke. The SSS-TOAST is an updated system that defines each subtype as being "evident," "probable," or "possible" [115]. Strokes may also be classified by the arteries and segments of the brains they impact. Notable arteries commonly impacted include the middle cerebral arteries, anterior cerebral arteries, and posterior inferior cerebral arteries.

With the burden of disease that stroke presents, prevention of recurrent events is significant. Antithrombotic therapy plays a significant role in the secondary prevention of ischemic stroke [113]. Several antiplatelet and anticoagulant options have been investigated for the secondary prevention of stroke. The choice of agent may also depend on the etiology of stroke. Aspirin has been demonstrated across many studies and meta-analyses to be an effective agent in the prevention of stroke [113]. The International Stroke Trial demonstrated a decrease in recurrent ischemic stroke and a composite outcome of nonfatal stroke and death with aspirin over placebo [116]. The CAST trial demonstrated a mortality benefit demonstrated a decrease in mortality at 4 weeks with aspirin after ischemic stroke [117]. The Antithrombotic Trialists' Collaboration has published several analyses describing the efficacy and safety of aspirin for this indication. A 2009 meta-analysis from the group demonstrated a 20% reduction in recurrent disease in patients taking aspirin compared to placebo [118], and a 2016 pooled analysis showed 58% reduction in recurrent disease in the first 6 weeks of treatment [119]. Doses of aspirin may range from 75 to 325 mg per day, with no apparent difference in safety or efficacy outcomes between higher and lower doses [113].

The use of clopidogrel and other P2Y12 inhibitors has been evaluated in the secondary prevention of ischemic stroke. The CAPRIE trial compared aspirin and clopidogrel in patients with recent stroke, MI, or peripheral arterial disease (PAD) [120]. Overall, there was a significant reduction in the composite outcome of recurrent disease with clopidogrel. However, there was not a significant difference in recurrent stroke, and the majority of difference between the two groups was observed in patients with PAD. Ticagrelor was compared with aspirin for ischemic stroke in the SOCRATES study [121]. However, in over 13,000 patients, there was no significant reduction in stroke, MI, or death in the ticagrelor arm.

Combination antiplatelet therapy with aspirin and a P2Y12 inhibitor has also been evaluated. The CHANCE trial compared clopidogrel plus aspirin to aspirin alone in a trial of over 5000 Chinese patients with either high risk TIA or ischemic stroke [122]. Overall, the study found a decrease in recurrent stroke in the combination therapy group, with no difference in major bleeding. However, two more recent trials, the MATCH trial [123] and CHARISMA [93] trial, have demonstrated no difference in efficacy with the combination of clopidogrel and aspirin over monotherapy with clopidogrel or aspirin. In the MATCH trial, DAPT was associated with an increased rate of major bleeding and intracranial hemorrhage compared to aspirin alone [123].

Dipyridamole is a phosphodiesterase inhibitor that exhibits antiplatelet effect through potentiation of prostacyclin. It is available as an immediate-release formulation and an extended-release formulation in combination with aspirin (Aggrenox®). In the largest trial evaluating the use of dipyridamole for recurrent stroke prevention, the ESPS-2 trial, enrolled patients with recent TIA or ischemic stroke to four groups: placebo, aspirin monotherapy (25 mg twice daily), dipyridamole monotherapy (200 mg extended release twice daily), or aspirin plus dipyridamole [124]. Both aspirin and dipyridamole monotherapy were superior to placebo, while the combination of dipyridamole and aspirin was superior to both individual components alone. However, in a subsequent meta-analysis of trials investigating dipyridamole, when ESPS-2 data were excluded from the trial, dipyridamole alone was not more effective to control groups [125].

Current guidelines from the AHA and the ACCP for the prevention of recurrent stroke or TIA recommend that for a non-cardioembolic event, an antiplatelet agent be prescribed [113]. There is no recommendation for any of the three agents described above over another. There may be potential benefit to the use of clopidogrel or dipyridamole, but with a possible increase in bleeding risk, and an added cost in comparison to aspirin alone [113]. For patients with cardioembolic stroke, anticoagulation is recommended over antiplatelet therapy. Cardioembolic stroke is most frequently a result of atrial fibrillation and should be treated utilizing treatment guidelines for this indication.

**Conclusion**

There are many indications that patients are utilizing antithrombotic medications. When assessing the need for these antithrombotic therapies, a careful assessment of the risk of thrombosis and the risk of bleeding must be undertaken. Utilization of risk scoring tools, when available, may aid in these decisions, as well discussion with a patient's cardiologist, primary care physician, and others involved in the patient's care.

## References

1. Baron TH, Kamath PS, McBane RD. Management of antithrombotic therapy in patients undergoing invasive procedures. N Engl J Med. 2013;368:2113–24.
2. Williams CD, Chan AT, Elman MR, et al. Aspirin use among adults in the U.S.: results of a national survey. Am J Prev Med. 2015;48(5):501–8.
3. Hsu JC, Maddox TM, Kennedy KF, et al. Oral anticoagulant therapy prescription in patients with atrial fibrillation across the spectrum of stroke risk: insights from the NCDR PINNACLE Registry. JAMA Cardiol. 2016;1(1):55–62.
4. Chugh SS, Havmoeller R, Narayanan K, et al. Worldwide epidemiology of atrial fibrillation: a global burden of disease 2010 study. Circulation. 2014;129(8):837–47.
5. Markides V, Schilling RJ. Atrial fibrillation: classification, pathophysiology, mechanisms and drug treatment. Heart. 2003;89(8):939–43.
6. Iwasaki YK, Nishida K, Kato T, Nattel S. Atrial fibrillation pathophysiology: implications for management. Circulation. 2011;124:2264–74.
7. Wann LS, Curtis AB, January CT, et al. 2011 ACCF/AHA/HRS focused update on the management of patients with atrial fibrillation (updating the 2006 guideline): a report of the American College of Cardiology Foundation/American Heart Association Task Force on Practice Guidelines. Circulation. 2011;123(1):104–23.
8. Fuster V, Rydn LE, Cannom DS, et al. ACC/AHA/ESC 2006 guidelines for the management of patients with atrial fibrillation: a report of the American College of Cardiology/American Heart Association Task Force on practice guidelines and the European Society of Cardiology Committee for Practice Guidelines (Writing Committee to revise the 2001 guidelines for the management of patients with atrial fibrillation): developed in collaboration with the European Heart Rhythm Association and the Heart Rhythm Society. Circulation. 2006;114(7):e257–354.
9. Kannel WB, Wolf PA, Benjamin EJ, Levy D. Prevalence, incidence, prognosis, and predisposing conditions for atrial fibrillation: population-based estimates. Am J Cardiol. 1998;82(8A):2N–9N.
10. Ferrari R, Bertini M, Blomstrom-Lundqvist C, et al. An update on atrial fibrillation in 2014: from pathophysiology to treatment. Int J Cardiol. 2016;203:22–9.
11. Akyürek O, Sayin T, Dinçer I, Karaoguz R, Güldal M, Oral D. Lengthening of intraatrial conduction time in atrial fibrillation and its relation with

early recurrence of atrial fibrillation. Jpn Heart J. 2001;42(5):575–84.

12. Lloyd-Jones DM, Wang TJ, Leip EP, Larson MG, Levy D, Vasan RS, et al. Lifetime risk for development of atrial fibrillation: the Framingham Heart Study. Circulation. 2004;110(9):1042–6.
13. van Walraven C, Hart RG, Connolly S, Austin PC, Mant J, Hobbs FD, Koudstaal PJ, Petersen P, Perez-Gomez F, Knottnerus JA, Boode B, Ezekowitz MD, Singer DE. Effect of age on stroke prevention therapy in patients with atrial fibrillation: the atrial fibrillation investigators. Stroke. 2009;40(4):1410–6.
14. Fox CS, Parise H, D'Agostino RB Sr, Lloyd-Jones DM, Vasan RS, Wang TJ, et al. Parental atrial fibrillation as a risk factor for atrial fibrillation in offspring. JAMA. 2004;291(23):2851–5.
15. Lubitz SA, Yin X, Fontes JD, Magnani JW, Rienstra M, Pai M, et al. Association between familial atrial fibrillation and risk of new-onset atrial fibrillation. JAMA. 2010;304(20):2263–9.
16. Wolf PA, Abbott RD, Kannel WB. Atrial fibrillation as an independent risk factor for stroke: the Framingham Study. Stroke. 1991;22(8):983–8.
17. Welles CC, Whooley MA, Na B, et al. The CHADS(2) score predicts ischemic stroke in the absence of atrial fibrillation among subjects with coronary heart disease: data from the Heart and Soul Study. Am Heart J. 2011;162(3):555–61.
18. Olesen JB, Lip GY, Hansen ML, Hansen PR, Tolstrup JS, Lindhardsen J, et al. Validation of risk stratification schemes for predicting stroke and thromboembolism in patients with atrial fibrillation: nationwide cohort study. BMJ. 2011;342:d124.
19. Gage BF, Waterman AD, Shannon W, et al. Validation of clinical classification schemes for predicting stroke: results from the National Registry of Atrial Fibrillation. JAMA. 2001;285(22):2864–70.
20. Kirchhof P, Benussi S, Kotecha D, et al. ESC guidelines for the management of atrial fibrillation. Eur Heart J. 2016;37(38):2893–962.
21. Gage BF, Yan Y, Milligan PE, Waterman AD, Culverhouse R, Rich MW, et al. Clinical classification schemes for predicting hemorrhage: results from the National Registry of Atrial Fibrillation (NRAF). Am Heart J. 2006;151(3):713–9.
22. Pisters R, Lane DA, Nieuwlaat R, et al. A novel user-friendly score (HAS-BLED) to assess 1-year risk of major bleeding in patients with atrial fibrillation: the Euro Heart Survey. Chest. 2010;138:1093–100.
23. Lane DA, Lip GYH. Use of the CHA2DS2-VASc and HAS-BLED scores to aid decision making for thromboprophylaxis in nonvalvular atrial fibrillation. Circulation. 2012;126:860–5.
24. Stroke Prevention in Atrial Fibrillation Investigators. Stroke prevention in atrial fibrillation study. Final results. Circulation. 1991;84:527–39.
25. The ACTIVE Writing Group on behalf of the ACTIVE Investigators. Clopidogrel plus aspirin versus oral anticoagulation for atrial fibrillation in the Atrial fibrillation Clopidogrel Trial with Irbesartan for prevention of Vascular Events (ACTIVE W): a randomised controlled trial. Lancet. 2006;367:1903–12.
26. Connolly SJ, Ezekowitz MD, Yusuf S, et al. Dabigatran versus warfarin in patients with atrial fibrillation. N Engl J Med. 2009;361:1139–51.
27. Patel MR, Mahaffey KW, Garg J, et al. Rivaroxaban versus warfarin in nonvalvular atrial fibrillation. N Engl J Med. 2011;365:883–91.
28. Granger CB, Alexander JH, McMurray JJV, et al. Apixaban versus warfarin in patients with atrial fibrillation. N Engl J Med. 2011;365:981–92.
29. Giugliano RP, Ruff CT, Braunwald E, et al. Edoxaban versus warfarin in patients with atrial fibrillation. N Engl J Med. 2013;369:2093–104.
30. Kirley K, Qato DM, Kornfield R, Stafford RS, Alexander GC. National trends in oral anticoagulant use in the United States, 2007 to 2011. Circ Cardiovasc Qual Outcomes. 2012;5(5):615–21.
31. Barnes GD, Lucas E, Alexander GC, Goldberger ZD. National trends in ambulatory oral anticoagulant use. Am J Med. 2015;128(12):1300–5.
32. Piazza G, Hohlfelder B, Goldhaber SZ. Handbook for venous thromboembolism. New York: Springer; 2015.
33. Office of the Surgeon General (US); National Heart, Lung, and Blood Institute (US). The surgeon general's call to action to prevent deep vein thrombosis and pulmonary embolism. Rockville, MD: Office of the surgeon general (US); 2008. Available from: https://www.ncbi.nlm.nih.gov/books/NBK44178/
34. Lang IM, Madani M. Update on chronic thromboembolic pulmonary hypertension. Circulation. 2014;130:508–18.
35. Vazquez SR, Kahn SR. Postthrombotic syndrome. Circulation. 2010;121:e217–9.
36. Kyrle PA, Eichinger S. Is Virchow's triad complete? Blood. 2009;114:1138–9.
37. Karcutskie CA, Meizoso JP, Ray JJ, et al. Association of mechanism of injury with risk for venous thromboembolism after trauma. JAMA Surg. 2017;152(1):35–40.
38. Creager MA, Luscher TF. Diabetes and vascular disease: pathophysiology, clinical consequences, and medical therapy: part I. Circulation. 2003;108:1527–32.
39. Kearon C, Kahn SR, Agnelli G, Goldhaber S, Raskob GE, Comerota AJ. Antithrombotic therapy for venous thromboembolic disease: American College of Chest Physicians Evidence-Based Clinical Practice Guidelines (8th edn). Chest. 2008;133(Suppl):454S–545S.
40. Schulman S, Kearon C, Kakkar AK, et al. Dabigatran versus warfarin in the treatment of acute venous thromboembolism. N Engl J Med. 2009;361: 2342–52.
41. The EINSTEIN-PE Investiagtors. Oral rivaroxaban for the treatment of symptomatic pulmonary embolism. N Engl J Med. 2012;366:1287–97.
42. Investigators TEINSTEIN. Oral rivaroxaban for symptomatic venous thromboembolism. N Engl J Med. 2010;363:2499–510.

43. Agnelli G, Butler HR, Cohen A, et al. Oral apixaban for the treatment of acute venous thromboembolism. N Engl J Med. 2013;369:799–808.
44. Investigators TH-VTE. Edoxaban versus warfarin for the treatment of symptomatic venous thromboembolism. N Engl J Med. 2013;369:1406–15.
45. Hutten BA, Prins MH, Gent M, Ginsberg J, Tijssen JG, Buller HR. Incidence of recurrent thromboembolic and bleeding complications among patients with venous thromboembolism in relation to both malignancy and achieved international normalized ratio: a retrospective analysis. J Clin Oncol. 2000;18:3078–83.
46. Prandoni P, Lensing AW, Piccioli A, et al. Recurrent venous thromboembolism and bleeding complications during anticoagulant treatment in patients with cancer and venous thrombosis. Blood. 2002;100:3484–8.
47. Lee AYY, Levine MN, Baker RI, et al. Low-molecular-weight heparin versus a coumarin for the prevention of recurrent venous thromboembolism in patients with cancer. N Engl J Med. 2003;349:146–53.
48. Lyman GH, Bohlke K, Khorana AA, et al. Venous thromboembolism prophylaxis and treatment in patients with cancer: american society of clinical oncology clinical practice guideline update 2014. J Clin Oncol. 2015;33(6):654–6.
49. Vedovati MC, Germini F, Agnelli G, Becattini C. Direct oral anticoagulants in patients with VTE and cancer: a systematic review and meta-analysis. Chest. 2015;147(2):475.
50. Kearon C, Akl EA, Omelas J, et al. Antithrombotic therapy for VTE disease: CHEST guideline and expert panel report. Chest. 2016;149:315–52.
51. Wells PS, Forgie MA, Rodger MA. Treatment of venous thromboembolism. JAMA. 2014;311(7):717–28.
52. Kearon C, Akl EA. Duration of anticoagulant therapy for deep vein thrombosis and pulmonary embolism. Blood. 2014;123(12):1794–801.
53. Nkomo VT, Gardin JM, Skelton TN, Gottdiener JS, Scott CG, Enriquez-Sarano M. Burden of valvular heart diseases: a population-based study. Lancet. 2006;368:1005–11.
54. Barreto-Filho JA, Wang Y, Dodson JA, et al. Contemporary trends in aortic valve surgery for elderly patients in the United States, 1999–2010. JAMA. 2013;310:2078–85.
55. Bonow RO. Improving outlook for elderly patients with aortic stenosis. JAMA. 2013;310:2045–7.
56. Nishimura RA, Otto CM, Bonow RO. 2014 AHA/ACC guideline for the management of patients with valvular heart disease: a report of the American College of Cardiology/American Heart Association Task Force on practice guidelines. J Am Coll Cardiol. 2014;63(22):e57.
57. Lindman BR, Clavel MA, Mathieu P, et al. Calcific aortic stenosis. Nat Rev Dis Primers. 2016;2:16006.
58. Jones EC, Devereux RB, Roman MJ, et al. Prevalence and correlates of mitral regurgitation in a population-based sample (the Strong Heart Study). Am J Cardiol. 2001;87(3):298.
59. Marijon E, Ou P, Celermajer DS, et al. Prevalence of rheumatic heart disease detected by echocardiographic screening. N Engl J Med. 2007;357(5):470.
60. Whitlock RP, Sun JC, Fremes SE, et al. Antithrombotic and thrombolytic therapy for valvular disease: antithrombotic therapy and prevention of thrombosis, 9th ed: American College of Chest Physicians Evidence-Based Clinical Practice Guidelines. Chest. 2012;141(2 Suppl):e576S.
61. Joint Task Force on the Management of Valvular Heart Disease of the European Society of Cardiology (ESC), European Association for Cardio-Thoracic Surgery (EACTS). Guidelines on the management of valvular heart disease (version 2012). Eur Heart J. 2451;33(19):2012.
62. Singhal P, Luk A, Butany L. Bioprosthetic heart valves: impact of implantation on biomaterials. ISRN Biomater. 2013;2013:728791.
63. Pibarot P, Dumesnil JG. Prosthetic heart valves: selection of the optimal prosthesis and long-term management. Circulation. 2009;119:1034–48.
64. Allou N, Piednoir P, Berroëta C, et al. Incidence and risk factors of early thromboembolic events after mechanical heart valve replacement in patients treated with intravenous unfractionated heparin. Heart. 2009;95(20):1694.
65. Puskas J, Gerdisch M, Nichols D, et al. Reduced anticoagulation after mechanical aortic valve replacement: interim results from the prospective randomized on-x valve anticoagulation clinical trial randomized Food and Drug Administration investigational device exemption trial. J Thorac Cardiovasc Surg. 2014;147:1202–10.
66. Eikelboom JW, Connolly SJ, Brueckmann M, et al. Dabigatran versus warfarin in patients with mechanical heart valves. N Engl J Med. 2013;369:1206–14.
67. Kitchens CS. Concept of hypercoagulability: a review of its development, clinical application, and recent progress. Semin Thromb Hemost. 1985;11:293–315.
68. Reiner AP, Siscovick DS, Rosendaal FR. Hemostatic risk factors and arterial thrombotic disease. Thromb Haemost. 2001;85:584–95.
69. Chan MY, Andreotti F, Becker RC. Hypercoagulable states in cardiovascular disease. Circulation. 2008;118:2286–97.
70. Zivelin A, Rosenberg N, Faier S, et al. A single genetic origin for the common prothrombotic G20210A polymorphism in the prothrombin gene. Blood. 1998;92:1119–24.
71. Seligsohn U, Lubetsky A. Genetic susceptibility to venous thrombosis. N Engl J Med. 2001;344:1222–31.
72. Aiach M, Borgel D, Gaussem P, et al. Protein C and protein S deficiencies. Semin Hematol. 1997;34:205–16.
73. Van Boven HH, Lane DA. Antithrombin and its inherited deficiency states. Semin Hematol. 1997;34:188–204.

74. Levine JS, Branch DW, Rauch J. The antiphospholipid syndrome. N Engl J Med. 2002;346:752–63.
75. Greinacher A. Heparin induced thrombocytopenia. N Engl J Med. 2015;373:252–61.
76. Hyers TM, Agnelli G, Hull RD, et al. Antithrombotic therapy for venous thromboembolic disease. Chest. 2001;119:176S–93S.
77. Piazza G. Thrombophilia testing, recurrent thrombosis, and women's health. Circulation. 2014;130:283–7.
78. Ornstein DL, Cushman M. Factor V Leiden. Circulation. 2003;107:e94–7.
79. Laslett LJ, Alagona P Jr, Clark BA III, et al. The worldwide environment of cardiovascular disease: prevalence, diagnosis, therapy, and policy issues: a report from the American College of Cardiology. J Am Coll Cardiol. 2012;60(25 Suppl):S1.
80. Roth GA, Huffman MD, Moran AE, et al. Global and regional patterns in cardiovascular mortality from 1990 to 2013. Circulation. 2015;132(17):1667.
81. Yusuf S, Hawken S, Ounpuu S, et al. Effect of potentially modifiable risk factors associated with myocardial infarction in 52 countries (the INTERHEART study): case-control study. Lancet. 2004;364(9438):937.
82. Dagostino RB Sr, Grundy S, Sullivan LM, Wilson P, CHD Risk Prediction Group. Validation of the Framingham coronary heart disease prediction scores: results of a multiple ethnic groups investigation. JAMA. 2001;286(2):180.
83. National Cholesterol Education Program (NCEP) Expert Panel on Detection, Evaluation, and Treatment of High Blood Cholesterol in Adults (Adult Treatment Panel III). Third Report of the National Cholesterol Education Program (NCEP) Expert Panel on Detection. Evaluation, and treatment of high blood cholesterol in adults (adult treatment panel III) final report. Circulation. 2002;106(25):3143.
84. Muntner P, Colantonio LD, Cushman M, et al. Validation of the atherosclerotic cardiovascular disease pooled cohort risk equations. JAMA. 2014;311(14):1406.
85. Vandvik PO, Lincoff AM, Gore JM, et al. Primary and secondary prevention of cardiovascular disease: antithrombotic therapy and prevention of thrombosis, 9th ed: American College of Chest Physicians Evidence-Based Clinical Practice Guidelines. Chest. 2012;141(2 Suppl):e637S.
86. Nansseau JRN, Noubiap JJN. Aspirin for primary prevention of cardiovascular disease. Thromb J. 2015;13:38.
87. Pignone M, Alberts MJ, Colwell JA, et al. Aspirin for primary prevention of cardiovascular events in people with diabetes: a position statement of the American Diabetes Association, a Scientific Statement of the American Heart Association, and an Expert Consensus Document of the American College of Cardiology Foundation. Circulation. 2010;121:2694–701.
88. Fox KA, Goodman SG, Klein W, et al. Management of acute coronary syndromes. Variations in practice and outcome; findings from the Global Registry of Acute Coronary Events (GRACE). Eur Heart J. 2002;23(15):1177.
89. Go AS, Mozaffarian D, Roger VL, et al. On Behalf of the American Heart Association Statistics Committee and Stroke Statistics Subcommittee. Heart disease and stroke statistics–2013 update: a report from the American Heart Association. Circulation. 2013;127(1):e6–e245.
90. Hasdai D, Behar S, Wallentin L, et al. A prospective survey of the characteristics, treatments and outcomes of patients with acute coronary syndromes in Europe and the Mediterranean basin; the Euro Heart Survey of Acute Coronary Syndromes (Euro Heart Survey ACS). Eur Heart J. 2002;23(15):1190.
91. Thygesen K, Alpert JS, Jaffe AS, et al. Third universal definition of myocardial infarction. Circulation. 2012;126(16):2020.
92. Fihn SD, Gardin JM, Abrams J, et al. 2012 ACCF/AHA/ACP/AATS/PCNA/SCAI/STS guideline for the diagnosis and management of patients with stable ischemic heart disease: a report of the American College of Cardiology Foundation/American Heart Association Task Force on Practice Guidelines, and the American College of Physicians, American Association for Thoracic Surgery, Preventive Cardiovascular Nurses Association, Society for Cardiovascular Angiography and Interventions, and Society of Thoracic Surgeons. Circulation. 2012;126:e354–245.
93. Bhatt DL, Fox KAA, Hacke W, et al. Clopidogrel and aspirin versus aspirin alone for the prevention of atherothrombotic events. N Engl J Med. 2006;354:1706–17.
94. Kulik A, Ruel M, Jneid H, et al. Secondary prevention after coronary artery bypass graft surgery: a scientific statement from the American Heart Association. Circulation. 2015;2015:CIR.0000000000000182.
95. The Clopidogrel in Unstable Angina to Prevent Recurrent Events Trial Investigators. Effects of clopidogrel in addition to aspirin in patients with acute coronary syndromes without ST-segment elevation. N Engl J Med. 2001;345:494–502.
96. Mehta SR, Yusuf S, Peters RJ, et al. Effects of pretreatment with clopidogrel and aspirin followed by long-term therapy in patients undergoing percutaneous coronary intervention: the PCI-CURE study. Lancet. 2001;358(9281):527–33.
97. Une D, Al-Atassi T, Kulik A, Voisine P, Le May M, Ruel M. Impact of clopidogrel plus aspirin versus aspirin alone on the progression of native coronary artery disease after bypass surgery: analysis from the Clopidogrel After Surgery for Coronary Artery DiseasE (CASCADE) randomized trial. Circulation. 2014;130(11 Suppl 1):S12–8.
98. Wiviott SD, Braunwald E, McCabe CH, et al. Prasugrel versus clopidogrel in patients with

acute coronary syndromes. N Engl J Med. 2007;357:2001–15.
99. Wallentin L, Becker RC, Budaj A, et al. Ticagrelor versus clopidogrel in patients with acute coronary syndromes. N Engl J Med. 2009;361:1045–57.
100. Morice MC, Urban P, Greene S, Schuler G, Chevalier B. Why are we still using coronary bare-metal stents? J Am Coll Cardiol. 2013;61(10):1121–3.
101. Ernst A, Bulum J. New generations of drug-eluting stents – a brief review. EMJ Int Cardiol. 2014;1:100–6.
102. Levine GN, Bates ER, Bittl JA, et al. ACC/AHA guideline update on duration of dual antiplatelet therapy in CAD patients. J Am Coll Cardiol. 2016;2016:CIR.0000000000000404.
103. Bhatt DL, Hulot JS, Moliterno DJ, Harrington RA. Antiplatelet and anticoagulation therapy for acute coronary syndromes. Circ Res. 2014;114:1929–43.
104. Sabatine MS, Cannon CP, Gibson CM, et al. Addition of clopidogrel to aspirin and fibrinolytic therapy for myocardial infarction with ST-segment elevation. N Engl J Med. 2005;352:1179–89.
105. Steinhubl SR, Berger PB, Mann JT III, et al. Early and sustained dual oral antiplatelet therapy following percutaneous coronary intervention: a randomized controlled trial. JAMA. 2002;288(19):2411–20.
106. Mehta SR, Tanguay JF, Eikelboom JW, et al. Double-dose versus standard-dose clopidogrel and high-dose versus low-dose aspirin in individuals undergoing percutaneous coronary intervention for acute coronary syndromes (CURRENT-OASIS 7): a randomised factorial trial. Lancet. 2010;376(9748):1233–43.
107. Bonaa KH, Mannsverk J, Wiseth R, et al. Drug-eluting or bare-metal stents for coronary artery disease. N Engl J Med. 2016;375:1242–52.
108. Butt M, Connolly D, Lip GY. Drug-eluting stents: a comprehensive appraisal. Futur Cardiol. 2009;5(2):141–57.
109. Iakovou I. Thrombosis after stent implantation: how much of a problem is there? Futur Cardiol. 2008;4(3):261–7.
110. Mauri L, Kereiakes DJ, Yeh RW, et al. Twelve or 30 months of dual antiplatelet therapy after drug-eluting stents. N Engl J Med. 2014;371:2155–66.
111. Van der Worp HB, van Gijn J. Acute ischemic stroke. N Engl J Med. 2007;357:572–9.
112. Ovbiagele B, Nguyen-Hyunh MN. Stroke epidemiology: advancing our understanding of disease mechanism and therapy. Neurotherapeutics. 2011;8(3):319–29.
113. Kernan WN, Ovbiagele B, Black HR, et al. Guidelines for the prevention of stroke in patients with stroke and transient ischemic attack: a guideline for healthcare professionals from the American Heart Association/American Stroke Association. Stroke. 2014;45:2160–236.
114. Adams HP, Bendixen BH, Kappelle LJ, et al. Classification of subtype of acute ischemic stroke: definitions for use in a multicenter clinical trial. Stroke. 1993;24:35–41.
115. Ay H, Furie KL, Singhal A, Smith WS, Sorensen AG, Koroshetz WJ. An evidence-based causative classification system for acute ischemic stroke. Ann Neurol. 2005;58(5):688–97.
116. International Stroke Trial Collaborative Group. The International Stroke Trial (IST): a randomised trial of aspirin, subcutaneous heparin, both, or neither among 19435 patients with acute ischaemic stroke. Lancet. 1997;349(9065):1569–81.
117. Pratt CM, Moye LA. The cardiac arrhythmia suppression trial. Circulation. 1995;91:245–7.
118. Antithrombotic Trialists' (ATT) Collaboration. Aspirin in the primary and secondary prevention of vascular disease: collaborative meta-analysis of individual participant data from randomised trials. Lancet. 2009;373(9678):1849–60.
119. Rothwell PM, Algra A, Chen Z, Diener HC, Norrving B, Mehta Z. Effects of aspirin on risk and severity of early recurrent stroke after transient ischaemic attack and ischaemic stroke: time-course analysis of randomised trials. Lancet. 2016;388(10042):365–75.
120. CAPRIE Steering Committee. A randomised, blinded, trial of clopidogrel versus aspirin in patients at risk of ischaemic events (CAPRIE). CAPRIE Steering Committee. Lancet. 1996;348(9038):1329–39.
121. Claiborne Johnston S, Amarenco P, Albers GW, et al. Ticagrelor versus aspirin in acute stroke or transient ischemic attack. N Engl J Med. 2016;375:35–43.
122. Wang Y, Wang Y, Zhao X, et al. Clopidogrel with aspirin in acute minor stroke or transient ischemic attack. N Engl J Med. 2013;369:11–9.
123. Diener HC, Bogousslavsky J, Brass LM, et al. Aspirin and clopidogrel compared with clopidogrel alone after recent ischaemic stroke or transient ischaemic attack in high-risk patients (MATCH): randomised, double-blind, placebo-controlled trial. Lancet. 2004;364(9431):331–7.
124. Diener HC, Cunha L, Forbes C, Sivenius J, Smets P, Lowenthal A. European stroke prevention study. 2. Dipyridamole and acetylsalicylic acid in the secondary prevention of stroke. J Neurol Sci. 1996;143(1–2):1–13.
125. Verro P, Gorelick PB, Nguyen D. Aspirin plus dipyridamole versus aspirin for prevention of vascular events after stroke or TIA: a meta-analysis. Stroke. 2008;39:1358–63.

# Review of Antiplatelet Agents

# 9

Jeremy R. DeGrado and Kevin E. Anger

**Abstract**

Development of thrombi can lead to various life-threatening cardiovascular and neurological events, and the role of platelets in thrombus formation is well known. Antiplatelet agents are used in the treatment, as well as both primary and secondary prevention, of various disease states or clinical scenarios. Mechanisms of action, reversibility, metabolism, drug interactions, duration of action, and other characteristics differ widely among the different classes of, and between individual, antiplatelet agents. An overview of the pharmacology, clinical indications, and monitoring considerations of antiplatelet drugs is included.

## 9.1 Introduction

Development of thrombi can lead to various life-threatening cardiovascular and neurological events, and the role of platelets in thrombus formation is well known [1–3]. Antiplatelet agents are used commonly for both the acute treatment and prevention of coronary artery disease (CAD) and stroke, as well as for prevention of venous thromboembolism (VTE) after orthopedic surgery, vascular disease, unstable angina, or in patients who have undergone percutaneous coronary intervention (PCI) or cardiac surgery. Mechanism of action, reversibility of binding to different receptors, degree of hepatic metabolism and renal clearance, duration of therapeutic effect, drug interactions, and monitoring of both efficacy and safety differ among available agents [3]. Understanding these key drug properties and differences between medications, along with patient-specific characteristics, is essential to appropriate monitoring in both the inpatient and outpatient setting [4].

This chapter focuses on the pharmacology, pharmacodynamics, clinical indications, and complications of specific antiplatelet agents. See Chaps. 8 and 12 for more information.

## 9.2 Antiplatelet Pharmacotherapy

### 9.2.1 Overview of Antiplatelet Pharmacotherapy

Platelet activation, adhesion, and aggregation are all affected by various antiplatelet agents. Pharmacological inhibitors of platelet function

J. R. DeGrado (✉) · K. E. Anger
Brigham and Women's Hospital, Boston, MA, USA
e-mail: jdegrado@bwh.harvard.edu; kanger@bwh.harvard.edu


R. P. Szumita, P. M. Szumita (eds.), *Hemostasis in Dentistry*, https://doi.org/10.1007/978-3-319-71240-6_9

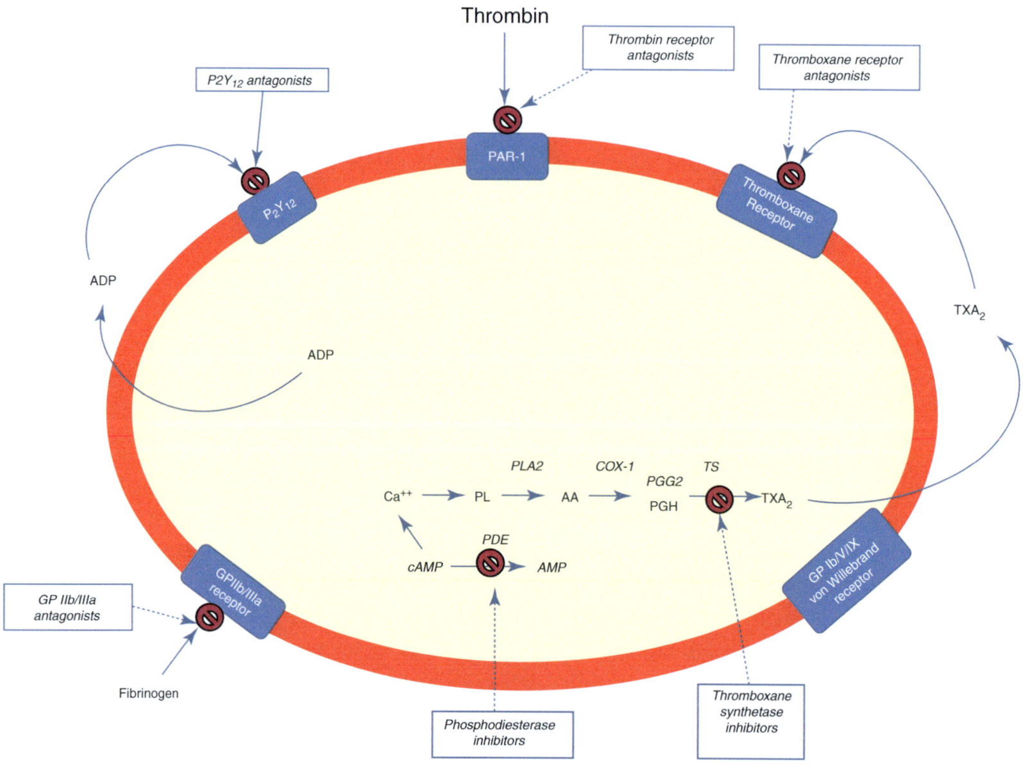


**Fig. 9.1** Mechanisms of platelet activation and pharmacological inhibition of platelet function. Pharmacological inhibitors of platelet function target adhesion, release, and aggregation mechanisms. Platelet adhesion occurs via binding of von Willebrand factor (VWF) to glycoprotein (GP) receptors. Platelet activation involves an intracellular signaling process that leads to the production of thromboxane $A_2$ ($TXA_2$) and adenosine diphosphate (ADP). Low dose aspirin inhibits cyclooxygenase 1 (COX-1) and consequently decreases production of $TXA_2$. $P2Y_{12}$ inhibitors diminish the effects of ADP, which is released in response to platelet adhesion and promotes platelet activation and release of prothrombotic factors. The stable adhesion phase involves the interaction of GP IIb/IIIa receptors with fibrinogen and VWF, which can be blocked with the use of GP IIb/IIIa inhibitors. Thrombin receptor antagonists block platelet aggregation by selectively blocking PAR-1 thrombin receptors

can be grouped as follows: thromboxane (TXA) inhibitors, antagonists of adenosine diphosphate (ADP)-mediated platelet activation, glycoprotein (GP) IIb/IIIa complex inhibitors, thrombin receptor antagonists, and phosphodiesterase inhibitors (Fig. 9.1).

Antiplatelet medications inhibit platelet function to varying degrees. The terms "resistance" and "nonresponse" describe a failure to prevent a thrombotic event due to inadequate platelet inhibition [5]. This may be due to underlying clinical, cellular, and genetic mechanisms, which can be confirmed by platelet function testing [5]. However, standard testing protocols have yet to be established [6].

## 9.2.2 Aspirin

### 9.2.2.1 Pharmacology, Pharmacodynamics, and Monitoring

Aspirin, or acetylsalicylic acid, is metabolized by esterases to its active form, salicylic acid, and subsequently blocks platelet activation. Aspirin irreversibly inhibits cyclooxygenase enzymes (COX-1, COX-2), therefore decreasing the conversion of arachidonic acid to prostaglandin and TXA by-products. Thromboxane $A_2$ stimulates platelet activation, aggregation, and recruitment and causes vasoconstriction [2, 7]. COX-1 enzymes are predominantly located in the GI

**Table 9.1** Aspirin and $P2Y_{12}$ inhibitor pharmacokinetics and pharmacodynamics

| | Aspirin | Cangrelor | Clopidogrel | Prasugrel | Ticagrelor | Ticlopidine |
|---|---|---|---|---|---|---|
| Route | Oral | IV | Oral | Oral | Oral | Oral |
| Receptor binding | Irreversible | Reversible | Irreversible | Irreversible | Reversible | Irreversible |
| Prodrug | Yes | No | Yes | Yes | No | Yes |
| Metabolism | Plasma esterase to salicylate (active); hepatic conjugation | Plasma esterase | CYP3A4, 2B6 | CYP3A4, 2B6, 2C9, 2C19 | CYP3A4 | CYP3A4 |
| Clearance | Renal 85% (75% metabolite) | Renal (58%) | Renal 50% Fecal 46% | Renal 68% Fecal 27% | Renal 1% (parent drug/ active metabolite) | Renal 60% Fecal 23% |
| Time to peak platelet inhibition | 30–60 min | 30 min | 300 mg LD: 6 h 600 mg LD: 2 h | 1–2 h | 2 h | 2–5 days |
| Duration of action | 7–10 days | 20–60 min | 7–10 days | 7–10 days | 3–5 days | 7–10 days |
| Genetic polymorphisms | Yes | Not reported | Yes | No | No | Yes |

*IV* intravenous, *CYP* cytochrome, *LD* loading dose

tract, kidneys, and on platelets. Aspirin's inhibition of COX-1 appears to be the primary mechanism of inhibition of hemostasis, and low doses of aspirin given daily can substantially block COX-1 production [2]. Aspirin irreversibly binds to platelets and therefore maintains its therapeutic effect for the life of the platelet (7–10 days) despite plasma concentrations quickly dropping due to a short half-life (Table 9.1). Aspirin may have its maximum antithrombotic effect at doses as low as 30–150 mg, while larger doses are required to fully inhibit COX-2 and produce systemic anti-inflammatory effects. Substantial variation exists between patients with regard to the daily doses required to suppress inflammation and inhibit platelet function [8].

Aspirin is available in various dosage forms and may be administered enterally or rectally. Chewable tablets can achieve peak concentrations within 30 minutes and platelet inhibition within 1 h [2]. Enteric-coated and delayed-release formulations have diminished bioavailability, delayed onset of action (approximately 3–4 h to reach peak plasma levels), and therefore delayed therapeutic effect. Rectal administration is associated with variable absorption (bioavailability of 20–60% over a 2- to 5-h retention time) [9]. For acute thrombosis, immediate-release enteral aspirin is always the preferred choice [2].

The optimal aspirin dose that maximizes efficacy and minimizes toxicity is unknown. Doses ranging from 75 to 325 mg daily are recommended, and the dose chosen may depend on various patient-specific factors, such as risk of bleeding, time from cardiovascular or neurologic event, type of stent placed, concomitant medications, and many more. Lower doses of aspirin (i.e., 81 mg/day) have not been shown to have diminished efficacy than higher doses in preventing clinical outcomes [2, 10].

Up to 5% of patients annually have vascular thrombotic events despite active prophylaxis with aspirin [11]. Aspirin resistance, potentially due to factors such as nonadherence, decreased absorption, smoking, receptor polymorphisms, upregulation of nontargeted pathways of platelet activation, and pharmacodynamic alterations, can occur in a wide range of patients. As would be expected, aspirin resistance has been correlated with an increased risk of death, acute coronary syndromes (ACS), and stroke [12].

#### 9.2.2.2 Clinical Indications

Aspirin is indicated for the treatment of ACS and stroke/TIA, as well as secondary prevention of arterial and venous thrombosis in patients with CAD or a history of ACS. Aspirin has been shown to reduce morbidity and mortality in acute coronary syndromes (ACS), stable angina, coronary bypass surgery, peripheral arterial disease (PAD), transient ischemic attack, acute ischemic stroke, and polycythemia vera. Aspirin is used as adjunctive therapy for thromboprophylaxis in patients on warfarin with prosthetic heart valves and in patients with nonvalvular atrial fibrillation [13]. Chapter 8 contains more information on the various indications of aspirin.

#### 9.2.2.3 Complications

Aspirin, in a dose-dependent manner, increases the incidence of major, gastrointestinal, and intracranial bleeding [2, 7]. The decision of whether to continue or discontinue aspirin prior to dental procedures is patient-specific. If warranted, discontinuation of aspirin prior to elective surgery or procedures is 7–10 days due to the irreversible binding to platelets. If holding therapy was indicated, resumption of aspirin approximately 24 h post-procedures is typically considered safe [14].

While the exact incidence of aspirin-induced bleeding is difficult to determine due to patient-specific risk factors, aspirin appears to increase bleeding risk in a dose-dependent manner. The mechanism of aspirin-induced bleeding is primarily due to inhibition of protective prostaglandin synthesis that may lead to gastrointestinal ulcerations. Aspirin, even when used at recommended doses, may increase the risk of gastrointestinal bleeding 1.5- to 3-fold by itself and possibly more when used with other antiplatelet or anticoagulant agents [15]. Due to the dose-dependent nature of aspirin-related bleeding, use of the lowest effective dose for each indication is encouraged, as this can reduce the risk by 30–40% [2]. Enteric-coated and buffered aspirin doses ≤325 mg seemingly do not reduce the incidence of gastrointestinal bleeding [16]. The risk of aspirin-induced gastric toxicity may be decreased with concurrent use of acid-suppressive therapy, especially proton pump inhibitors [15]. Serious side effects, such as intracranial hemorrhage, are thought to occur in <1% of patients.

### 9.2.3 $P2Y_{12}$ Inhibitors

#### 9.2.3.1 Pharmacology, Pharmacodynamics, and Monitoring

$P2Y_{12}$ inhibitors decrease platelet activation by blocking adenosine diphosphate (ADP) binding to $P2Y_{12}$ receptors, thereby blocking activation of the GP IIb/IIIa receptor complex on the platelet surface [2]. These $P2Y_{12}$ are divided into thienopyridines (clopidogrel, prasugrel, and ticlopidine) and non-thienopyridines (ticagrelor and cangrelor). Thienopyridines are prodrugs that require hepatic metabolism via the cytochrome P450 (CYP450) isoenzyme system in order to have a therapeutic effect (Table 9.1). Each agent has differing onset of action, potency, duration of effect, and drug interaction profile [17, 18]. Loading doses of all three agents are administered in order to quickly achieve therapeutic concentrations and a rapid onset of action. The metabolism of clopidogrel and ticlopidine is a two-step activation process via CYP450. Prasugrel's active metabolite reaches peak concentrations within 30 minutes, compared to 2–4 h for clopidogrel [2]. Additionally, prasugrel undergoes one-step oxidation by multiple CYP450 isoenzyme pathways which may contribute to its more predictable pharmacokinetics.

While the actual half-life of the active metabolites of thienopyridines is short (1–8 h), their irreversible binding to $P2Y_{12}$ receptors leads to a duration of effect that is significantly longer (7–10 days). Newer agents are being developed in an attempt to improve in areas such as onset of action, duration of effect, and predictability of platelet inhibition [19]. Ticagrelor is a non-thienopyridine $P2Y_{12}$ inhibitor that is not a prodrug and therefore does not require hepatic metabolism for therapeutic effect. This results in a more rapid and predictable inhibition of platelet activation and aggregation [20]. Ticagrelor binds reversibly at $P2Y_{12}$ receptors, resulting in a shorter duration of antiplatelet activity compared to thienopyridines [20]. Ticagrelor's reversible binding and short half-life make for a potentially easier transition for procedures that require prior discontinuation of antiplatelet therapy; however, patients may be at increased risk of thrombosis compared to other longer acting agents if a few doses are held due to its shorter duration of action (see Table 9.1). It is given twice daily, so patients must be compliant to ensure therapeutic levels maintained. Cangrelor is a new, intravenous (IV), non-thienopyridine with a very short half-life and rapid onset that may have a role in select patients undergoing PCI who cannot tolerate enteral P2Y12 inhibitors or in situations where it is desirable to be able to quickly remove the antiplatelet effect [21].

Resistance to clopidogrel occurs in a wide range of patients and depends on both patient-specific variables, such as genetic polymorphisms and comorbidities, and various factors related to the platelet function test [18]. Genetic and drug-induced alterations of CYP3A4 and CYP2C19 enzymes, the pathways responsible for thienopyridine activation, appear to be of great importance in determining resistance [19]. Specifically, polymorphisms that involve a loss of function with CYP2C19 enzymes have been linked with an increased incidence of clopidogrel failure. Clopidogrel resistance is estimated to occur in up to one third of patients and may lead to up to a fivefold increase in risk of thrombosis leading to death, myocardial infarction, and stroke [22]. There is still no consensus on how to routinely monitor the antiplatelet effect of $P2Y_{12}$ inhibitors using platelet function testing [6]. Available data do not demonstrate superior outcomes when platelet function monitoring is routinely performed [23]. Higher maintenance dosing has not shown to improve antiplatelet activity in all patients with established CYP450 polymorphisms [6, 10]. Availability of newer agents with more favorable and predictable pharmacokinetics and pharmacodynamics, combined with general unavailability and unclear utility of platelet function testing, may push clinicians to switch to agents such as prasugrel and ticagrelor.

#### 9.2.3.2 Clinical Indications

$P2Y_{12}$ inhibitors are indicated for primary and secondary thrombosis prevention in a variety of disease states. Ticlopidine has been shown to reduce thrombotic events in patients with stroke but is associated with neutropenia, thrombocytopenia, and thrombotic thrombocytopenic purpura [19]. Clopidogrel, typically with aspirin, is used for primary and secondary prevention of ischemic events in ACS, PAD, stroke, and coronary artery disease. Prasugrel, also usually with aspirin, is indicated for the prevention of thrombotic cardiovascular events, including in-stent thrombosis, in ACS patients after percutaneous coronary intervention (PCI) [18]. Ticagrelor is indicated in combination with aspirin for primary and secondary prevention of ischemic events in patients experiencing ACS and may be preferred over clopidogrel in patients with ACS undergoing early invasive reperfusion procedures [24]. Cangrelor is indicated for the reduction of cardiovascular (CV) events in select patients undergoing PCI [25]. Patients requiring cangrelor are typically transitioned to enteral $P2Y_{12}$ inhibitors as soon as able. Please see Chap. 8 for more information.

#### 9.2.3.3 Complications

The incidence of major bleeding with $P2Y_{12}$ inhibitors is different among the agents and may depend on other factors such as dosing, patient-specific risk factors, and concomitant antithrombotic therapies. Gastrointestinal hemorrhage is a relatively common complication of $P2Y_{12}$ inhibitor therapy [15]. $P2Y_{12}$ inhibitors should be avoided in patients undergoing neuraxial analgesia due to the risk of subdural hematoma [26]. Clopidogrel and prasugrel may need to be discontinued 7–10 days prior to elective surgery or invasive procedure, while it is recommended ticagrelor be stopped 5 days prior if discontinuation is warranted. Therapy usually is resumed approximately 24 h or the next morning after surgery. See Chap. 12.

Due to the unique structure of ticagrelor and possibly its ability to delay adenosine metabolism, it has been associated with adverse effects not seen with thienopyridine derivatives. An increased rate of dyspnea, ventricular pauses, and hyperuricemia have been reported [20].

### 9.2.4 Other Antiplatelet Targets

#### 9.2.4.1 Pharmacology, Pharmacodynamics, and Monitoring

Aspirin and P2Y12 inhibitors are utilized by the overwhelming majority of patients receiving antiplatelet therapy. Other agents, however, are used in specific disease states or clinical scenarios. Abciximab, eptifibatide, and tirofiban are IV agents that inhibit the GP IIb/IIIa receptor on the platelet surface and prevent platelet activation, aggregation, and fibrinogen-mediated platelet-to-platelet bridging [2, 27]. These agents have been shown to rapidly suppress approximately 80–90% of ADP-induced platelet aggregation [27, 28]. Eptifibatide and tirofiban quickly dissociate from the GP IIb/IIIa receptor, and normal platelet function is achieved within 8 h, while the effects of abciximab may persist for weeks due to its affinity for the receptor [28]. The main receptor for thrombin binding, protease-activated receptor-1 (PAR-1), appears to play an important role in thrombin-stimulated platelet activation and inflammatory responses, possibly leading to events such as myocardial infarction and arterial thrombosis. Vorapaxar is a PAR-1 antagonist that inhibits platelet aggregation mediated by thrombin and thrombin receptor agonist peptide (TRAP) [29]. Cilostazol, through selective inhibition of phosphodiesterase 3 (PDE 3), increases cAMP. An increase in cAMP leads to an increase in the active form of protein kinase A, which is directly related to both inhibition of platelet aggregation and vasodilation [30]. Cilostazol is extensively metabolized by CYP 450-3A4 and therefore has many drug-drug interactions that may require dose adjustments or selection of an alternative in patients taking strong inhibitors of this enzyme [31]. Dipyridamole inhibits adenosine deaminase and phosphodiesterase, leading to an increase in adenosine and cAMP. These mediators then increase platelet aggregation, as well as possibly vasodilation. Dipyridamole is metabolized through glucuronidation via the liver and has a half-life of approximately 10 h [2].

#### 9.2.4.2 Clinical Indications

GP IIb/IIIa inhibitors may be used as adjunctive therapy for patients with ACS and those undergoing PCI. The decision to use these agents must weigh various factors, including patient-specific risk factors, utilization of other antiplatelet and antithrombotic agents, and required duration [24, 28]. Vorapaxar is indicated for the reduction of CV events in patients with a myocardial infarction or peripheral arterial disease [29]. Cilostazol is indicated for treatment of intermittent claudication and has been shown to improve pain-free walking distance [31]. In patients who have undergone heart valve replacement surgery, dipyridamole may be indicated as adjunctive therapy for the prevention of thromboembolism. Dipyridamole, in combination with aspirin, has been shown to reduce the incidence of major vascular events in patients with a history of cerebrovascular accidents and TIA and therefore is indicated for secondary prevention [2, 32].

#### 9.2.4.3 Complications

The frequency of major bleeding with GP IIb/IIIa therapy ranges from 1% to 14% of patients and depends on the specific agent, concomitant therapies, and other factors related to ACS or PCI [27, 28]. Eptifibatide and tirofiban require dose adjustment in patients with renal dysfunction in order to decrease risk of drug accumulation and bleeding [33]. Vorapaxar has a long half-life (165–311 h) and may still cause up to 50% inhibition of platelet aggregation for as long as 4 weeks after discontinuation of therapy [19, 29]. Headache is the most common adverse effect caused by both dipyridamole and cilostazol. However, while hemorrhage is rare with both agents, patients should be monitored for signs and symptoms of bleeding [31].

## 9.3 Summary

The list of antiplatelet medications available for patients has grown dramatically in recent times. Aspirin is still used as the backbone of antiplatelet therapy, but the introduction of new, potent classes of medications such as $P2Y_{12}$ inhibitors, GP IIb/IIIa antagonists, and PAR-1 antagonists demonstrates that the landscape is continuing to change. Understanding the pharmacology of these classes of drugs, and the differences between each of the medications, is essential for the management of these patients.

## References


1. Siller-Matula JM, Krumphuber J, Jilma B. Pharmacokinetic, pharmacodynamic and clinical profile of novel antiplatelet drugs targeting vascular diseases. Br J Pharmacol. 2010;159(3):502–17.
2. Eikelboom JW, Hirsh J, Spencer FA, Baglin TP, Weitz JI. Antiplatelet drugs: antithrombotic therapy and prevention of thrombosis, 9th ed: American College of Chest Physicians evidence-based clinical practice guidelines. Chest. 2012;141(2 Suppl):e89S–119S.
3. Packard KA, Campbell JA, Knezevich JT, Davis EM. Emerging antiplatelet therapy for coronary artery disease and acute coronary syndrome. Pharmacotherapy. 2012;32(3):244–73.
4. Smith BS, Yogaratnam D, Levasseur-Franklin KE, Forni A, Fong J. Introduction to drug pharmacokinetics in the critically ill patient. Chest. 2012;141(5):1327–36.
5. Airee A, Draper HM, Finks SW. Aspirin resistance: disparities and clinical implications. Pharmacotherapy. 2008;28(8):999–1018.
6. Gurbel PA, Tantry US. Do platelet function testing and genotyping improve outcome in patients treated with antithrombotic agents?: platelet function testing and genotyping improve outcome in patients treated with antithrombotic agents. Circulation. 2012;125(10):1276–87. discussion 87
7. Fuster V, Sweeny JM. Aspirin: a historical and contemporary therapeutic overview. Circulation. 2011;123(7):768–78.
8. Patrono C, Rocca B. Aspirin, 110 years later. J Thromb Haemost. 2009;7(Suppl 1):258–61.
9. Nowak MM, Brundhofer B, Gibaldi M. Rectal absorption from aspirin suppositories in children and adults. Pediatrics. 1974;54(1):23–6.
10. Mehta SR, Bassand JP, Chrolavicius S, Diaz R, Eikelboom JW, Fox KA, et al. Dose comparisons of clopidogrel and aspirin in acute coronary syndromes. N Engl J Med. 2010;363(10):930–42.
11. Sanderson S, Emery J, Baglin T, Kinmonth AL. Narrative review: aspirin resistance and its clinical implications. Ann Intern Med. 2005;142(5):370–80.
12. Krasopoulos G, Brister SJ, Beattie WS, Buchanan MR. Aspirin "resistance" and risk of cardiovascular morbidity: systematic review and meta-analysis. BMJ. 2008;336(7637):195–8.
13. Loualidi A, Bredie SH, Janssen MC. Indications of combined vitamin K antagonists and aspirin therapy. J Thromb Thrombolysis. 2009;27(4):421–9.
14. Douketis JD, Spyropoulos AC, Spencer FA, Mayr M, Jaffer AK, Eckman MH, et al. Perioperative management of antithrombotic therapy: antithrombotic therapy and prevention of thrombosis, 9th ed: American College of Chest Physicians evidence-based clinical practice guidelines. Chest. 2012;141(2 Suppl):e326S–50S.
15. Cryer B. Management of patients with high gastrointestinal risk on antiplatelet therapy. Gastroenterol Clin N Am. 2009;38(2):289–303.
16. Kelly JP, Kaufman DW, Jurgelon JM, Sheehan J, Koff RS, Shapiro S. Risk of aspirin-associated major upper-gastrointestinal bleeding with enteric-coated or buffered product. Lancet. 1996;348(9039):1413–6.
17. Cattaneo M. New P2Y(12) inhibitors. Circulation. 2010;121(1):171–9.
18. Reinhart KM, White CM, Baker WL. Prasugrel: a critical comparison with clopidogrel. Pharmacotherapy. 2009;29(12):1441–51.
19. Mega JL, Simon T. Pharmacology of antithrombotic drugs: an assessment of oral antiplatelet and anticoagulant treatments. Lancet. 2015;386:281–91.
20. Dobesh PP, Oestreich JH. Ticagrelor: pharmacokinetics, pharmacodynamics, clinical efficacy, and safety. Pharmacotherapy. 2014;34(10):1077–90.
21. Waite LH, Phan YL, Spinler SA. Cangrelor: a novel intravenous antiplatelet agent with a questionable future. Pharmacotherapy. 2014;34(10):1061–76.
22. Bonello L, Tantry US, Marcucci R, Blindt R, Angiolillo DJ, Becker R, et al. Consensus and future directions on the definition of high on-treatment platelet reactivity to adenosine diphosphate. J Am Coll Cardiol. 2010;56(12):919–33.
23. Collet JP, Cuisset T, Range G, Cayla G, Elhadad S, Pouillot C, et al. Bedside monitoring to adjust antiplatelet therapy for coronary stenting. N Engl J Med. 2012;367(22):2100–9.
24. Amsterdam EA, Wenger NK, Brindis RG, Casey DE Jr, Ganiats TG, Holmes DR Jr, et al. 2014 AHA/ACC guideline for the management of patients with non-ST-elevation acute coronary syndromes: executive summary: a report of the American College of Cardiology/American Heart Association Task Force on practice guidelines. Circulation. 2014;130(25):2354–94.
25. Kengreal™ (Cangrelor). 2015. Available from: http://www.accessdata.fda.gov/drugsatfda_docs/label/2015/204958lbl.pdf
26. Horlocker TT, Wedel DJ, Rowlingson JC, Enneking FK, Kopp SL, Benzon HT, et al. Regional anesthesia in the patient receiving antithrombotic or thrombolytic therapy: American Society of Regional Anesthesia and Pain Medicine evidence-based guidelines (third edition). Reg Anesth Pain Med. 2010;35(1):64–101.
27. Crouch MA, Nappi JM, Cheang KI. Glycoprotein IIb/IIIa receptor inhibitors in percutaneous coronary intervention and acute coronary syndrome. Ann Pharmacother. 2003;37(6):860–75.

28. Atwater BD, Roe MT, Mahaffey KW. Platelet glycoprotein IIb/IIIa receptor antagonists in non-ST segment elevation acute coronary syndromes: a review and guide to patient selection. Drugs. 2005;65(3):313–24.
29. Frampton JE. Vorapaxar: a review of its use in the long-term secondary prevention of atherothrombotic events. Drugs. 2015;75(7):797–808.
30. Ansara AJ, Shiltz DL, Slavens JB. Use of cilostazol for secondary stroke prevention: an old dog with new tricks? Ann Pharmacother. 2012;46(3):394–402.
31. Jacoby D, Mohler ER III. Drug treatment of intermittent claudication. Drugs. 2004;64(15):1657–70.
32. Sacco RL, Diener HC, Yusuf S, Cotton D, Ounpuu S, Lawton WA, et al. Aspirin and extended-release dipyridamole versus clopidogrel for recurrent stroke. N Engl J Med. 2008;359(12):1238–51.
33. Alexander KP, Chen AY, Roe MT, Newby LK, Gibson CM, Allen-LaPointe NM, et al. Excess dosing of antiplatelet and antithrombin agents in the treatment of non-ST-segment elevation acute coronary syndromes. JAMA. 2005;294(24):3108–16.

# Review of Anticoagulants

# 10

David P. Reardon and Christopher Zemaitis

**Abstract**

Anticoagulation therapy is utilized for many thromboembolic indications with oral therapy being the first-line therapy choice for long-term management of many of these disorders. Warfarin has been utilized for decades as the primary oral anticoagulant, and more recently, oral direct thrombin inhibitors and factor Xa inhibitors have emerged as alternative therapies. Subcutaneous and intravenous therapies are also often utilized in clinical practice most commonly as short-term therapies for bridging or the ability to initiate long-term anticoagulation. Dentists should be familiar with these agents and also be aware of potential drug interactions that may increase or decrease anticoagulant serum concentrations and alter clinical efficacy. Concomitant use with antiplatelet agents and the perioperative management of these agents, including the need for anticoagulation reversal, are discussed in other chapters of this book.

D. P. Reardon (✉)
Vizient Pharmacy Member Services, Vizient, Inc., Irving, TX, USA
e-mail: david.reardon@vizientinc.com

C. Zemaitis
Yale New Haven Hospital, New Haven, CT, USA
e-mail: christopher.zemaitis@ynhh.org

## 10.1 Introduction

Pharmacological disruption and prolongation of the coagulation cascade is of therapeutic benefit in patients with thromboembolic disorders such as atrial fibrillation (AF), venous thromboembolism (VTE), and acute coronary syndromes (ACS) [1]. The current rate of atrial fibrillation in the adult population is estimated between one and two percent and a stroke risk stratification tool, such as the $CHADS_2$ score, should be utilized to determine appropriateness of anticoagulation [2, 3]. VTE, such as deep vein thrombosis (DVT) and pulmonary embolism (PE), has many known risk factors, and it is a serious but preventable cause of death in hospitalized and postsurgical patients [4, 5]. ACS has traditionally been treated with dual antiplatelet therapy although new evidence may suggest a role for anticoagulation as well [1]. Dentists should be familiar with these indications for anticoagulation to help identify patients that may be at higher risk for thromboembolic and bleeding complications peri-procedure.

The most appropriate agent to treat one of the aforementioned disorders is dependent on both drug and patient characteristics [6]. From the drug standpoint, the onset of action and possible need for "bridging" parenteral therapy, absorption, distribution, metabolism, excretion, and Food and Drug Administration (FDA)-approved indications should be taken into account.



R. P. Szumita, P. M. Szumita (eds.), *Hemostasis in Dentistry*, https://doi.org/10.1007/978-3-319-71240-6_10

Medications with a prolonged onset of action, such as vitamin K antagonists, may require overlap or "bridging" with another, faster acting agent until therapeutic anticoagulation with the chronic agent can be confirmed. For most dental procedures, discontinuation of anticoagulation therapy prior to procedure(s) and subsequent bridging is not needed. This is determined by patient specific factors, the invasiveness of the dental procedure and is outlined in more detail in Chaps. 13 and 14. Metabolism and excretion are of particular importance due to the potential for adverse effects or treatment failure with worsening or improving hepatic or renal function as well as the potential for drug-drug interactions.

Patient characteristics to consider include comorbities such as renal dysfunction, obesity and age, medication and follow-up adherence, and concomitant medication therapies. The length of therapy (i.e., prophylaxis versus chronic therapy) should also be taken into account to help increase compliance with the prescribed therapy. Patients at high risk for VTE due to a reversible cause such as total hip or knee arthroplasty should be considered for a short course of prophylactic anticoagulation while those with active VTE or another high risk chronic thromboembolic disorder should be consider for prolonged therapy [7, 8]. This chapter will focus on currently available anticoagulants and their role in clinical practice.

## 10.2 Pharmacologic Agents

### 10.2.1 Oral Agents

#### 10.2.1.1 Vitamin K Antagonists, Warfarin (Coumadin®)

Warfarin continues to be the most widely prescribed anticoagulant in North America. Warfarin was discovered in the early 1940s at the University of Wisconsin as researchers were investigating deaths in cattle that ate spoiled sweet clover in the 1920s. The agent responsible for these deaths was identified as bishydroxycoumarin. A more potent agent, *W*isconsin *A*lumni *R*esearch *F*oundation, coum*arin* derivative, was introduced as an effective rodenticide in 1948 [9]. Warfarin is FDA approved for the prophylaxis and treatment of deep vein thrombosis (DVT) and pulmonary embolisms (PE), along with treatment and prevention of thromboembolic complications associated with atrial fibrillation and/or cardiac valve replacement. It is also indicated for reduction in the risk of death, recurrent myocardial infarction, and thromboembolic events after myocardial infarctions [10]. Though it has been in use since the 1950s and is studied in most clotting disorders, its use is complicated by its narrow therapeutic window and its many drug and food interactions. These issues necessitate close patient monitoring and education to ensure effectiveness and safety.

#### 10.2.1.2 Mechanism of Action, Pharmacodynamics, and Pharmacokinetics

Warfarin exerts its effects by inhibiting the synthesis of activated vitamin K-dependent coagulation factors (II, VII, IX, X, proteins C and S) but has no effect on factors currently circulating in the body [11]. This leads warfarin to have delayed onset of action as vitamin K-dependent coagulation factors have half-lives ranging from 6 h to 3 days with factor II or prothrombin having the longest half-life of about 60–72 h. The full anticoagulant effect of warfarin is not seen for 3–5 days which requires the use of a parenteral anticoagulant, heparin, or low molecular weight heparin (LMWH), for at least 5 days after starting warfarin for treatment of DVT or PE as "bridging" therapy [12]. Additional dosing and pharmacokinetic information for warfarin and other oral anticoagulants are available in Table 10.1.

#### 10.2.1.3 Monitoring, Precautions for Use, and Specific Considerations

Due to its narrow therapeutic window, many food and drug interactions, and genetic variation among patients, warfarin requires close monitoring to ensure safety. It is monitored using the international normalized ratio (INR). The INR is calculated from the prothrombin time (PT) or PT

**Table 10.1** Common oral anticoagulant's dosing and kinetics [10, 17, 22, 25, 28]

| | Warfarin (Coumarin®) | Dabigatran (Pradaxa®) | Rivaroxaban (Xarelto®) | Apixaban (Eliquis®) | Edoxaban (Savaysa®) |
|---|---|---|---|---|---|
| Class | Vitamin K epoxide reductase inhibitor (II, VII, IX, X, C/S) | Direct thrombin inhibitor | Factor Xa inhibitor | Factor Xa inhibitor | Factor Xa inhibitor |
| Dosing for DVT/PE and NVAF | Individualized, 2–10 mg+ | 150 mg BID | 20 mg once daily with dinner | 5 mg BID | 60 mg daily |
| Loading dose (DVT/PE treatment) | +/– | N/A | 15 mg BID × 21 days | 10 mg BID × 7 days | N/A |
| Dose adjustments (NVAF) | INR = 2–3 | CrCl 15–30: 75 mg BID<br>Avoid <15 ml/min | CrCl 15–50: 15 mg once daily<br>Avoid <15 ml/h | SCr ≥1.5 and ≥ 80 years old/≤60 kg: 2.5 mg BID | CrCl 15–50 mL/min:<br>30 mg orally once daily<br>Avoid >95 or < 15 ml/h |
| Dosing for other indications | N/A | Prophylaxis DVT/PE after hip surgery<br>220 mg daily × 28–35 days | Prophylaxis DVT/PE after knee/hip surgery<br>10 mg daily × 12 days (knee), 35 days (hip) | Prophylaxis DVT/PE after knee/hip surgery<br>2.5 mg daily × 12 days (knee), 35 days (hip) | N/A |
| Elimination | 92% renal as metabolites | 80% renal; 20% fecal | 66% renal; 33% fecal | 27% renal; 66% fecal | 50% renal |
| Peak effect | 72–96 h | 2 h | 2–4 h | 3–4 h | 1–2 h |
| Half-life | 40 h | 14–17 h | 5–9 h | 10–14 h | 10–14 h |
| Interactions | CYP2C9, antibiotics, dietary, highly protein bound drugs | P-glycoprotein inducers/inhibitors | CYP3A4, P-glycoprotein inducers/inhibitors | CYP3A4, P-glycoprotein inducers/inhibitors | P-glycoprotein inducers/inhibitors |
| Specific reversal agent[a] | Vitamin K | Idarucizumab (Praxbind®) | None[b] | None[b] | None[b] |

*DVT* deep vein thrombosis, *PE* pulmonary embolism, *NVAF* nonvalvular atrial fibrillation, *CrCl* Cockcroft-Gault calculated creatinine clearance

[a]Please refer to Chap 13 for more information about pharmacological reversal of anticoagulants

[b]Andexanet alfa is a reversal agent of both direct and indirect factor Xa inhibitors currently in development but was not FDA approved at the time of publication of this text

observed/PT control which is a measure of bleeding time. For most indications the desired INR range is 2–3 and for patients with mechanical valves in the mitral position the goal range is 2.5–3.5. Though with less supporting evidence in literature, some clinicians will aim for a range of 1.5–2 or 2.5 in patients with a lower risk for clotting and a higher risk for bleeding such as pulmonary hypertension or VTE prophylaxis. INR needs to be monitored frequently when warfarin is initiated, whenever interacting medications are added or discontinued, or if there is a change in the patient's diet. Once the INR is stable within the desired range, it should be monitored every 4 weeks with the CHEST guidelines stating longer intervals are appropriate in certain situations [12].

Patients should also be monitored for signs of bleeding. Anything from a greater propensity for nosebleeds to hemorrhage is possible while receiving warfarin. Patients should be counseled on what to watch out for such as black tarry stools, which can indicate a lower GI bleed, or vomit that looks like coffee grounds which may indicate an upper GI bleed. They should also be instructed to seek medical care if they fall and hit their head or have a headache that doesn't go away because of the possibility of intracranial bleeds.

Warfarin is contraindicated in pregnancy and is considered a category X, except in patients with mechanical heart valves where it is classified a category D. It is teratogenic weeks 6–12 of pregnancy and can cause maternal or fetal hemorrhage during the third trimester.

#### 10.2.1.4 Drug/Food Interactions

Warfarin has many interactions with food and other medications [13]. These interactions are mediated through various mechanisms. Substrates, inducers and inhibitors of the cytochrome P450 liver enzymes responsible for metabolism of warfarin, especially CYP2C9, will have an impact on the degree of anticoagulation and INR [14]. Enzyme inducers such as rifampin, carbamazepine, or chronic alcohol consumption can significantly lower the INR leading to an increased risk of clotting. Whereas, enzyme inhibitors like metronidazole, trimethoprim/sulfamethoxazole, ciprofloxacin, fluconazole, and acute alcohol consumption (binge drinking) will lead to increases in the INR. Medications that are highly plasma protein bound such as valproic acid can displace warfarin from albumin in the blood stream and lead to higher INRs. Lastly, changes dietary consumption of or supplement with vitamin K will impact the INR. For example, if a patient increases consumption of leafy greens which are high in vitamin K, an increase in vitamin K-dependent clotting factors will result followed by a decrease in the INR. In patients who have a decrease in oral intake due to acute illness or procedural intervention, a decrease in vitamin K intake may result in an increase in INR. Other medications, like many antibiotics, affect gut absorption of vitamin K which can lead to a raise in INR. Herbal medications can interact in various ways including affecting liver enzymes like St. John's Wort or increase the risk of bleeding by acting as blood thinners like ginkgo biloba.

#### 10.2.1.5 Direct Thrombin Inhibitor, Dabigatran (Pradaxa®)

The first of the direct oral anticoagulants (DOACs), dabigatran, was approved for use in the United States by the FDA in fall of 2010. It offered a new option for the prevention of venous thromboembolism in nonvalvular atrial fibrillation (NVAF) and treatment of VTE [15, 16]. It is also indicated for the prophylaxis of DVT and PE in patients after hip replacement surgery [17].

#### 10.2.1.6 Mechanism of Action, Pharmacodynamics, and Pharmacokinetics

Dabigatran is a direct thrombin inhibitor, inhibiting both free and clot-bound thrombin as well as thrombin-induced platelet aggregation. In clinical studies it was proven non-inferior for extended treatment of atrial fibrillation and VTE. From a safety standpoint, there was decreased overall bleeding but increased risk of gastrointestinal bleeds (GI) versus warfarin. Dabigatran should be used with caution in patients with renal dysfunction as it is cleared 80% by the kidneys. Table 10.1 below has the dose adjustments based on estimated creatinine clearance and indication. Dabigatran requires an acidic environment for absorption and the capsules formulated with tartaric acid core [17].

#### 10.2.1.7 Monitoring, Precautions for Use, and Specific Considerations

One of the advantages of dabigatran and the other DOACs is that they do not require routine monitoring of coagulation tests [18]. A complete blood count (CBC) with differential and renal function should be done prior to initiation and periodically throughout treatment. Coagulation assays such as activated partial thromboplastin time (aPTT) and thrombin time (TT) or dilute thrombin time (dTT) may be used to determine the presence or absence of circulating dabigatran. Table 10.2 summarizes commonly available laboratory monitoring techniques that can be used to assess for the presence of circulating DOACs. The clinical utility of laboratory monitoring has not been fully determined, and coagulation assays should not be used for the adjustment of therapy but may be useful in determining the presence or absence of an anticoagulant in a patient needing an urgent or emergent procedure or actively bleeding [18, 19].

**Table 10.2** Laboratory coagulation assays for DOACs [18, 19]

| | Oral direct thrombin inhibitors (dabigatran) | Oral direct factor Xa inhibitors (rivaroxaban, apixaban, edoxaban) |
|---|---|---|
| Coagulation assays | Able to determine presence of circulating anticoagulant?[a] | |
| Activated partial thromboplastin time (aPTT) | Yes | No |
| Prothrombin time (PT) | No | Yes |
| Thrombin time (TT) | Yes | No |
| Dilute thrombin time (dTT) | Yes | No |
| Chromogenic anti-factor Xa assay | No | Yes |

[a]Qualitative measure for presence of medication, but not quantitative measure

Dabigatran is dosed twice daily with a rapid onset of action. If stopped abruptly, due to the short half-life of the medication, there will be an increased risk of clotting. For the treatment of VTE, 5–10 days of parenteral anticoagulation must be given prior to initiation of dabigatran. It is contraindicated for patients with mechanical prosthetic heart valves due to significantly more thromboembolic events and bleeding [20]. Common side effects include GI distress up to 25–35% in clinical trials and bleeding. Dabigatran must be stored in the original bottle and once opened the capsules are good for 30 days, and capsules cannot be crushed or opened as this can lead to a 75% increase in absorption and increased risk of bleeding [17]. Finally, due to low protein binding of approximately 35%, dabigatran is the only DOAC that can be successfully removed through hemodialysis [21].

#### 10.2.1.8 Drug/Food Interactions

Dabigatran is minimally affected by food and cytochrome P450 interactions. It is affected by the permeability glycoprotein (P-gp) efflux pump on the cell membrane which removes foreign substances from the cells. The concomitant use of dabigatran with P-gp inducers like rifampin reduces the exposure to dabigatran and should generally be avoided. Medications that inhibit P-gp mediated transport (dronedarone, verapamil) will increase exposure to dabigatran. This is especially important in patients with impaired renal function which may further increase exposure to dabigatran [17].

#### 10.2.1.9 Direct Factor Xa Inhibitors

The oral direct factor Xa inhibitors where first introduced with rivaroxaban, which was approved by the FDA in July 2011 [22]. They work by selectively inhibiting factor Xa, an important step in the coagulation cascade. They, like dabigatran, don't require routine monitoring of coagulation tests. Prothrombin time and chromogenic anti-factor Xa assays may be utilized for the director factor Xa inhibitors to determine the presence of anticoagulation [18, 19]. Refer to Table 10.2 for more details. All are cleared to varying degrees by the kidneys and liver. Specific dosing based renal function and indications are listed below in Table 10.1. Like dabigatran, if these medications are abruptly stopped or if patients are nonadherent, there is an increased risk of clotting. Because it has not been studied, the oral factor Xa inhibitors are not recommended for use for patients with prosthetic heart valves.

#### 10.2.1.10 Specific Considerations

**Rivaroxaban (Xarelto®)**

Rivaroxaban was the first oral direct factor Xa inhibitor brought to the market. In clinical trials it was non-inferior to warfarin for prevention of reoccurrence of VTE and for prevention of stroke and systemic embolism in nonvalvular atrial fibrillation [23, 24]. It is also indicated for the prophylaxis of VTE after hip or knee replacement surgery. In clinical trials rivaroxaban had similar major bleeds compared to warfarin.

The 15 and 20 mg tablets that are used in atrial fibrillation and DVT/PE treatment should be taken with food according to the package insert [22]. Doing so increases bioavailability and increased the area under the curve by 39% in trials. The tablets may be crushed and administered via a nasogastric (NG) tube but not a nasojejunal (NJ) tube because rivaroxaban is absorbed in the stomach.

Unlike warfarin or dabigatran, rivaroxaban does not require treatment with a parenteral anticoagulant prior to initiating treatment for VTE. The loading dose for VTE is listed below in Table 10.1. Rivaroxaban is dosed once daily for maintenance dosing which may result in improved patient compliance. A dose reduction is necessary for renal dysfunction and concomitant therapies that affect CYP3A4, and P-gp will affect clearance of rivaroxaban.

**Apixaban (Eliquis®)**

Apixaban was the next oral direct factor Xa inhibitor approved by the FDA in 2012 [25]. In clinical trials it demonstrated mortality benefit verses warfarin for prevention of stroke in nonvalvular atrial fibrillation [26]. It is also FDA indicated for the prophylaxis of VTE in patients who after hip or knee replacement surgery and for the treatment of VTE and reduction of reoccurrence [25]. Apixaban had less major bleeding then warfarin for VTE treatment in clinical trials [27]. Apixaban does not require the use of a parenteral anticoagulant prior to starting treatment for DVT or PE. Apixaban is dosed twice daily and can be administered via a NG or a NJ tube. Renal clearance of apixaban is only about 27% making it the least affected by renal dysfunction of the DOACs. Clearance of apixaban, like rivaroxaban, is affected by medications that act on liver enzyme CYP3A4 and P-gp.

**Edoxaban (Savaysa®)**

Edoxaban was approved in 2015 for thromboembolism/stroke prophylaxis in patients with nonvalvular atrial fibrillation [28]. In clinical trials it was non-inferior to warfarin for the prevention of VTE in nonvalvular atrial fibrillation, and there was no difference in major bleeding [29, 30]. Edoxaban is also indicated for the treatment of VTE following 5–10 days of initial therapy with a parenteral anticoagulant. This like dabigatran and warfarin makes treatment of DVT or PE a little more burdensome. Edoxaban is highly dependent on renal clearance and should be dose adjusted for renal dysfunction and should not be used for treatment of nonvalvular atrial fibrillation if the patient's CrCL is greater than 95 mL/min because of an increased risk of ischemic stroke during the trials. It is dosed once a day making it easier for some patients, and there is currently no data on crushing edoxaban.

### 10.2.2 Subcutaneous Agents

#### 10.2.2.1 Unfractionated Heparin

Therapeutic anticoagulation with heparin is typically given by continuous infusion, which will be discussed later, but historically has been given subcutaneously [12]. Therapeutic dosing of subcutaneous heparin is given as a 333 units/kg loading dose followed by 250 units/kg every 12 h [13]. In clinical practice, subcutaneous heparin is most commonly used for VTE prophylaxis at a dose of 5000 units every 8 or 12 h.

#### 10.2.2.2 Low Molecular Weight Heparin

LMWH are produced by either chemical or enzymatic depolymerization of unfractionated heparin (UFH). They work by inactivating Factor Xa and to a lesser extent thrombin through potentiation of antithrombin. They have been extensively evaluated and used in the treatment of acute coronary syndromes, PE, DVT, as well as the prevention of VTE in high risk populations including cancer patients [13]. Common LMWHs include enoxaparin (Lovenox®) and dalteparin (Fragmin®) which are dosed empirically based on weight and are administered subcutaneously on a fixed schedule once to twice daily based on the particular drug and indication. They need to be dose adjusted for renal dysfunction.

#### 10.2.2.3 Monitoring, Precautions for Use, and Specific Considerations

The pharmacokinetics of LMWHs are more predictable than their predecessor, UFH, so levels are not typically followed for short term use. For outlier patients or situations such as overweight, underweight, severe burns, pregnancy, and extended use or for individuals with renal dysfunction, a peak anti-Xa level is used to monitor [31]. Prior to starting therapy, it is recommended to check the patient's serum creatinine and CBC with platelet count [13].

LMWHs should be avoided in patients with a history of heparin induced thrombocytopenia (HIT). LMWHs also should also be avoided in patients undergoing spinal/epidural anesthesia or spinal puncture. These procedures while receiving LMWHs increase the risk of spinal or epidural hematoma which has led to long-term or permanent paralysis in some patients [12].

#### 10.2.2.4 Fondaparinux (Arixtra®)

Fondaparinux is a fully synthetic pentasaccharide. It is a five saccharide molecular piece of heparin. It acts by indirectly inhibiting factor Xa and but no activity on thrombin. It is dosed as a once daily subcutaneous injection based on patient weight [13]. Fondaparinux is FDA approved for the treatment of DVT/PE when administered in conjunction with warfarin. It is also approved for DVT prophylaxis after knee, hip, or abdominal surgery [32].

#### 10.2.2.5 Monitoring, Precautions for Use, and Specific Considerations

Fondaparinux displays predictable pharmacokinetics and levels are not typically followed. For outliers an anti-Xa concentration can be drawn. As with LMWHs, patient's Scr and CBC should be monitored. Fondaparinux is renal cleared and is contraindicated with CrCl < 30 ml/min. Adverse drug reactions to fondaparinux are similar to those found in LMWHs.

Fondaparinux shows no cross-reactivity with heparins so may be useful in patients with or with a history of HIT. For the treatment of HIT, fondaparinux offers an easier option to bridge to warfarin compared to intravenous direct thrombin inhibitors as it does not have any impact on INR like argatroban or bivalirudin. Lastly, fondaparinux is a fully synthetic moiety so can be used for patients that unable to use pork products unlike heparin or LMWHs which are derivatives of porcine gut mucosa.

### 10.2.3 Intravenous Agents

#### 10.2.3.1 Unfractionated Heparin

Unfractionated heparin (UFH) is extracted from porcine and bovine mucosa with most products used in clinical practice today of porcine origin. It indirectly inactivates clotting factors IIa and Xa by binding to and promoting the activity of antithrombin [31]. It is indicated for the prevention and treatment of VTE and PE, prevention and treatment of thromboembolic complications associated with atrial fibrillation, and treatment of acute and chronic coagulopathies and is commonly used in blood transfusions, extracorporeal circulation, and dialysis procedures. It is metabolized by the reticuloendothelial system after binding to endothelial cells and also undergoes renal clearance.

#### 10.2.3.2 Monitoring, Precautions for Use, and Specific Considerations

Due to patient specific differences in pharmacokinetics, intravenous UFH should be monitored utilizing either anti-Xa activity or aPTT. The standard loading dose of UFH is 75–100 units/kg followed by a continuous infusion of 18–20 units/kg/h for the treatment of most acute thrombotic events or highly prothrombotic conditions such as atrial fibrillation or mechanical heart valves. Lower doses such as a loading dose of 60 units/kg (maximum of 5000 units) followed by 12 units/kg/h (maximum of 1000 units/h) may be utilized for patients with acute coronary syndromes [31, 33]. Platelet count should also be assessed at the initiation of heparin and monitored throughout therapy due to the risk of developing HIT. Platelet factor 4 (PF4) is a protein released by platelets that has antagonistic activity against heparin and when bound, heparin-dependent IgG antibodies may be produced against this complex [31]. These antibodies may cause platelets activation and consumption through their Fc receptors which may also propagate clot formation [34]. Treatment of suspected or confirmed HIT should include discontinuation of any heparin or heparin-containing product and initiation of a non-heparin anticoagulant to mitigate the risk of thrombosis [34].

#### 10.2.3.3 Direct Thrombin Inhibitors

Intravenous direct thrombin inhibitors (DTI) offer an alternative to UFH in patients requiring anticoagulation through the intravenous route. These medications bind directly to thrombin without the need of an antithrombin intermediary. The two DTIs commonly used in clinical practice today include bivalirudin and argatroban. They have been studied and are used for multiple indications including ACS with or without percutaneous coronary intervention, acute stroke, and coronary artery bypass surgery. Due to their short half-lives of 25–45 min, both medications are initiated at a weight-based infusion without the need for a loading dose [35].

#### 10.2.3.4 Monitoring, Precautions for Use, and Specific Considerations

Argatroban is currently FDA approved for the treatment of HIT and has been shown to decrease the incidence of new thrombotic events and as well as bleeding episodes [36, 37]. Monitoring of argatroban and bivalirudin should be done with aPTT, and special care should be taken when bridging patients from these agents to warfarin as they may falsely elevate the INR leading to premature discontinuation of the parenteral agent or inappropriate dose adjustments to warfarin [38].

**Conclusion**

Anticoagulation is a mainstay of treatment for many disease states including but not limited to atrial fibrillation, VTE, and mechanical heart valves. There are multiple agents available for both short-term and long-term use. Oral agents are used most commonly for chronic therapy with warfarin being the most prevalent agent and the oral direct thrombin and factor Xa inhibitors playing a larger role. Subcutaneous and intravenous agents are typically reserved for acute, short-term therapy and may be used as bridging therapy in patients that need interruption in anticoagulation therapy at the initiation of therapy or around the time of an applicable procedure. Of the oral agents, warfarin is the only medication that requires routine coagulation assay monitoring, and routine monitoring of the other agents is not recommended. For more information regarding antiplatelet agents, please refer to Chap. 11, and for perioperative management of patients receiving anticoagulants or the need for anticoagulation reversal, please refer to Chaps. 13–17.

## References

1. Cove CL, Hylek EM. An updated review of target specific oral anticoagulants used in stroke prevention in atrial fibrillation, venous thromboembolic disease, and acute coronary syndrome. J Am Heart Assoc. 2013;2:e000136. https://doi.org/10.1161/JAHA.113.000136.

2. DeWilde S, Carey IM, Emmas C, Richards N, Cook DG. Trends in the prevalence of diagnosed atrial fibrillation, its treatment with anticoagulation and predictors of such treatment in UK primary care. Heart. 2006;92:1064–70. https://doi.org/10.1136/hrt.2005.069492.
3. Gage BF, Waterman AD, Shannon W, Boechler M, Rich MW, Radford MJ. Validation of clinical classification schemes for predicting stroke: results from the National Registry of Atrial Fibrillation. JAMA. 2001;285:2864–70. https://doi.org/10.1001/jama.285.22.2864.
4. Hirsh J, Guyatt G, Albers GW, Harrington R, Schunemann HJ. Antithrombotic and thrombolytic therapy: American College of Chest Physicians evidence based clinical practice guidelines. Chest. 2008;133:110S–2S. https://doi.org/10.1378/chest.08-0652.
5. Alikhan R, Peters F, Wilmott R, Cohen AT. Fatal pulmonary embolism in hospitalised patients: a necropsy review. J Clin Pathol. 2004;57:1254–7. https://doi.org/10.1136/jcp.2003.013581.
6. Schaefer JK, McBane RD, Wysokinski WE. How to choose appropriate direct oral anticoagulant for patient with nonvalvular atrial fibrillation. Ann Hematol. 2016;95:437–49. https://doi.org/10.1007/s00277-015-2566-x.
7. Geerts WH, Bergqist D, Pineo GF, Heit JA, Samama CM, Lassen MR, et al. Prevention of thromboembolism: American College of Chest Physicians evidence-based clinical practice guidelines (8th edition). Chest. 2008;133(6):381S–453S. https://doi.org/10.1378/chest.08-0656.
8. Kearon C, Akl EA, Comerota AJ, Prandoni P, Bounameaux H, Goldhaber SZ, et al. Antithrombotic therapy for VTE disease. Antithrombotic therapy and prevention of thrombosis, 9th ed. American College of Chest Physicians evidence-based practice guidelines. Chest. 2012;141(2 Suppl):e419–94S. https://doi.org/10.1378/chest.11-2301.
9. Ansell JE. Oral anticoagulant therapy-50 years later. Arch Intern Med. 1993;153:586–96. https://doi.org/10.1001/archinte.1993.00410050024005.
10. Bristol-Myers Squibb. Coumadin (warfarin) prescribing information. 2016. http://packageinserts.bms.com/pi/pi_coumadin.pdf. Accessed 23 Dec 2016.
11. Hirsh J, Dalen JE, Anderson DR, Poller L, Bussey H, Ansell J, et al. Oral anticoagulants: mechanism of action, clinical effectiveness, and optimal therapeutic range. Chest. 2001;119:8S–21S. https://doi.org/10.1378/chest.119.1_suppl.8S.
12. Kearon C, Akl EA, Ornelas J, Blaivas A, Jimenez D, Bounameaux H, et al. Antithrombotic therapy for VTE disease: chest guideline and expert panel report. Chest. 2016;149(2):315–52. https://doi.org/10.1016/j.chest.2015.11.026.
13. Witt DM, Clark NP. Venous thromboembolism. In: DiPiro JT, Talbert RL, Yee GC, Matzke GR, Wells BG, Posey LM, editors. Pharmacotherapy: a pathophysiologic approach. 9th ed. New York, NY: McGraw-Hill; 2014. p. 245–78.
14. Holbrook AM, Pereira JA, Labris R, McDonald H, Douketis JD, Crowther M, et al. Systematic overview of warfarin and its drug and food interactions. Arch Intern Med. 2005;165:1095–106. https://doi.org/10.1001/archinte.165.10.1095.
15. Connolly SJ, Ezekowitz MD, Yusuf S, Eikelboom J, Oldgren J, Parekh A, et al. Dabigatran versus warfarin in patients with atrial fibrillation. N Engl J Med. 2009;361:1139–51. https://doi.org/10.1056/NEJMoa0905561.
16. Schulman S, Kearon C, Kakkar AK, Schellong S, Eriksson H, Baanstra D, et al. Extended use of dabigatran, warfarin, or placebo in venous thromboembolism. N Engl J Med. 2013;368:709–18. https://doi.org/10.1056/NEJMoa1113697.
17. Boehringer-Ingelheim. Pradaxa (dabigatran) prescribing information. 2017. http://docs.boehringer-ingelheim.com/Prescribing%20Information/PIs/Pradaxa/Pradaxa.pdf. Accessed 18 Jan 2017.
18. Samama MM, Guinet C. Laboratory assessment of new anticoagulants. Clin Chem Lab Med. 2011;49(5):761–72. https://doi.org/10.1515/CCLM.2011.134.
19. Conway SE, Hwang AY, Ponte CD, Gums JG. Laboratory and clinical monitoring of director acting oral anticoagulants: what clinicians need to know. Pharmacotherapy. 2017;37(2):236–48.
20. Eikelboom JW, Connolly SJ, Brueckmann M, Granger CB, Kappetein AP, Mack MJ, et al. Dabigatran versus warfarin in patients with mechanical heart valves. N Engl J Med. 2013;369:1206–14. https://doi.org/10.1056/NEJMoa1300615.
21. Liesenfel KH, Staab A, Hartter S, Fromella S, Clemens A, Lehr T. Pharmacometric characterization of dabigatran hemodialysis. Clin Pharmacokinet. 2013;52:453–62. https://doi.org/10.1007/s40262-013-0049-6.
22. Janssen Pharmaceuticals. Xarelto (rivaroxaban) prescribing information. 2017. http://www.accessdata.fda.gov/drugsatfda_docs/label/2011/202439s001lbl.pdf. Accessed 18 Jan 2017.
23. Investigators EINSTEIN, Bauersachs R, Berkowitz SD, Brenner B, Buller HR, Decousus H, Gallus AS, et al. Oral rivaroxaban for symptomatic venous thromboembolism. N Engl J Med. 2010;363:2499–510. https://doi.org/10.1056/NEJMoa1007903.
24. Patel MR, Mahaffey KW, Garg J, Pan G, Singer DE, Hacke W, et al. Rivaroxaban versus warfarin in nonvalvular atrial fibrillation. N Engl J Med. 2011;365:883–91. https://doi.org/10.1056/NEJMoa1009638.
25. Bristol-Myers Squibb Company and Pfizer Inc. Eliquis (apixaban) prescribing information. 2017. http://packageinserts.bms.com/pi/pi_eliquis.pdf. Accessed 18 Jan 2017.
26. Granger CB, Alexander JH, McMurray JJ, Lopes RD, Hylek EM, Hanna M, et al. Apixaban versus warfarin in patients with atrial fibrillation. N Engl J Med. 2011;365:981–92. https://doi.org/10.1056/NEJMoa1107039.

27. Agnelli G, Buller HR, Cohen A, Curto M, Gallus AS, Johnson M, et al. Apixaban for extended treatment of venous thromboembolism. N Engl J Med. 2013;368:699–708. https://doi.org/10.1056/NEJMoa1207541.
28. Daiichi Sankyo. Savaysa (edoxaban) prescribing information. 2017. http://dsi.com/prescribing-information-portlet/getPIContent?productName=Savaysa&inline=true. Accessed 19 Jan 2017.
29. Buller HR, Decousus H, Grosso MA, Mercuri M, Middeldorp S, Prins MH, et al. Edoxaban versus warfarin for the treatment of symptomatic venous thromboembolism. N Engl J Med. 2013;369(15):1406. https://doi.org/10.1056/NEJMoa1306638.
30. Giugliano RP, Ruff CT, Braunwald E, Murphy SA, Wiviott SD, Halperin JL, et al. Edoxaban versus warfarin in patients with atrial fibrillation. N Engl J Med. 2013;369:2093–104. https://doi.org/10.1056/NEJMoa1310907.
31. Baglin T, Barrowcliffe TW, Cohen A, Greaves M. Guidelines for the use and monitoring of heparin. Br J Haematol. 2006;133(1):19–34. https://doi.org/10.1111/j.1365-2141.2005.05953.x.
32. GlaxoSmithKline. Arixtra (fondaparinux) prescribing information. 2017. http://www.accessdata.fda.gov/drugsatfda_docs/label/2010/021345s023lbl.pdf. Accessed 19 Jan 2017.
33. Spinler SA, Wittowsky AK, Nutescu E, Smythe MA. Anticoagulation monitoring part 2: unfractionated heparin and low-molecular-weight-heparin. Ann Pharmacother. 2005;39:1275–85. https://doi.org/10.1345/aph.1E524.
34. Greinacher A. Heparin-induced thrombocytopenia. N Engl J Med. 2015;373:252–61. https://doi.org/10.1056/NEJMoa1411910.
35. Nisio MD, Middeldorp S, Buller HR. Direct thrombin inhibitors. N Engl J Med. 2005;353:1028–40. https://doi.org/10.1056/NEJMoa044440.
36. Lewis BE, Wallis DE, Berkowitz SD, Matthai WH, Fareed J, Walenga JM, et al. Argatroban anticoagulant therapy in patients with heparin-induced thrombocytopenia. Circulation. 2001;103:1838–43. https://doi.org/10.1161/01.CIR.103.14.1838.
37. Lewis BE, Wallis DE, Leya F, Hursting MJ, Kelton JG. Argatroban anticoagulation in patients with heparin-induced thrombocytopenia. Arch Intern Med. 2003;163:1849–56. https://doi.org/10.1001/archinte.163.15.1849.
38. Hafner G, Roser M, Nauck M. Methods for the monitoring of direct thrombin inhibitors. Semin Thromb Hemost. 2002;28(5):425–30. https://doi.org/10.1055/s-2002-35282.

# 11 Pharmacologic Reversal Agents

James F. Gilmore, Michael J. Schontz,
and Kenneth E. Lupi Jr.

**Abstract**

Management of antithrombotic and anticoagulant therapy in patients undergoing dental procedures involves balancing the risks of thrombosis and bleeding. Variability in mechanism of action of commonly employed outpatient anticoagulant medications has increased over the past several years. While many patients may be able to have dental procedures performed on therapeutic anticoagulant therapy, providers must be aware of specific supportive care and reversal techniques to match each patient's individual scenario. An overview of commonly employed and anticipated FDA-approved anticoagulant reversal agents, including indications and dosing, is provided.

J. F. Gilmore (✉)
Department of Pharmacy, Cedars-Sinai Medical Center, Los Angeles, CA, USA

M. J. Schontz · K. E. Lupi Jr.
Department of Pharmacy, Brigham and Women's Hospital, Boston, MA, USA
e-mail: Mschontz@bwh.harvard.edu; lupi@bwh.harvard.edu

## 11.1 Introduction

Antiplatelet and antithrombotic agents are commonly prescribed for a number of medical conditions. Patients on oral anticoagulants undergoing invasive dental treatments may be at higher risk of bleeding than those who are not depending on patient- and procedure-specific factors [1]. The most effective strategy for prevention of anticoagulant- or antiplatelet-induced bleeding during a dental procedure is an appropriate assessment of the patient and the procedure being conducted for the need of medication cessation prior to intervention. This requires a thorough history and communication between specialists and the patient's primary care provider, a process that may take preparation weeks in advance of intervention. Often dental procedures are able to be carried out in patients on anticoagulants, and if determined that changes are warranted, in many cases medication changes to short-acting agents for an appropriate period of time is an achievable solution. In the event an acute intervention is required in a patient on anticoagulant therapy, rarely pharmacologic reversal of anticoagulation is desired to minimize bleeding risks. This chapter will review pharmacologic reversal agents for commonly prescribed anticoagulant medications, indications for use, dosing, and monitoring strategies. In-depth discussion on clinical perioperative management of patients on antiplatelets and anticoagulants will be discussed in Chaps. 12 and



R. P. Szumita, P. M. Szumita (eds.), *Hemostasis in Dentistry*, https://doi.org/10.1007/978-3-319-71240-6_11

13, respectively. For in-depth discussion of perioperative management of dental patients on anticoagulants, refer to Chap. 14.

## 11.2 Blood Products

Blood products are some of the oldest products that have been considered to reverse pharmacologic coagulopathy. In addition to transfusing all components together as whole blood, one to four transfusable products can be produced from each donation. These are red cells, platelets, plasma, and cryoprecipitate. By utilizing only the components, several patients are able to be treated with each donation [2]. Whole blood and red cells do not have a role in reversal, while plasma, platelets, cryoprecipitate, and concentrated fibrinogen will assist in either reversal or attenuation of clinical bleeding caused by pharmacologic coagulopathy.

As a reversal agent, fresh frozen plasma (FFP) has been used to replace factors II, VII, IX, and X and is included in warfarin reversal guidelines although prothrombin complex concentrate (PCC) is now generally the preferred agent if emergent reversal is desired [3–5]. A more in-depth look at PCC is provided later in this chapter. When used in conjunction with vitamin K, FFP will rapidly reverse the INR until endogenous factors can be produced which can take up to 24 h after vitamin K administration. The effect of FFP is sustained for about 12–24 h, while vitamin K duration can be days [6]. Vitamin K is discussed in greater detail later in the chapter. Several disadvantages prohibit FFP usage for emergent use in certain patient populations compared to PCC, making PCC preferred in those clinical scenarios. PCC advantages include efficacy, speed of reversal, and reduced volume administration (approximately 250 mL per unit of FFP). The total amount of FFP administered will vary patient to patient depending on the INR value and desired goal. Additionally, the INR of FFP is approximately 1.6 (will vary from unit to unit) and will therefore not lower the INR of a patient below that value consistently unlike PCC [6, 7].

Platelets can be used to help attenuate the effects of agents that inhibit the effects of platelets such as aspirin and thienopyridines. These medications inhibit platelet function for the lifespan of the platelet [8]. The pharmacology of antiplatelet medication is provided in Chap. 9. Platelet transfusion will not reverse the effects but provide additional, functional platelets. As with all transfusions, risks and benefit needs to be weighed against the urgency of the procedure. This should include platelet-specific risks; they should not be used when the patient has thrombotic thrombocytopenic purpura or heparin-induced thrombocytopenia unless the bleed is life threatening [9].

Cryoprecipitate contains high levels of fibrinogen and factor VIII [9]. Its role, as well as concentrated fibrinogen (RiaSTAP), in reversal is limited to recombinant tissue plasminogen activator (tPA). Recombinant tPA is used to dissolve clots by converting plasminogen to plasmin, which in turn, cleaves fibrin polymers [10]. Fibrinogen replacement helps to promote hemostasis. Similar to FFP, there are disadvantages to cryoprecipitate (thawing, blood matching, higher volume than fibrinogen concentrate) [9]. Additionally, cryoprecipitate dose per unit is not standardized like the concentrated fibrinogen product [11]. Although clinically useful, reversal of tPA is not likely to be encountered during dental procedures. Cryoprecipitate and concentrated fibrinogen have a bigger role in congenital or acquired fibrinogen deficiency as well as severe postpartum hemorrhage.

The risks of transfusion should be considered before utilizing any blood product (Table 11.1). These complications can be acute, occurring between minutes and up to 24 h, or delayed, greater than 24 h and up to years later. Acute complications include hemolytic reactions, allergic reactions, transfusion-related acute lung injury (TRALI), transfusion-associated circulatory overload (TACO), febrile nonhemolytic transfusion reactions (FNHTR), and metabolic disturbances. Delayed complications include hemolytic reactions, iron overload, transfusion-related immunomodulation (TRIM), infection, posttransfusion purpura, and transfusion-associated graft-versus-host disease [9].

**Table 11.1** Indications and monitoring of blood products [3, 9, 12, 13]

| | FFP | Cryoprecipitate | Concentrated fibrinogen | Platelets |
|---|---|---|---|---|
| Uses | VKA reversal | Supportive in tPA-induced bleeding | Supportive in tPA-induced bleeding | Supportive in antiplatelet-induced bleeding |
| Dose | 15–30 ml/kg | 10 pooled units (1000–2000 mg fibrinogen) | Unknown fibrinogen: 70 mg/kg<br>Dose (mg/kg) = (Target level-measured)/1.7 | 5 units |
| Monitoring | Hemostasis, INR | Hemostasis, goal fibrinogen > 100 mg/dl | Hemostasis, goal fibrinogen >100 mg/dl | Hemostasis, can consider platelet reactivity assay |

## 11.3 Desmopressin

Desmopressin (DDAVP) is a synthetic analog of the natural antidiuretic hormone vasopressin. Desmopressin is used to prevent or control the symptoms of central diabetes insipidus and is also indicated for the management of bleeding episodes in patients with mild to moderate hemophilia A or von Willebrand's disease type 1 [14]. Refer to Chap. 3 for full discussion on von Willebrand's disease and perioperative management in dentistry. The chemical substitutions made to desmopressin are responsible for its enhanced antidiuretic effect, reduced vasopressor effect, and prolonged duration of action [15, 16].

Desmopressin acts similarly to native vasopressin. Vasopressin exerts its effect through two receptor subtypes: the vasopressin 1 (V1) subtype, which mediates smooth muscle contraction in the peripheral vasculature, and the vasopressin 2 (V2) subtype, which regulates water reabsorption in the collecting duct [14, 17]. Additionally, the hemostatic effects of desmopressin are mediated through agonism at the V2 receptor [17]. DDAVP is a strong V2 agonist with no effect on V1 receptors. DDAVP increases the plasma concentrations of factor VIII and von Willebrand factor, with possible direct effects on platelet reactivity [18–20]. Increases in factor VIII and von Willebrand factor levels are thought to be due to their release from endogenous reservoirs and not via increased synthesis due to the rapidity in response [17]. The increased levels of factor VIII and von Willebrand factor subsequently stimulate glycoprotein IIb/IIIa-mediated platelet aggregation [21].

Desmopressin has also been used in acquired bleeding disorders, including drug-induced platelet dysfunction [17]. Bleeding is the major side effect of inhibitors of platelet aggregation, and there are conflicting data on the clinical efficacy of desmopressin in reversing antiplatelet agents [19]. Desmopressin has been shown to improve drug-induced bleeding related to heparin, ticlopidine, hirudin, dextran, and aspirin [19, 22]. A single dose of desmopressin was successfully used to prevent procedure-related bleeding in patients with uremia receiving aspirin and was also shown to shorten bleeding time in patients with platelet dysfunction due to cirrhosis or aspirin use [23, 24]. DDAVP was also shown to normalize platelet dysfunction from clopidogrel and acetylsalicylic acid, in healthy volunteers and in vitro studies, respectively [19, 25, 26]. However, another study evaluating the use of DDAVP in healthy volunteers treated with ticagrelor determined that desmopressin is unlikely to be of therapeutic value for the control of bleeding events associated with ticagrelor [19]. A recent review of strategies to reverse antiplatelet therapy suggests consideration of desmopressin administration in individual cases, such as patients that will undergo neurosurgical evaluation, or life-threatening bleeding refractory to standard hemostatic techniques [21].

Desmopressin can be administered by oral, intranasal, or parenteral (IV or SC) routes; the oral route is utilized for central diabetes insipidus and primary nocturnal enuresis [14]. The maximal dose-response increase in factor VIII activity occurs at 0.3–0.4 μg/kg of intravenous desmopressin. There is no increase in activity with doses greater than 0.4 μg/kg, likely due to saturation at receptor sites. Factor VIII activity is increased 30 min after IV or intranasal administration, with a peak activity at 90 min to 2 h. Peak plasma concentrations are noted within 40–45 min. Intranasal desmopressin, at a dose of 300 μg, results in maximal factor VIII and von Willebrand factor activity levels of 150–200% of normal. The terminal half-life for desmopressin is approximately 90 min to 3 h [27]. In patients with renal dysfunction receiving single doses of desmopressin injection, the terminal half-life was significantly increased of a mean of 3.4 h to a mean of 7.2 h in patients with moderate renal impairment and 10 h in patients with severe renal impairment [27].

The dose of desmopressin for the management of spontaneous bleeding or for bleeding prophylaxis in patients with drug-induced platelet dysfunction is 0.3–0.4 μg/kg IV or SC as a single dose [28–31]. Repeat dosing is not recommended due to tachyphylaxis [29]. Preoperatively, give desmopressin 30 min prior to surgery. Due to short duration of action, many patients will see bleeding times return to baseline within 24 h [29, 31]. Caution is advised in patients with cardiac disease, especially hypertension, heart failure, or coronary artery disease [14, 32–34].

## 11.4 Protamine

Protamine sulfate is a protein derived from fish sperm that is effective for reversal of unfractionated heparin and low molecular weight heparin. When protamine is administered alone, it possesses weak and clinically insignificant anticoagulant effects. When protamine makes contact with a heparin molecule, it forms a salt, neutralizing the anticoagulant effect of both drugs by forming a protamine-heparin complex and disrupting the heparin-antithrombin III complex. The onset of action is rapid, with neutralization of heparin evident within 5 min [35].

Dosing of protamine will depend on the dose of heparin product the patient has received and the timeframe of the administration. For unfractionated heparin, the protamine dose will be calculated based on the amount of heparin administered in the last 3 h accounting for any bolus doses administered (Table 11.2). For heparin exposure less than 1 h, 1 mg protamine for every 100 units of heparin should be administered. For heparin exposure between 1 and 2 h, 0.5 mg protamine for every 100 units heparin should be administered. For heparin exposure more than 2 h, 0.25 mg protamine for every 100 units of heparin should be administered [35].

For patients on a low molecular weight heparin such as enoxaparin, time since dose is also a factor in determining protamine dose (Table 11.3) [35, 36]. If enoxaparin has been administered within 8 h, administer 1 mg of protamine for every 1 mg of enoxaparin. If enoxaparin was administered between 8 and 12 h prior, administer 0.5 mg of protamine for every 1 mg of enoxaparin. If greater than 12 h from enoxaparin exposure, protamine administration may not be necessary unless there is continued bleeding or renal dysfunction. If second dose of protamine is needed (prolonged aPTT at 2–4 h after protamine), give 0.5 mg IV for every 1 mg of enoxaparin.

**Table 11.2** Protamine dosing for reversal of unfractionated heparin [35]

| Time from heparin exposure | Protamine dose |
|---|---|
| Less than 1 h | 1 mg protamine for every 100 units heparin |
| 1–2 h | 0.5 mg protamine for every 100 units heparin |
| More than 2 h | 0.25 mg protamine for every 100 units heparin |

**Table 11.3** Protamine dosing for reversal of enoxaparin [35, 36]

| Time from enoxaparin exposure | Protamine dose |
|---|---|
| Less than 8 h | 1 mg protamine for every 1 mg enoxaparin |
| 8–12 h | 0.5 mg protamine for every 1 mg enoxaparin |
| More than 12 h | Protamine may not be necessary unless continued bleeding or renal dysfunction |

### 11.4.1 Example Patient Case

Patient has been receiving a heparin infusion at 1400 units/h without any recent bolus doses. To calculate the total amount of heparin received in the last 3 h:

1. 100% heparin in last hour: 1400 units.
2. 50% heparin in preceding hour: 700 units.
3. 25% heparin in hour before that: 350 units.
4. Total heparin: 1400 + 700 + 350 units = 245 0 units.
5. Protamine dose to be administered: 24.5 mg.

Protamine can be administered undiluted via slow IV push, not to exceed 5 mg/min. Severe hypotension, cardiovascular collapse, and anaphylactoid reactions associated with rapid administration of protamine. Other risk factors for developing a hypersensitivity reaction include high doses or overdose of protamine, previous exposure, current or previous use of protamine-containing drugs (e.g., neutral protamine Hagedorn insulin), fish hypersensitivity, vasectomy, and severe left ventricular dysfunction [35]. The risks and benefits of administration of protamine should be carefully considered, and resuscitation equipment should be immediately available in case of a severe reaction.

Another important consideration with protamine is to not simultaneously administer with perioperative antibiotics, as protamine has exhibited incompatibilities with several penicillins and cephalosporins and should not be administered through the same infusion line [35].

## 11.5 Phytonadione (Vitamin K)

Phytonadione stimulates synthesis of the vitamin K-dependent clotting factors, II, VII, IX, and X, and can be administered via the oral, IM, IV, or SC route to reverse vitamin K antagonists such as warfarin [21, 37–39]. Due to this mechanism, reversal of the INR takes several hours. High doses of phytonadione (>10 mg), although effective, can lead to warfarin resistance for 1 week or more after administration.

The oral route is effective for lowering the INR and is the preferred route unless rapid reversal of the INR is critical [40, 41]. In emergent settings, the IV route is recommended due to its faster onset of action (within 2–4 h) [42–44]. The IV route also has a more appreciable effect in 6–12 h when compared to oral therapy. Following IV administration a normal prothrombin time may be observed in 12–24 h [38–40, 45]. A meta-analysis showed similar efficacy and safety between oral and intravenous vitamin K in patients taking vitamin K antagonists with a supratherapeutic INR, but not actively bleeding [21, 46]. After PO administration, the effect may not be seen for 12–24 h. Subcutaneous administration can result in erratic absorption, and effects may be delayed for upward of 24 h. Additionally, this route has been shown to be inferior to both IV and PO administration and similar to placebo [40, 47–49]. IV and IM administration may cause anaphylactoid reactions. The reactions are reported frequently; however the true incidence of this complication is approximately 3 out of 100,000 doses administered. The anaphylactoid reactions may be more likely related to the vehicle previously used to keep vitamin K in solution, polyethoxylated castor oil. When administered IV, a slow infusion over at least 20 min of diluted phytonadione is recommended to mitigate the already very low risk of potentially fatal reactions [21, 38, 39, 42, 50].

The American College of Chest Physicians (ACCP) clinical practice guidelines for anticoagulant management and reversal of warfarin were updated in 2012 (Table 11.4). In summary, the guidelines concluded that excessively elevated INR values have an increased risk of bleeding, particularly at INR values greater than 5.0. However, the short-term major bleeding risk is low for patients with an INR value less than 10 [40, 43]. The current guidelines recommend against routine vitamin K administration in patients with an INR of 4.5–10 and no bleeding. In patients who need an elective procedure or have an elevated INR but are asymptomatic and at low risk for bleeding, holding warfarin therapy may be sufficient. It takes approximately 2.5 days for an INR between 6.0 and 10.0 to fall

**Table 11.4** Management strategies for elevated INRs in patients on warfarin [40–42, 51, 52]

| INR | Bleeding status | Phytonadione recommendation | Additional considerations |
|---|---|---|---|
| <4.5 | No evidence of bleeding | Phytonadione not recommended<br>If pre-procedural in patient whom warfarin has been held, consider PO 1–2.5 mg day prior to procedure with repeat INR on day of procedure or surgery | Lower or skip a dose of warfarin; monitor more frequently; no dose modifications may be needed if only slightly above range |
| 4.5–10 | No evidence of bleeding | Phytonadione not routinely recommended. Consider PO 1–2.5 mg if at increased bleeding risk<br>If patient and procedural factors warrant reversal therapy, ≤5 mg PO can be given (expect INR reduction in 24 h); additional 1–2 mg PO if INR still elevated | Skip 1–2 doses of warfarin and resume when INR is therapeutic |
| >10 | No evidence of bleeding | Phytonadione PO 2.5–5 mg | Expect INR to be reduced within 24–48 h, additional dose may be given after 24 h |
| Any INR | Major bleeding | Phytonadione 5–10 mg by slow IV infusion | Phytonadione administration recommended in addition to 4-factor prothrombin complex concentrate (PCC) |

to <4.0 [40, 42, 53]. When administering PO phytonadione in conjunction with a temporary interruption of warfarin therapy, approximately 1.4 days are required for an INR between 6.0 and 10.0 to decline to <4.0 [42, 53]. For patients with an INR of >10 and no bleeding, oral vitamin K is recommended [40]. At 24 h, 5 mg of PO and 1 mg IV phytonadione produce similar effects on the INR [42, 51, 54]. For major bleeding at any INR, IV vitamin K at a dose of 5–10 mg should be administered, in combination with 4-factor PCC [40]. Due to the short half-lives of PCC, FFP, and recombinant factor VIIa, vitamin K is given in the setting of major bleeding to sustain the coagulant effects of these agents [40]. When given at higher doses for the management of the bleeding, IV administration works more rapidly than either PO or SC. Reduction of the INR begins within 2 h, with a correction to within the normal range usually achieved within 24 h (depending on if hepatic function is normal and a sufficiently large dose was administered) [42, 44, 45]. Refer to Chap. 13 for a more in-depth discussion of perioperative management of patients on anticoagulants and Chap. 14 for more information regarding perioperative management of dental patients on anticoagulants. In the peri-procedural or surgical setting, one strategy for INR normalization in patients receiving warfarin (in which holding therapy was not completely effective) is to administer 1–2.5 mg of oral phytonadione the day prior to the procedure, with an INR check on the day of procedure or surgery [51, 55].

## 11.6 Recombinant Factor VIIa (NovoSeven RT)

Initially approved in 1999, activated recombinant factor VII (rFVIIa) was FDA approved as an orphan drug for use in the treatment of bleeding episodes and perioperative management in hemophilia A or B patients with inhibitors to factor VIII or factor IX. Chapter 4 of this book provides a more hemophilia A and B and perioperative management in dentistry. Additional approvals have been added for treatment of bleeding episodes and perioperative management with acquired hemophilia, congenital factor VII deficiency, and Glanzmann's thrombasthenia with refractoriness to platelet transfusions, with or without antibodies to platelets [56, 57].

Mechanistically, rFVIIa has the same effect as endogenous factor VIIa and complexes with tissue factor although the concentration after injection is up to 1000 times the physiological levels.

This will activate the extrinsic clotting pathway ultimately resulting in thrombin formation and a hemostatic plug [56].

Although approved for specific indications, recombinant factor VIIa has been frequently used off-label in the clinical setting [58]. As more specific reversal agents (aPCC, idarizumab, adexanet, etc.) have become available, the role that recombinant factor VIIa plays in anticoagulant reversal has lessened.

The use of recombinant factor VIIa in addition to vitamin K and 3-factor PCC (or FFP) has been used to correct warfarin-related bleeding [21, 59–61]. As a sole agent, rFVIIa does not result in a complete reversal of warfarin due to half-life of rFVIIa (2.3 h) and lack of warfarin depleted factors [56]. When combined with vitamin K and 3-factor PCC, the combination will provide sufficient replacement of the vitamin K-dependent factors II, VII, IX, and X to rapidly reverse the INR, while vitamin K leads to a sustained response. In current guidelines, 4-factor PCC is preferred which provides the same factors [40, 62].

In vitro and in vivo studies of rFVIIa on anti-Xa inhibitors have shown variable effects on coagulation tests [63–67]. Even though these tests may be corrected, there was no effect on anti-Xa activity which was induced specifically by rivaroxaban. Without more data showing efficacy and reliability to reverse anti-Xa inhibitors, it is not recommended [63, 64]. Coagulation tests and evidence of a hemostatic effect should be monitored for both warfarin and anti-Xa reversal although the coagulation tests may not correlate with clinical response.

As is expected with rFVIIa, thrombosis is the biggest safety concern. One risk factor for events appears to be patients who are not hemophiliacs receiving rFVIIa for an off-label use due to their intact clotting cascade and a more pronounced response to rFVIIa. An earlier meta-analysis which included clinical trials, case series, and case reports found a low thrombotic incidence of 1–2% [68]. However, the risk of off-label use is as high as 9% in randomized controlled trials [69]. The risk also is higher for higher doses of rFVIIa [58, 69, 70].

The use of rFVIIa as a reversal agent for anticoagulation agents is limited, and its use will likely be replaced as newer agents are available.

## 11.7 Prothrombin Complex Concentrate (PCC)

For clinical scenarios where pharmacologic reversal or other coagulopathy correction is required quickly, it is warranted to consider reversal using prothrombin complex concentrate (PCC) with or without the addition of phytonadione. PCCs are characterized as 3-factor, 4-factor, or activated PCCs. 3-Factor PCCs (Profilnine SD) contain therapeutic amounts of vitamin K-dependent factors II, IX, and X, as well as nontherapeutic amounts of factor VII. 4-Factor PCCs (Kcentra, Beriplex) contain therapeutic amounts of vitamin K-dependent factors II, VII, IX, and X, as well as proteins C and S and a small amount of heparin. 4-Factor PCC is the recommended agent for rapid reversal of anticoagulation according to the most recent guidelines from several medical communities [40, 71]. Dosing for 4-factor PCC depends on the patient's INR (Table 11.5) [72]. Clinical trial data in patients with major bleeding has demonstrated 4-factor PCCs to be non-inferior to FFP in achieving hemostasis. Patients receiving PCC developed less volume overload than patients receiving FFP [73]. In patients on a VKA requiring reversal before surgery, 4-factor PCC has demonstrated superiority over FFP [74, 75]. Safety and efficacy of 4-factor PCCs has been confirmed in several observational analyses [76–78]. PCC has been shown to work faster to lower the INR than both FFP and phytonadione [6, 79–82]. As 4-factor

**Table 11.5** 4-Factor prothrombin complex concentrate dosing based on INR [72]

| Pretreatment INR | $<4$ | 4–6 | $>6$ |
|---|---|---|---|
| Dose of 4-factor PCC units/kg actual body weight | 25 | 35 | 50 |
| Maximum dose (units of factor IX) | Not to exceed 2500 | Not to exceed 3500 | Not to exceed 5000 |

4-Factor PCC is dosed in units of factor IX

PCCs contain heparin, they should not be administered to patients with active or a recent history of heparin-induced thrombocytopenia.

3-Factor PCCs containing factors II, IX, and X must be coadministered with FFP because they lack factor VII and on their own only are able to achieve partial reversal of VKA anticoagulation [83]. The combination of 3-factor PCC and FFP demonstrated efficacy and safety in reversal of warfarin-related bleeding and prior to surgery [59, 84–87]. The use of 4-factor PCC is more cost effective than the combination of 3-factor PCC and FFP together [21, 88–90]. As 3-factor PCC does not contain heparin, it may be appropriate for use in patients with active or a recent history of HIT. Activated PCCs (aPCC, factor VIII inhibitor bypassing activity, FEIBA) have been used to reverse warfarin and direct oral anticoagulant (DOAC)-related bleeding, but is not considered first line for these indications [91, 92].

There is a small risk of thrombosis with the use of all PCCs [93]. This risk is higher with the use of aPCC. Case reports and case series suggest utility in different dosing regimens of PCC to reverse DOACs, though as more targeted antidotes are developed and become commercially available, PCC use for this indication will decline. As the DOACs have markedly shorter half-lives than VKAs, holding for procedure should be achievable for most patients prior to their dental procedure [94–96].

## 11.8 Idarucizumab

Idarucizumab is a monoclonal antibody for the reversal of dabigatran for emergency or urgent procedures or for life-threatening or uncontrolled bleeding. It was approved under accelerated approval based on data which showed a reduction of unbound dabigatran and normalization of coagulation parameters in healthy volunteers, and continued approval may be contingent on results of an ongoing cohort case series study [97, 98]. Idarucizumab was FDA approved in October of 2015.

Idarucizumab is a humanized monoclonal antibody fragment that binds to dabigatran and its acyl glucuronide metabolites with higher affinity (>350 times) than the binding affinity of dabigatran to thrombin, thus neutralizing their anticoagulant effect within minutes and lasting over 24 h [97–99]. Idarucizumab is a reversal agent specific only for dabigatran and has no impact on the effect of other anticoagulants or antithrombotic therapies. In healthy subjects aged 45–64 years, the plasma concentrations of unbound dabigatran were decreased to the lower limit of quantification immediately after administration of 5 g of idarucizumab. The diluted thrombin time, ecarin clotting time, activated partial thromboplastin time, thrombin time, and activated clotting time returned to baseline. The reduction in dabigatran plasma concentration was seen over the entire observation period of at least 24 h. Idarucizumab is rapidly eliminated with an initial half-life of 47 min and a terminal half-life of 10.3 h [97, 98].

The Reversal of Dabigatran Anticoagulant Effect with Idarucizumab (REVERSE-AD) is an ongoing open-label, single-arm, phase III trial of idarucizumab administration in patients who are taking dabigatran that present with overt, life-threatening, or uncontrollable bleeding or require emergent surgery [100]. In the interim analysis of 90 patients, idarucizumab reversed hemostatic parameters, as measured by ecarin clotting time or dilute thrombin time in the first 4 h after administration, in 100% of cases, and in 88–98% of them, the reversal occurred within minutes [21, 100]. Also from the interim analysis, thrombosis was reported in five patients. Thrombosis occurred 2 days after idarucizumab in one patient and 7 days or more after idarucizumab treatment in the remaining four patients. None of the patients were receiving antithrombotic therapy when the events occurred [97, 100]. Administration of idarucizumab in the absence of dabigatran was shown to have no effect on coagulation parameters, suggesting it is unlikely to be prothrombotic [101].

For dabigatran reversal during emergency surgery, for urgent procedures, or for life-threatening or uncontrolled bleeding, the dose of idarucizumab is 5 g intravenously once. In the REVERSE-AD study, 6 patients had a rebound of dabigatran concentrations at 12 h and 16 patients had a rebound in concentrations at 24 h. The subsequent increases in concentrations were associated with increases in clotting times. This observation may be explained by a redistribution of dabigatran into the intravascular space. Data supporting the administration of an additional 5 g dose is limited, and the safety and effectiveness of repeat treatment have not been established. If reappearance of clinically relevant bleeding together with elevated coagulation parameters (e.g., activated partial thromboplastin time or ecarin clotting time) is observed or a patient requires a second emergency surgery/urgent procedure and has elevated coagulation parameters, administration of an additional 5 g dose of idarucizumab may be considered. Dabigatran may be reinitiated 24 h after idarucizumab administration [98].

## 11.9 Coagulation Factor Xa (Recombinant), Inactivated-zhzo

Direct oral anticoagulants (DOACs) are an important advancement in anticoagulation therapy. DOACs include the medications dabigatran, rivaroxaban, apixaban, and edoxaban. The reversal of dabigatran was previously discussed. Coagulation factor Xa (recombinant), inactivated-zhzo (trade name Andexxa, also sometimes referred to as andexanet alfa) is a novel antidote which is being studied to reverse direct and indirect factor Xa (fXa) inhibitors which were previously discussed in Chap. 10. Specifically, these include rivaroxaban, apixaban, edoxaban, and enoxaparin [102–104].

Coagulation factor Xa (recombinant), inactivated-zhzo is a recombinant protein that has been designed to be a universal antidote for fXa inhibitors. It is a modified fXa molecule with a serine mutation in the catalytic site which maintains the protein's structure but eliminates any fXa anticoagulant activity. An additional deletion of the membrane binding γ-carboxyglutamic acid (GLA) domain prevents the antidote's potential to competitively bind factor Va which assists in cleaving prothrombin to thrombin. By effectively binding the medication and becoming a "decoy," endogenous fXa retains its procoagulant activity and promotes hemostasis via the coagulation cascade [105]. Coagulation factor Xa (recombinant), inactivated-zhzo dosing consists of a bolus and infusion dose and depends on the agent requiring reversal and time of last ingestion (Table 11.6).

**Table 11.6** Coagulation factor Xa (recombinant), inactivated-zhzo dosing by indication [102, 106–108]

| | Bolus dose, mg | Infusion dose (over 2 h), mg |
|---|---|---|
| Apixaban or rivaroxaban >7 h ago | 400 | 480 |
| Edoxaban, enoxaparin, or rivaroxaban <7 h ago | 800 | 960 |
| Unknown time of last dose of anticoagulant | 800 | 960 |

A multicenter, prospective, open-label, single-group study involving 67 patients with acute major bleeding within 18 h of a dose of fXa inhibitor administration were evaluated for pharmacokinetic and pharmacodynamic data. Anti-Xa activity decreases from baseline were 89% after bolus and 86% after 2 h infusion for rivaroxaban, while apixaban showed decreases of 93% and 92%. Hemostatic efficacy was evaluated and adjudicated by an independent committee for each case 12 h after coagulation factor Xa (recombinant), inactivated-zhzo infusion with objective definitions based upon location of bleed. Of the 47 patients included in the hemostatic efficacy population, 37 patients had either excellent ($n = 31$) or good hemostasis ($n = 6$) (79%; 95% CI, 64–89). Nine patients had poor or no hemostasis [106].

The safety of coagulation factor Xa (recombinant), inactivated-zhzo was evaluated in several trials [102, 105, 107–109]. It is well tolerated with minimal adverse effects. One of the main concerns for anticoagulant reversal is thrombosis. In the ANNEXA-4 study, thrombotic events occurred in 12/67 (18%) of the safety population within the 30-day follow-up period. Of the 12 patients, 4 had an event occur within 3 days after infusion. Therapeutic anticoagulation was restarted in 1 of the 12 patients prior to the thrombotic event [106].

**Table 11.7** Summary of available pharmacologic reversal agents [4, 5, 8, 40, 42, 55, 73, 110–112]

| Medication | Half-life/duration of action | Available reversal options |
|---|---|---|
| Aspirin | $T_{1/2}$ = 20 min, but effect up to 5–7 days | Platelet transfusion ± desmopressin |
| Clopidogrel, ticagrelor, prasugrel | $T_{1/2}$ = 6–15 h, but effect up to 5–7 days | Platelet transfusion |
| Warfarin | $T_{1/2}$ = 20–60 h, significant variability between patients | Phytonadione ± 4-factor PCC Or phytonadione ± 3-factor PCC + FFP |
| Dabigatran | $T_{1/2}$ = 11–17 h | Idarucizumab |
| Apixaban, rivaroxaban, edoxaban, betrixaban | $T_{1/2}$ = 5-27 h | Coagulation factor Xa (recombinant), inactivated-zhzo (where available) or 4-factor PCC ± rFVIIa |
| Unfractionated heparin | $T_{1/2}$ = 30–90 min | Protamine |
| Enoxaparin, dalteparin | $T_{1/2}$ = 4–7 h | Protamine (partial reversal) + FFP or PCC |
| Fondaparinux | $T_{1/2}$ = 17–20 h | aPCC ± rFVIIa |

One key exclusion criteria of the ANNEXA-4 was the scheduling of surgery within less than 12 h after presentation, although this does not include minimally invasive surgery or procedure. Additionally, these patients presented with acute bleeds which may be rare when presenting for evaluation [106]. This may preclude a subset of patients with potential for dental surgery. The risks and benefits should be weighed when deciding to reverse a fXa inhibitor emergently or allowing the medication's effects to subside by holding before surgery.

### Conclusion

Pharmacologic reversal agents are a rapidly expanding area of research, due to the substantial need to balance the risks of bleeding and thrombotic events. There are several pharmacologic reversal agents available to practitioners; these are summarized in Table 11.7. This chapter summarizes the available pharmacologic reversal agents and their place in therapy. As will be discussed further in upcoming Chaps. 12 and 13, patient- and procedure-specific factors will drive the perioperative management of anticoagulant and antiplatelet therapy. In cases where pharmacologic reversal of an anticoagulant is desired, it is important for dental practitioners to be comfortable with selecting and dosing the appropriate reversal agent based on the anticoagulant, as well as monitoring and reinitiating of the medication being reversed.

## References


1. Perry DJ, Noakes TJ, Helliwell PS. Guidelines for the management of patients on oral anticoagulants requiring dental surgery. Br Dent J. 2007;203(7):389–93.
2. American Red Cross (2017) Blood facts and statistics. Available from: http://www.redcrossblood.org/learn-about-blood/blood-facts-and-statistics
3. Garcia DA, Crowther MA. Reversal of warfarin: case-based practice recommendations. Circulation. 2012;125(23):2944–7.
4. Ansell J, Hirsh J, Hylek E, Jacobson A, Crowther M, Palareti G. Pharmacology and management of the vitamin K antagonists: American College of Chest Physicians evidence-based clinical practice guidelines (8th edition). Chest. 2008;133(6 Suppl):160S–98S.
5. Guyatt GH, Akl EA, Crowther M, Gutterman DD, Schuunemann HJ. Executive summary: antithrombotic therapy and prevention of thrombosis, 9th ed: American College of Chest Physicians evidence-based clinical practice guidelines. Chest. 2012;141(2 Suppl):7S–47S.
6. Vigue B. Bench-to-bedside review: optimising emergency reversal of vitamin K antagonists in severe haemorrhage – from theory to practice. Crit Care. 2009;13(2):209.
7. Holland LL, Brooks JP. Toward rational fresh frozen plasma transfusion: the effect of plasma transfusion on coagulation test results. Am J Clin Pathol. 2006;126(1):133–9.
8. Eikelboom JW, Hirsh J, Spencer FA, Baglin TP, Weitz JI. Antiplatelet drugs: antithrombotic therapy and prevention of thrombosis, 9th ed: American College of Chest Physicians evidence-based clinical practice guidelines. Chest. 2012;141(2 Suppl):e89S–119S.
9. Sharma S, Sharma P, Tyler LN. Transfusion of blood and blood products: indications and complications. Am Fam Physician. 2011;83(6):719–24.

10. Lee K, Istl A, Dubois L, DeRose G, Forbes TL, Wiseman D, et al. Fibrinogen level and bleeding risk during catheter-directed thrombolysis using tissue plasminogen activator. Vasc Endovasc Surg. 2015;49(7):175–9.
11. Warmuth M, Mad P, Wild C. Systematic review of the efficacy and safety of fibrinogen concentrate substitution in adults. Acta Anaesthesiol Scand. 2012;56(5):539–48.
12. Behring CLS. RiaSTAP® [prescribing information]. Kankakee, IL: Behring CLS; 2016.
13. Aiyagari V. Counteracting the effects of anticoagulants and antiplatelet agents during neurosurgical emergencies. Neurosurgery. 2006;59(5):E1152. author reply E
14. Desmopressin [database on the Internet]. Gold Standard, Inc. Available from: http://www.clinicalpharmacology.com.
15. Gahart B. Intravenous medications. St. Louis, MO: Mosby; 1999.
16. McEnvoy G. American hospital formulary service. American Society of Hospital Pharmacists: Bethesda, MD; 2000.
17. Lethagen S. Desmopressin (DDAVP) and hemostasis. Ann Hematol. 1994;69(4):173–80.
18. Baglin T. Drugs and haemostasis. In: Bowes JCF, editor. Clinical pharmacology. 11th ed. London: Churchill Livingstone; 2012. p. 482–95.
19. Teng R, Mitchell PD, Butler K. The effect of desmopressin on bleeding time and platelet aggregation in healthy volunteers administered ticagrelor. J Clin Pharm Ther. 2014;39(2):186–91.
20. Galvez A, Gomez-Ortiz G, Diaz-Ricart M, Escolar G, Gonzalez-Sarmiento R, Zurbano MJ, et al. Desmopressin (DDAVP) enhances platelet adhesion to the extracellular matrix of cultured human endothelial cells through increased expression of tissue factor. Thromb Haemost. 1997;77(5):975–80.
21. Raimondi P, Hylek EM, Aronis KN. Reversal agents for oral antiplatelet and anticoagulant treatment during bleeding events: current strategies. Curr Pharm Des. 2016;23(9):1406–23.
22. Mannucci PM. Desmopressin: a nontransfusional form of treatment for congenital and acquired bleeding disorders. Blood. 1988;72(5):1449–55.
23. Mannucci PMVV, Vianello L, et al. Controlled trial of desmopressin in liver cirrhosis and other conditions associated with a prolonged bleeding time. Blood. 1986;67:1148–53.
24. Kim JH, Baek CH, Min JY, Kim JS, Kim SB, Kim H. Desmopressin improves platelet function in uremic patients taking antiplatelet agents who require emergent invasive procedures. Ann Hematol. 2015;94(9):1457–61.
25. Leithauser B, Zielske D, Seyfert UT, Jung F. Effects of desmopressin on platelet membrane glycoproteins and platelet aggregation in volunteers on clopidogrel. Clin Hemorheol Microcirc. 2008;39(1-4):293–302.
26. Reiter RA, Mayr F, Blazicek H, Galehr E, Jilma-Stohlawetz P, Domanovits H, et al. Desmopressin antagonizes the in vitro platelet dysfunction induced by GPIIb/IIIa inhibitors and aspirin. Blood. 2003;102(13):4594–9.
27. Agerso H, Seiding Larsen L, Riis A, Lovgren U, Karlsson MO, Senderovitz T. Pharmacokinetics and renal excretion of desmopressin after intravenous administration to healthy subjects and renally impaired patients. Br J Clin Pharmacol. 2004;58(4):352–8.
28. Mannucci PM, Remuzzi G, Pusineri F, Lombardi R, Valsecchi C, Mecca G, et al. Deamino-8-D-arginine vasopressin shortens the bleeding time in uremia. N Engl J Med. 1983;308(1):8–12.
29. Hedges SJ, Dehoney SB, Hooper JS, Amanzadeh J, Busti AJ. Evidence-based treatment recommendations for uremic bleeding. Nat Clin Pract Nephrol. 2007;3(3):138–53.
30. Kohler M, Hellstern P, Tarrach H, Bambauer R, Wenzel E, Jutzler GA. Subcutaneous injection of desmopressin (DDAVP): evaluation of a new, more concentrated preparation. Haemostasis. 1989;19(1):38–44.
31. Watson AJ, Keogh JA. Effect of 1-deamino-8-D-arginine vasopressin on the prolonged bleeding time in chronic renal failure. Nephron. 1982;32(1):49–52.
32. Ferring Pharmaceuticals I. DDAVP (desmopressin acetate) injection [prescribing information]. Parsippany, NJ: Ferring Pharmaceuticals I; 2014.
33. Sanofi-Aventis. DDAVP nasal spray (desmopressin acetate) [prescribing information]. Bridgewater, NJ: Sanofi-Aventis; 2015.
34. CLS Behring. Stimate (desmopressin acetate) intranasal [prescribing information]. King of Prussia, PA: CLS Behring; 2013.
35. Pharmaceuticals A. Protamine sulfate IV injection [prescribing information]. Schaumburg, IL: Pharmaceuticals A; 2008.
36. Sanofi-Aventis US L. LOVENOX(R) IV, SC injection, enoxaparin sodium IV, SC injection [prescribing information]. Bridgewater, NJ: Sanofi-Aventis US L; 2008.
37. Phytonadione, Vitamin K1 [database on the Internet]. Gold Standard, Inc. [cited February 8th, 2017]. Available from: http://www.clinicalpharmacology.com
38. Merck. AquaMephyton (phytonadione, vitamin K1) [prescribing information]. Whitehouse Station, NJ: Merck; 2002.
39. Merck. Mephyton (phytonadione, vitamin K1) [prescribing information]. Whitehouse Station, NJ: Merck; 2004.
40. Holbrook A, Schulman S, Witt DM, Vandvik PO, Fish J, Kovacs MJ, et al. Evidence-based management of anticoagulant therapy: antithrombotic therapy and prevention of thrombosis, 9th ed: American College of Chest Physicians evidence-based clinical practice guidelines. Chest. 2012;141(2 Suppl):e152S–84S.

41. Ansell J, Hirsh J, Poller L, Bussey H, Jacobson A, Hylek E. The pharmacology and management of the vitamin K antagonists: the seventh ACCP conference on antithrombotic and thrombolytic therapy. Chest. 2004;126(3 Suppl):204S–33S.
42. Ageno W, Gallus AS, Wittkowsky A, Crowther M, Hylek EM, Palareti G. Oral anticoagulant therapy: antithrombotic therapy and prevention of thrombosis, 9th ed: American College of Chest Physicians evidence-based clinical practice guidelines. Chest. 2012;141(2 Suppl):e44S–88S.
43. Wilson MD, Davis JE. Antithrombotic reversal agents. Emerg Med Clin North Am. 2014;32(3):715–25.
44. Dentali F, Ageno W, Crowther M. Treatment of coumarin-associated coagulopathy: a systematic review and proposed treatment algorithms. J Thromb Haemost. 2006;4(9):1853–63.
45. Watson HG, Baglin T, Laidlaw SL, Makris M, Preston FE. A comparison of the efficacy and rate of response to oral and intravenous Vitamin K in reversal of over-anticoagulation with warfarin. Br J Haematol. 2001;115(1):145–9.
46. Dezee KJ, Shimeall WT, Douglas KM, Shumway NM, O'Malley PG. Treatment of excessive anticoagulation with phytonadione (vitamin K): a meta-analysis. Arch Intern Med. 2006;166(4):391–7.
47. Crowther MA, Douketis JD, Schnurr T, Steidl L, Mera V, Ultori C, et al. Oral vitamin K lowers the international normalized ratio more rapidly than subcutaneous vitamin K in the treatment of warfarin-associated coagulopathy. A randomized, controlled trial. Ann Intern Med. 2002;137(4):251–4.
48. Whitling AM, Bussey HI, Lyons RM. Comparing different routes and doses of phytonadione for reversing excessive anticoagulation. Arch Intern Med. 1998;158(19):2136–40.
49. Raj G, Kumar R, McKinney WP. Time course of reversal of anticoagulant effect of warfarin by intravenous and subcutaneous phytonadione. Arch Intern Med. 1999;159(22):2721–4.
50. Fiore LD, Scola MA, Cantillon CE, Brophy MT. Anaphylactoid reactions to vitamin K. J Thromb Thrombolysis. 2001;11(2):175–83.
51. Patriquin C, Crowther M. Treatment of warfarin-associated coagulopathy with vitamin K. Expert Rev Hematol. 2011;4(6):657–65. quiz 66–7
52. Woods K, Douketis JD, Kathirgamanathan K, Yi Q, Crowther MA. Low-dose oral vitamin K to normalize the international normalized ratio prior to surgery in patients who require temporary interruption of warfarin. J Thromb Thrombolysis. 2007;24(2):93–7.
53. Patel RJ, Witt DM, Saseen JJ, Tillman DJ, Wilkinson DS. Randomized, placebo-controlled trial of oral phytonadione for excessive anticoagulation. Pharmacotherapy. 2000;20(10):1159–66.
54. Lubetsky A, Yonath H, Olchovsky D, Loebstein R, Halkin H, Ezra D. Comparison of oral vs intravenous phytonadione (vitamin K1) in patients with excessive anticoagulation: a prospective randomized controlled study. Arch Intern Med. 2003;163(20):2469–73.
55. Douketis JD, Spyropoulos AC, Spencer FA, Mayr M, Jaffer AK, Eckman MH, et al. Perioperative management of antithrombotic therapy: antithrombotic therapy and prevention of thrombosis, 9th ed: American College of Chest Physicians evidence-based clinical practice guidelines. Chest. 2012;141(2 Suppl):e326S–50S.
56. NovoNordisk. NovoSeven® RT (recombinant factor VIIa) [prescribing information]. Plainsboro, NJ: NovoNordisk; 2014.
57. American Society of Health-System Pharmacists. AHFS drug information. Bethesda, MD: American Society of Health-System Pharmacists; 2010.
58. Yank V, Tuohy CV, Logan AC, Bravata DM, Staudenmayer K, Eisenhut R, et al. Systematic review: benefits and harms of in-hospital use of recombinant factor VIIa for off-label indications. Ann Intern Med. 2011;154(8):529–40.
59. Barton CA, Johnson NB, Case J, Warden B, Hughes D, Zimmerman J, et al. Risk of thromboembolic events after protocolized warfarin reversal with 3-factor PCC and factor VIIa. Am J Emerg Med. 2015;33(11):1562–6.
60. DeLoughery E, Avery B, DeLoughery TG. Retrospective study of rFVIIa, 4-factor PCC, and a rFVIIa and 3-factor PCC combination in improving bleeding outcomes in the warfarin and non-warfarin patient. Am J Hematol. 2016;91(7):705–8.
61. Brody DL, Aiyagari V, Shackleford AM, Diringer MN. Use of recombinant factor VIIa in patients with warfarin-associated intracranial hemorrhage. Neurocrit Care. 2005;2(3):263–7.
62. Dixit D, Thomas Z. Letter by Dixit and Thomas regarding article, "Guidelines for the management of spontaneous intracerebral hemorrhage: a guideline for healthcare professionals from the American Heart Association/American Stroke Association". Stroke. 2015;46(11):e236.
63. Siegal DM. Managing target-specific oral anticoagulant associated bleeding including an update on pharmacological reversal agents. J Thromb Thrombolysis. 2015;39(3):395–402.
64. Herrmann R, Thom J, Wood A, Phillips M, Muhammad S, Baker R. Thrombin generation using the calibrated automated thrombinoscope to assess reversibility of dabigatran and rivaroxaban. Thromb Haemost. 2014;111(5):989–95.
65. Marlu R, Hodaj E, Paris A, Albaladejo P, Cracowski JL, Pernod G. Effect of non-specific reversal agents on anticoagulant activity of dabigatran and rivaroxaban: a randomised crossover ex vivo study in healthy volunteers. Thromb Haemost. 2012;108(2):217–24.
66. Perzborn E, Gruber A, Tinel H, Marzec UM, Buetehorn U, Buchmueller A, et al. Reversal of rivaroxaban anticoagulation by haemostatic agents in rats and primates. Thromb Haemost. 2013;110(1):162–72.

67. Martin AC, Le Bonniec B, Fischer AM, Marchand-Leroux C, Gaussem P, Samama CM, et al. Evaluation of recombinant activated factor VII, prothrombin complex concentrate, and fibrinogen concentrate to reverse apixaban in a rabbit model of bleeding and thrombosis. Int J Cardiol. 2013;168(4):4228–33.
68. Levi M, Peters M, Buller HR. Efficacy and safety of recombinant factor VIIa for treatment of severe bleeding: a systematic review. Crit Care Med. 2005;33(4):883–90.
69. Levi M, Levy JH, Andersen HF, Truloff D. Safety of recombinant activated factor VII in randomized clinical trials. N Engl J Med. 2010;363(19):1791–800.
70. Lin Y, Stanworth S, Birchall J, Doree C, Hyde C. Use of recombinant factor VIIa for the prevention and treatment of bleeding in patients without hemophilia: a systematic review and meta-analysis. CMAJ. 2011;183(1):E9–19.
71. Frontera JA, Lewin JJ 3rd, Rabinstein AA, Aisiku IP, Alexandrov AW, Cook AM, et al. Guideline for reversal of antithrombotics in intracranial hemorrhage: a statement for healthcare professionals from the Neurocritical Care Society and Society of Critical Care Medicine. Neurocrit Care. 2016;24(1):6–46.
72. Behring CLS. KCENTRA(R) intravenous injection lyophilized powder for solution, prothrombin complex concentrate human intravenous injection lyophilized powder for solution [prescribing information]. Kankakee, IL: Behring CLS; 2014.
73. Sarode R, Milling TJ Jr, Refaai MA, Mangione A, Schneider A, Durn BL, et al. Efficacy and safety of a 4-factor prothrombin complex concentrate in patients on vitamin K antagonists presenting with major bleeding: a randomized, plasma-controlled, phase IIIb study. Circulation. 2013;128(11):1234–43.
74. Demeyere R, Gillardin S, Arnout J, Strengers PF. Comparison of fresh frozen plasma and prothrombin complex concentrate for the reversal of oral anticoagulants in patients undergoing cardiopulmonary bypass surgery: a randomized study. Vox Sang. 2010;99(3):251–60.
75. Goldstein JN, Refaai MA, Milling TJ Jr, Lewis B, Goldberg-Alberts R, Hug BA, et al. Four-factor prothrombin complex concentrate versus plasma for rapid vitamin K antagonist reversal in patients needing urgent surgical or invasive interventions: a phase 3b, open-label, non-inferiority, randomised trial. Lancet. 2015;385(9982):2077–87.
76. Joseph R, Burner J, Yates S, Strickland A, Tharpe W, Sarode R. Thromboembolic outcomes after use of a four-factor prothrombin complex concentrate for vitamin K antagonist reversal in a real-world setting. Transfusion. 2016;56(4):799–807.
77. Preston FE, Laidlaw ST, Sampson B, Kitchen S. Rapid reversal of oral anticoagulation with warfarin by a prothrombin complex concentrate (Beriplex): efficacy and safety in 42 patients. Br J Haematol. 2002;116(3):619–24.
78. Pabinger I, Brenner B, Kalina U, Knaub S, Nagy A, Ostermann H. Prothrombin complex concentrate (Beriplex P/N) for emergency anticoagulation reversal: a prospective multinational clinical trial. J Thromb Haemost. 2008;6(4):622–31.
79. Huttner HB, Schellinger PD, Hartmann M, Kohrmann M, Juettler E, Wikner J, et al. Hematoma growth and outcome in treated neurocritical care patients with intracerebral hemorrhage related to oral anticoagulant therapy: comparison of acute treatment strategies using vitamin K, fresh frozen plasma, and prothrombin complex concentrates. Stroke. 2006;37(6):1465–70.
80. Fredriksson K, Norrving B, Stromblad LG. Emergency reversal of anticoagulation after intracerebral hemorrhage. Stroke. 1992;23(7):972–7.
81. Goldstein JN, Thomas SH, Frontiero V, Joseph A, Engel C, Snider R, et al. Timing of fresh frozen plasma administration and rapid correction of coagulopathy in warfarin-related intracerebral hemorrhage. Stroke. 2006;37(1):151–5.
82. Makris M, Greaves M, Phillips WS, Kitchen S, Rosendaal FR, Preston EF. Emergency oral anticoagulant reversal: the relative efficacy of infusions of fresh frozen plasma and clotting factor concentrate on correction of the coagulopathy. Thromb Haemost. 1997;77(3):477–80.
83. Holland L, Warkentin TE, Refaai M, Crowther MA, Johnston MA, Sarode R. Suboptimal effect of a three-factor prothrombin complex concentrate (Profilnine-SD) in correcting supratherapeutic international normalized ratio due to warfarin overdose. Transfusion. 2009;49(6):1171–7.
84. Tilton R, Michalets EL, Delk B, Sutherland SE, Ramming SA. Outcomes associated with prothrombin complex concentrate for international normalized ratio reversal in patients on oral anticoagulants with acute bleeding. Ann Pharmacother. 2014;48(9):1106–19.
85. Imberti D, Magnacavallo A, Dentali F, Condoleo E, Gallerani M, Benedetti R, et al. Emergency reversal of anticoagulation with vitamin K antagonists with 3-factor prothrombin complex concentrates in patients with major bleeding. J Thromb Thrombolysis. 2013;36(1):102–8.
86. Switzer JA, Rocker J, Mohorn P, Waller JL, Hughes D, Bruno A, et al. Clinical experience with three-factor prothrombin complex concentrate to reverse warfarin anticoagulation in intracranial hemorrhage. Stroke. 2012;43(9):2500–2.
87. Kantorovich A, Fink JM, Militello MA, Wanek MR, Smedira NG, Soltesz EG, et al. Low-dose 3-factor prothrombin complex concentrate for warfarin reversal prior to heart transplant. Ann Pharmacother. 2015;49(8):876–82.
88. Mangram A, Oguntodu OF, Dzandu JK, Hollingworth AK, Hall S, Cung C, et al. Is there a difference in efficacy, safety, and cost-effectiveness between 3-factor and 4-factor prothrombin complex concentrates among trauma patients on oral anticoagulants? J Crit Care. 2016;33:252–6.

89. Jones GM, Erdman MJ, Smetana KS, Mohrien KM, Vandigo JE, Elijovich L. 3-Factor versus 4-factor prothrombin complex concentrate for warfarin reversal in severe bleeding: a multicenter, retrospective, propensity-matched pilot study. J Thromb Thrombolysis. 2016;42(1):19–26.
90. Al-Majzoub O, Rybak E, Reardon DP, Krause P, Connors JM. Evaluation of warfarin reversal with 4-factor prothrombin complex concentrate compared to 3-factor prothrombin complex concentrate at a tertiary academic medical center. J Emerg Med. 2016;50(1):7–13.
91. Stewart WS, Pettit H. Experiences with an activated 4-factor prothrombin complex concentrate (FEIBA) for reversal of warfarin-related bleeding. Am J Emerg Med. 2013;31(8):1251–4.
92. Wojcik C, Schymik ML, Cure EG. Activated prothrombin complex concentrate factor VIII inhibitor bypassing activity (FEIBA) for the reversal of warfarin-induced coagulopathy. Int J Emerg Med. 2009;2(4):217–25.
93. Dentali F, Marchesi C, Giorgi Pierfranceschi M, Crowther M, Garcia D, Hylek E, et al. Safety of prothrombin complex concentrates for rapid anticoagulation reversal of vitamin K antagonists. A meta-analysis. Thrombosis and haemostasis. 2011;106(3):429–38.
94. Levi M, Eerenberg E, Kamphuisen PW. Bleeding risk and reversal strategies for old and new anticoagulants and antiplatelet agents. J Thromb Haemost. 2011;9(9):1705–12.
95. DeWald TA, Becker RC. The pharmacology of novel oral anticoagulants. J Thromb Thrombolysis. 2014;37(2):217–33.
96. Curto A, Albaladejo A, Alvarado A. Dental management of patients taking novel oral anticoagulants (NOAs): dabigatran. J Clin Exp Dent. 2017;9(2):e289–e93.
97. Idarucizumab [database on the Internet]. Gold Standard, Inc. [cited 8 Feb 2017]. Available from: http://www.clinicalpharmacology.com
98. Boehringer Ingelheim Pharmaceuticals I. Praxbind (Idarucizumab) injection [prescribing information]. Ridgefield, CT: Boehringer Ingelheim Pharmaceuticals I; 2015.
99. Schiele F, van Ryn J, Canada K, Newsome C, Sepulveda E, Park J, et al. A specific antidote for dabigatran: functional and structural characterization. Blood. 2013;121(18):3554–62.
100. Pollack CV Jr, Reilly PA, Eikelboom J, Glund S, Verhamme P, Bernstein RA, et al. Idarucizumab for dabigatran reversal. N Engl J Med. 2015;373(6):511–20.
101. Glund S, Moschetti V, Norris S, Stangier J, Schmohl M, van Ryn J, et al. A randomised study in healthy volunteers to investigate the safety, tolerability and pharmacokinetics of idarucizumab, a specific antidote to dabigatran. Thromb Haemost. 2015;113(5):943–51.
102. Siegal DM, Curnutte JT, Connolly SJ, Lu G, Conley PB, Wiens BL, et al. Andexanet alfa for the reversal of factor Xa inhibitor activity. N Engl J Med. 2015;373(25):2413–24.
103. Curto A, Albaladejo A. Implications of apixaban for dental treatments. J Clin Exp Dent. 2016;8(5):e611–e4.
104. Curto A, Curto D, Sanchez J. Managing patients taking edoxaban in dentistry. J Clin Exp Dent. 2017;9(2):e308–e11.
105. Lu G, DeGuzman FR, Hollenbach SJ, Karbarz MJ, Abe K, Lee G, et al. A specific antidote for reversal of anticoagulation by direct and indirect inhibitors of coagulation factor Xa. Nat Med. 2013;19(4):446–51.
106. Connolly SJ, Milling TJ Jr, Eikelboom JW, Gibson CM, Curnutte JT, Gold A, et al. Andexanet alfa for acute major bleeding associated with factor Xa inhibitors. N Engl J Med. 2016;375(12):1131–41.
107. Crowther MLG, Lu G, et al. A phase 2 randomized, double-blind, placebo-controlled trial demonstrating reversal of edoxaban-induced anticoagulation in healthy subjects by andexanet alfa (PRT064445), a universal antidote for factor Xa (fXa) inhibitors. Blood. 2014;124(21):4269.
108. Crowther MVM, Kitt M, et al. A phase 2 randomized, double-blind, placebo-controlled trial demonstrating reversal of rivaroxaban-induced anticoagulation in healthy subjects by andexanet alfa (PRT064446), an antidote for fXa inhibitors. Blood. 2013;122:3636.
109. Crowther MLT, Mathur V, et al. A phase 2 randomized double-blind, placebo-controlled trial of PRT064445, a novel, universal antidote for direct and indirect factor Xa inhibitors. J Thromb Haemost. 2013;11(suppl):1322.
110. Greinacher A, Thiele T, Selleng K. Reversal of anticoagulants: an overview of current developments. Thromb Haemost. 2015;113(5):931–42.
111. Ortel TL. Perioperative management of patients on chronic antithrombotic therapy. Hematology Am Soc Hematol Educ Program. 2012;2012:529–35.
112. Kor DJ, Gajic O. Blood product transfusion in the critical care setting. Curr Opin Crit Care. 2010;16(4):309–16.

# Part III

# Management of the Dental Patient on Antithrombotic Therapy

# 12 Perioperative Management of Dental Patients on Antiplatelet Medications

Michael J. Wahl

**Abstract**

When dental patients on continuous antiplatelet medications present for dental surgery, a decision must be made to continue antiplatelet therapy with potential increased bleeding risks or to interrupt therapy with potential increased embolic risks. But dental surgery is unlike other types of surgery in that major vessels are unlikely to be encountered and most bleeding complications are easy to access without additional surgeries both perioperatively and postoperatively. Of more than 3522 dental patients undergoing more than 6265 dental surgical procedures without interrupting antiplatelet therapy reported in the medical and dental literature, no more than 86 patients (a 2.4% minor bleeding incidence) required additional local measures for hemostasis, and still only two patients (in separate reports) suffered bleeding complications requiring more than local measures for hemostasis, a remarkably low incidence of serious bleeding complications of 0.06%. A close look at these two cases, one over 30 years old and the other over 50 years old, shows that they do not support interrupting antiplatelet therapy for dental surgery. Of 702 patients undergoing at least 752 interruptions of antiplatelet therapy for dental procedures, there were at least 19 embolic complications (2.5% of cessations). These embolic complications included myocardial infarction, stent thrombosis, coronary artery syndrome, and cerebrovascular strokes. Since the review of the literature of antiplatelet interruption for dental procedures includes some case reports and some studies that were not prospective, randomized, and controlled, it is virtually certain that the actual incidence of embolic complications with antiplatelet interruption for dental procedures is significantly lower than 2.5%, but there certainly is an increased embolic risk, regardless of the reason for the interruption. As a result, antiplatelet therapy should not be interrupted for dental surgery.

The history of antiplatelet drugs can be traced to antiquity. Hippocrates recommended chewing on willow leaves, which contain salicylic acid, to ease the pain of childbirth, but it wasn't until the late 1890s that Felix Hoffman, a chemist at the Bayer Company isolated pure acetylsalicylic acid (ASA), calling it "aspirin." Since then, aspirin has been used by millions of people for its antipyretic, anti-inflammatory, analgesic, and antithrombotic effects, earning its name as a "wonder drug." When aspirin is used for its antithrombotic effects, the usual dose of this antiplatelet drug is 75–325 mg once daily [1]. There are also newer

M. J. Wahl
Christiana Care Health System,
Wilmington, DE, USA


R. P. Szumita, P. M. Szumita (eds.), *Hemostasis in Dentistry*, https://doi.org/10.1007/978-3-319-71240-6_12

**Table 12.1** Antiplatelet medications

| |
|---|
| Cilostazol (Pletal) |
| Clopidogrel (Plavix) |
| Dipyridamole (Persantine, Aggrenox) |
| Prasugrel (Effient) |
| Ticagrelor (Brilinta) |
| Ticlopidine (Ticlid) |

**Table 12.2** Antiplatelet medication indications

| |
|---|
| History of transient ischemic attack or stroke |
| Atrial fibrillation |
| History of angina or myocardial infarction |
| History of coronary bypass surgery |
| History of coronary artery disease |
| History of myocardial infarction |
| History of peripheral vascular disease |
| Primary prevention of cardiovascular disease |

antiplatelet drugs, including dipyridamole (Persantine, Aggrenox), clopidogrel (Plavix), ticagrelor (Brilinta), prasugrel (Effient), cilostazol (Pletal), and ticlopidine (Ticlid) (see Table 12.1). Continuous antiplatelet therapy is used for atrial fibrillation, history of angina or myocardial infarction, prevention of coronary artery disease, history of coronary bypass surgery, history of transient ischemic attack or stroke, and asymptomatic carotid artery disease (see Table 12.2) When patients on continuous antiplatelet therapy present for dental treatment, a decision must be made to continue therapy and increase the risk of bleeding complications or interrupt therapy and increase the risk of thromboembolic complications like myocardial infarction or stroke.

## 12.1 Controlled Studies of Antiplatelet Drugs and Dental Surgery

Most controlled studies of dental surgical patients have shown no significant difference in bleeding complications between those whose antiplatelet medications are continued versus those not on antiplatelet medications or whose medications are interrupted. A 2000 study by Ardekian et al. [2] consisted of 39 dental extraction patients, randomly assigned into one of two groups: a study group (19 patients whose aspirin therapy was continued) or a control group (20 patients whose aspirin therapy was interrupted for 7 days before and restarted the day after the procedure). There were no bleeding complications requiring more than local hemostatic methods in either group, leading the authors to conclude, "Low-dose aspirin should not be stopped before oral surgery. Local hemostasis is sufficient to control bleeding."

In a study first described by Valerin et al. [3] in 2006 and then by Brennan et al. [4] in 2008, 36 healthy dental extraction patients were randomly divided into two groups: 17 on 325 mg daily aspirin for 4 days and 19 on a placebo. There were no bleeding complications requiring more than local measures for hemostasis in either group, and there were no differences in bleeding time between the two groups. The authors concluded that "there is no indication to discontinue aspirin for persons requiring single-tooth extraction."

In 2008, Krishnan et al. [5] studied 82 dental extraction patients divided into three groups: group 1 consisted of 25 patients whose antiplatelet therapy was interrupted between 1 and 10 days (mean 4.7 days) before the procedure; group 2 consisted of 32 patients whose antiplatelet therapy was continued; and group 3 comprised 25 healthy patients not on antiplatelet therapy. There were no bleeding complications requiring more than local measures for hemostasis in any group, and the authors concluded, "Routine dental extractions can be safely performed in patients on long-term antiplatelet medication, with no interruption or alteration of their medication. Such patients do not have an increased risk of prolonged or excessive postoperative bleeding."

In 2011, Medeiros et al. [6] studied 63 patients on 100 mg daily aspirin divided into two groups: 31 patients whose aspirin therapy was interrupted for 7 days before extraction and 32 patients whose aspirin therapy was continued for the procedure. There were no bleeding complications requiring more than local hemostatic methods, and there was no difference in the amount of postoperative bleeding between the two groups. The authors concluded that there is no need to interrupt aspirin therapy for dental patients undergoing single extractions.

In 2015, Varghese et al. [7] studied 190 dental extraction patients on antiplatelet medications and randomly assigned 2 patients to 2 groups: 1 group of 95 patients continued their antiplatelet medications for the procedure and the other group of 95 patients interrupted antiplatelet therapy for 5 days before the procedure. No patient in either group had any bleeding complications requiring more than local measures for hemostasis. The authors concluded that antiplatelet therapy should not be interrupted for single dental extractions.

In 2016, Eapen et al. [8] studied 80 dental extraction patients on low-dose aspirin, divided into two groups—those who continued aspirin and those whose aspirin therapy was interrupted for 5 days before the procedure. Although the bleeding time was longer in the aspirin group, there were no bleeding complications requiring more than local measures for hemostasis in either group, and the authors concluded that "dental extraction procedures in patients on low-dose [aspirin] therapy can be safely carried out without stopping the antiplatelet therapy."

Even for full mouth extractions, antiplatelet medications should not be interrupted. In a 2015 retrospective study [9], Omar et al. studied patients on antiplatelet medications undergoing full mouth extractions. There were 68 patients studied, divided into four groups: 25 using aspirin, 12 using clopidogrel, 9 using both aspirin and clopidogrel, and 22 had interrupted antiplatelet therapy at least 5 days before the procedure. There were no bleeding complications requiring more than local measures for hemostasis in any patient, and the authors concluded, "Clopidogrel therapy during full-mouth extraction is not associated with significant bleeding complications and may be continued in patients who have a high risk of experiencing a cardiac event."

## 12.2 Controlled Studies of Dual Antiplatelet Therapy and Dental Surgery

Although dual antiplatelet therapy can theoretically increase the risk of bleeding after, controlled studies have repeatedly and consistently shown that dental surgery in such patients is safe. In a 2009 retrospective study of 43 patients on single or dual antiplatelet therapy undergoing invasive dental procedures (extractions, gingival surgery, scaling and root planing, and subgingival scaling), Napeñas et al. [10] reported that there were no bleeding complications or prolonged bleeding in any patient. They concluded, "The risks of altering or discontinuing use of antiplatelet medications far outweigh the low risk of postoperative oral bleeding complications resulting from dental procedures."

Lillis et al. in 2011 [11] studied 111 dental extraction patients on antiplatelet medications (aspirin and/or clopidogrel) of whom 33 were on dual aspirin-clopidogrel medication and 532 patients not on antiplatelet medications in a control group. No patient in the study or control groups required more than local measures for hemostasis. Minor postoperative bleeding complications were higher in the single antiplatelet groups than in the control groups. Although minor postoperative bleeding was higher in the dual antiplatelet group than in the single antiplatelet or control groups, the authors concluded, "[D]ental extractions may be safely performed in patients receiving single or dual antiplatelet therapy when appropriate local hemostatic measures are taken, thus averting thrombotic risk of temporary antiplatelet discontinuation."

Dudek et al. in 2011 [12] studied 55 oral surgical patients on dual antiplatelet therapy with aspirin and clopidogrel and compared with 33 patients not on antiplatelet medications in the control group. There was no excessive bleeding in any patient in either group, and the authors concluded, "Therapy with clopidogrel and aspirin after acute coronary syndromes does not seem to increase the risk of real-life bleeding following oral surgery, regardless of the platelet activity response to dual antiplatelet therapy."

Girotra et al. in 2014 [13] studied 546 oral surgical patients on antiplatelet medications (aspirin or clopidogrel) including 139 on aspirin-clopidogrel dual therapy and a control group of 575 healthy patients. Prolonged bleeding was greatest in the dual therapy group, followed by the single antiplatelet group, and least in the control group, but no patient in any group required more than local measures for hemostasis. The authors recommended that "patients on dual therapy require higher levels of hemostatic measures, thus suturing should be the first line of control to arrest bleeding." Their conclusion was that with these additional local hemostatic measures, "there is no need to expose the patient to the risk of thromboembolism, cerebrovascular accidents, or myocardial or renal infarction by discontinuing anti-platelet therapy before minor oral surgical procedures, which could cost the patient his or her life."

In 2016, Lu et al. [14] studied 183 patients on antiplatelet therapy, including 42 patients on dual aspirin-clopidogrel therapy undergoing 24 surgical appointments and a control group of 1088 patients not on antiplatelet or anticoagulant therapy. No patient in the study or control groups required more than local measures for hemostasis. There was a higher incidence of minor bleeding in the study group than in the control group and a slightly higher incidence in the dual antiplatelet group than the single antiplatelet group, but the differences in bleeding complications were not significant. The authors concluded, "These findings indicate that there is no need to interrupt antiplatelet drugs before dental extraction."

## 12.3 Controlled Study of Combination Antiplatelet-Anticoagulant Therapy and Dental Surgery

Dental surgery has been shown to be safe in patients on combination antiplatelet and anticoagulant therapy (e.g., warfarin), provided their international normalized ratio (INR) is not above therapeutic levels (INR $\leq 3.5$). In a 2012 prospective study of 213 dental extraction patients, Bajkin et al. [15] studied 213 dental extraction patients divided into three groups of 71 patients each: those on aspirin therapy, those on vitamin K antagonist anticoagulant therapy, and those on combined aspirin and anticoagulant therapy. No patient in any of three groups required more than local measures for hemostasis, and there was no statistical difference in minor postoperative bleeding between groups. The authors concluded, "Tooth extractions can be performed safely while patients continue to receive combined anticoagulant-aspirin therapy."

## 12.4 Systematic and Narrative Reviews of Dental Surgery in Patients on Antiplatelet Therapy

In a 2015 systematic review and meta-analysis of dental patients on long-term aspirin therapy undergoing extractions, there were three randomized controlled trials and seven controlled trials that met the inclusion criteria for a total of 1752 patients (529 on aspirin therapy and 1223 not on aspirin) [16]. The results showed that although "bleeding time is prolonged or hemorrhage is exacerbated by long-term use of aspirin," aspirin should be continued for dental extractions with local measures for hemostasis. In a systematic review of dental extractions on patients on dual antiplatelet therapy, Nathwani and Martin concluded, "Patients on dual antiplatelet therapy—although at an increased risk of postoperative bleeding complications—can be managed safely with local haemostatic measures and without the need to discontinue antiplatelet therapy" [17].

In a narrative review in 2014, [18] this author found that of more than 1282 patients undergoing more than 2343 dental surgical procedures, no more than 35 patients (2.7% of patients and 2.6% of visits) suffered bleeding complications requiring additional local hemostatic measures and only two patients (0.16% of patients and 0.15% of visits) suffered bleeding complications requiring more than additional local hemostatic measures.

Since then, there have been more studies identified. Of more than 3522 dental patients undergoing more than 6265 dental surgical procedures without interrupting antiplatelet therapy reported in the medical and dental literature [2–15, 19–54] (see Table 12.3), no more than 86 patients required additional local measures for hemostasis

**Table 12.3** Dental surgery in patients on continuous antiplatelet drugs

| Source | No. of patents treated | No. of extractions (surgical procedures) | Antiplatelet medications | Comment | Postoperative bleeding requiring treatment with local measures (other than immediately postoperative) | Bleeding complications requiring more than local measures |
|---|---|---|---|---|---|---|
| Ardekian et al. [2] | 19 | 29 (29) | Aspirin 100 mg/day | | 0 | 0 |
| Bajkin et al. [15] | 71 | 119 (119) | Aspirin 100 mg/day | | 0 | 0 |
| Bajkin et al. [19] | 160 | 342 (342) | Aspirin, clopidogrel, ticlopidine as single therapy, or a combination of aspirin and clopidogrel, ticlopidine, or prasugrel as dual therapy | Postoperative bleeding incidence not statistically different between single antiplatelet, dual antiplatelet, or control groups | 1 | 0 |
| Brennan et al. [4] Valerin et al. [3] | 17 | 17 (17) | Aspirin 325 mg/day | | 0 | 0 |
| Broekema et al. [20] | 71 | ≥58 ≤ 71 (≥58 ≤ 71) | Thrombocyte aggregation inhibitors (generally aspirin or clopidogrel) | | 4 | 0 |
| Cañigral et al. [21] | 51 | 51 (51) | ASA, clopidogrel, NSAIDS dosages not reported | | 5 | 0 |
| Cardona-Tortajada et al. [22] | 155 | 222 (222) | Aspirin 100–300 mg/day, clopidogrel 75 mg/day, ticlopidine 250 mg/day, or triflusal 300 mg/day | | 1 | 0 |
| Clemm et al. [23] | 63 | 0 (63) | Type of platelet inhibitors not specified; 21 were on dual antiplatelet therapy | Implant surgical procedures | 1 | 0 |
| Darawade et al. [24] | 100 | 100 (100) | 81 mg aspirin | No bleeding problems in either continuation or interruption group | 0 | 0 |
| Dézsi et al. [25] | 129 | 129 (129) | Dual platelet (clopidogrel-aspirin and prasugrel-aspirin) | | 2 | 0 |
| Dudek D et al. [12] | 55 | 124 (134) | Dual antiplatelet aspirin (81–150 mg) and clopidogrel 75 mg | No excessive bleeding in study or control group | 0 | 0 |
| Duygu et al. [26] | 25 | 50 (50) | Aspirin 75–300 mg/day | | 0 | 0 |
| Eapen et al. [8] | 40 | ≥42 ≤ 120 (≥42 ≤ 120) | 75 mg aspirin | No bleeding complications in study or control group | 0 | 0 |

(continued)

**Table 12.3** (continued)

| Source | No. of patents treated | No. of extractions (surgical procedures) | Antiplatelet medications | Comment | Postoperative bleeding requiring treatment with local measures (other than immediately postoperative) | Bleeding complications requiring more than local measures |
|---|---|---|---|---|---|---|
| Flanagan [27] | 1 | 2 (4) | Dual clopidogrel 75 mg and aspirin 81 mg | Patient seen twice; once for two extractions and implant placement with no complications; then for implant uncovering surgery with some postoperative bleeding treated with local measures for hemostasis including tranexamic acid | 1 | 0 |
| Garnier et al. [28] | 52 | 218 (218) | | | 1 | 0 |
| Girotra et al. [13] | 546 | ≥511 (≥975) | Aspirin, clopidogrel, or dual | No significant bleeding in bleeding between single antiplatelet and control groups. Dual antiplatelet group had more prolonged bleeding, but in no case did bleeding require more than local measures for hemostasis | 4 | 0 |
| Hanken et al. [29] | 195 | 297 (297) | Aspirin 100 mg/day | Surgical extractions; the difference in postoperative bleeding was not significant between the antiplatelet group and the control group (on no antiplatelet medications) of 165 patients and 179 procedures | 5 (procedures of the 297) | 0 |
| Hemelik et al. [30] | 65 | 151 (151) | Aspirin 100 mg | No excessive bleeding in study or control group | 1 | 0 |
| Hepsö et al. [31] | 23 | 46 (46) | Aspirin 1 g night before surgery and then 2 g day for 3 days | Each patient underwent 2 extractions of impacted wisdom teeth | 5 | 0 |
| Jimson et al. [32] | 76 | ≥76 ≤ 228 | Aspirin, clopidogrel, or dual | | 4 | 0 |
| Kale et al. [33] | 40 | 80 (80) | Aspirin, clopidogrel, or ticlopidine dosage not reported | | 0 | 0 |
| Krishnan et al. [5] | 32 | 40 (40) | Aspirin 75–150 mg/day | | 0 | 0 |

| | | | | | | |
|---|---|---|---|---|---|---|
| Lemkin et al. [34] | 1 | 18 (18) | 12–20 daily aspirin tablets (dosage unreported) | Uncontrolled bleeding after 18 extractions. Hemostasis achieved after platelet transfusion | 1 | 1 |
| Lillis et al. [11] | 111 | 169 (169) | Aspirin, clopidogrel, aspirin-clopidogrel, dosage unreported | | 0 | 0 |
| Lu et al. [14] | 183 (274 occasions) | 548 (548) | Aspirin, clopidogrel, dual antiplatelet | No significant difference in postoperative bleeding between antiplatelet and control groups | 12 | 0 |
| Madan et al. [35] | 51 | ≥46 (≥57) | Aspirin 75–100 mg/day | | 0 | 0 |
| McGaul [36] | 1 | 0 (2) | Postoperative aspirin 600 mg: 1 dose; 3 doses | | 2 | 0 |
| Medeiros et al. [6] | 32 | 32 (32) | Aspirin 100 mg/day | | 0 | 0 |
| Morimoto et al. [37, 38] | 87 (93 visits) | 144 (144) | 78 patients on aspirin 115.4 ± 48.2 mg/day, 8 on ticlopidine 218.2 ± 60.3 mg/day, 8 on cilostazol 135.7 ± 62.7 mg/day, 4 on dipyridamole 250.0 ± 100 mg/day | | 2 | 0 |
| Morimoto et al. [39] | ≥7 ≤ 15 | 0 (15) | Aspirin 81–243 mg/day; ticlopidine 100–200 mg/day, cilostazol 200 mg/day | | 1 on patient on combined warfarin-aspirin therapy | 0 |
| Napeñas et al. [10] | ≥25 (≥70 visits) | 213 (≥213) | A total of 43 patients, but some were receiving deep subgingival scaling and root planing: of the 43 patients, 14 patients on single antiplatelet and 29 on dual antiplatelet: 88 invasive procedure visits; 70 extraction visits; various novel antiplatelet medication dosages not reported | | 0 | 0 |
| Nooh [40] | 102 | ≥102 (≥102) | Aspirin 81 mg/day | ≥49 surgical extractions | 1 | 0 |
| Olmos-Carrasco et al. [41] | 181 | 217 (217) | Dual antiplatelet aspirin 100 mg and either clopidogrel 75 mg or prasugrel 10 mg | | 15 (more than 30 min) | 0 |
| Omar et al. [9] | 46 | 880 (≥880) | 81 or 325 mg aspirin, 75 mg clopidogrel, or dual | Full mouth extractions. No significant difference in blood loss between single, dual, or interruption groups based on number of teeth extracted | 0 | 0 |

(continued)

**Table 12.3** (continued)

| Source | No. of patents treated | No. of extractions (surgical procedures) | Antiplatelet medications | Comment | Postoperative bleeding requiring treatment with local measures (other than immediately postoperative) | Bleeding complications requiring more than local measures |
|---|---|---|---|---|---|---|
| Park et al. [42] | 100 | 176 (176) | Aspirin 100–200 mg/day with clopidogrel 75 mg/day and if needed cilostazol 100 mg two times per day | | 2 | 0 |
| Partridge et al. [43] | 27 | 38 (38) | Clopidogrel, aspirin, NSAIDs, at "therapeutic dosages" | | 0 | 0 |
| Pawalk et al. [44] | 20 | 20 (20) | Aspirin 2600 mg the day before and 2600 mg the day after surgery | | 0 | 0 |
| Pereira et al. [45] | 10 | ≥10 (≥10) | 9 patients combined warfarin-aspirin, 1 aspirin only, aspirin dosages not reported | | ≤1 | 0 |
| Sadhasivam et al. [46] | 100 | >116 (>116) | Aspirin, clopidogrel, and dual | No bleeding complications after 1 h in study or control groups | 0 after 60 min | 0 |
| Sammartino et al. [47] | 84 | 330 (330) | Clopidogrel, ticlopidine, aspirin dosages not reported | Combined warfarin-antiplatelet therapy. Some patients had warfarin withdrawn preoperatively; some did not | 6 | 0 |
| Sánchez-Palomino et al. [48] | 32 | >32 < 128 (> 32 < 128) | Dual antiplatelet aspirin and clopidogrel | | 0 | 0 |
| Shah et al. [49] | 127 | 127 (127) | Aspirin 75–150 mg | | 1 at 12 h | 0 |
| Sung et al. [50] | 5 | 32 (32) | Aspirin, warfarin, heparin, clopidogrel | 3 patients on aspirin and warfarin; 1 patient on aspirin, warfarin, heparin, and argatroban; 1 patient on heparin, aspirin, and clopidogrel | 0 | 0 |
| Svensson et al. [51] | 11 | ≥11 (≥11) | ASA dosage not reported | Warfarin continued | ≤5 | 0 |

| | | | | | | |
|---|---|---|---|---|---|---|
| Thomason et al. [52] | 1 | 0 (2) | Aspirin 150 mg day | Hemostasis achieved with local measures after upper gingivectomy. Excessive hemorrhage uncontrolled with local measures after lower gingivectomy | 1 | 1 |
| Varghese et al. [7] | 95 | 95 (95) | Aspirin, clopidogrel, and dual | | 0 | 0 |
| Wahl and Schmitt [53] | 1 | 1 (1) | Aspirin 81 mg and apixaban 10 mg | | 1 | 0 |
| Zirk et al. [54] | 96 | >96 ≤ 666 (>96 ≤ 666) | Aspirin, clopidogrel, dipyridamole, and dual antiplatelet | | 0 | 0 |
| Totals | ≥3522 patients (≥3613 visits) | ≥6157 (≥6265) | | | ≤86 (2.4% of patients or visits) | 2 (0.06% of patients or visits) |

Adapted and updated from Table 1 the *American Journal of Medicine,* Vol. 127, "Dental surgery and antiplatelet agents: bleed or die," pages 260–267, Copyright 2014, with permission from Elsevier (a 2.4% minor bleeding incidence), and still only two patients (in separate reports) suffered bleeding complications requiring more than local measures for hemostasis, a remarkably low incidence of serious bleeding complications of 0.06%. A close look at these two cases, one over 30 years old and the other over 50 years old, shows that they do not support interrupting antiplatelet therapy for dental surgery.

## 12.5 Analysis of Cases of Bleeding Complications Requiring More Than Local Hemostatic Methods

In 1974, Lemkin et al. reported a case of significant bleeding after 18 extractions that could not be controlled with local measures for hemostasis. On hospital admission, a platelet transfusion was administered. The patient had a history of ethanol abuse but denied recent ethanol ingestion and was taking 12–20 aspirin tablets daily (dosage unreported)—significantly more than the single daily dose typically prescribed today for antithrombosis [34]. In 1997, Thomason et al. reported on a kidney transplant patient who received a platelet transfusion after local measures for hemostasis were unsuccessful following an upper anterior gingivectomy [52]. The patient was taking 150 mg daily aspirin as well as cyclosporine, azathioprine, and amlodipine, any or all of which could have independently contributed to the postoperative bleeding and/or platelet function reduction. As a result, it is not certain that the aspirin ingestion caused the postoperative bleeding.

## 12.6 Embolic Risk with Antiplatelet Therapy Interruption

In a narrative review from 2014 [18], there were at least 17 cases (5%) of embolic complications of 324 patients whose antiplatelet therapy was interrupted at least 374 times for dental procedures (see Table 12.4). In an update of this review, there have been more studies and case reports

**Table 12.4** Antiplatelet withdrawal for dental procedures

| Source | No. of patents treated | No. of cessations | No. of extractions | Antiplatelet medications | Comment | Days of withdrawal | Thrombotic complications |
|---|---|---|---|---|---|---|---|
| Ardekian et al. [2] | 20 | 34 | 34 | Aspirin | | 7 | 0 |
| Bajkin et al. [19] | 19 | 19 | ≥19 | Usually aspirin | | Not reported | None reported |
| Candemir et al. [55] | 1 | 1 | 1 | Clopidogrel | Warfarin was continued | 10 | 1 myocardial infarction due to very late stent thrombosis |
| Collet et al. [56] | 1 | 1 | Not reported | Aspirin | | 8 | Myocardial infarction 10 days after aspirin withdrawal for dental surgery |
| Darawade et al. [24] | 100 | 100 | 100 | 81 mg aspirin | | 7 | 0 |
| Duygu et al. [26] | 19 | 48 | 48 | Aspirin | | 7 | None reported |
| Eapen et al. [8] | 40 | 40 | ≥40 ≤ 120 | 75 mg aspirin | | 5 | 0 |

**Table 12.4** (continued)

| Source | No. of patents treated | No. of cessations | No. of extractions | Antiplatelet medications | Comment | Days of withdrawal | Thrombotic complications |
|---|---|---|---|---|---|---|---|
| Ferrari et al. [57] | 13 | ≥13 | ≥13 | Aspirin | | Not reported | 13 cases of acute coronary syndrome |
| Ferreira-González et al. [58] | 17 | 17 | Not reported | Aspirin, clopidogrel, or both | | Not reported | Not reported |
| Gagneja et al. [59] | 1 | 1 | 6 | ASA | Warfarin was continued | 10 | 0 |
| Kovacic et al. [60] | 197 | ≥197 | ≥197 | Aspirin, clopidogrel, aspirin, and clopidogrel | | Not reported | ≥2 cases of stent thrombosis and/or acute myocardial infarction (personal communication 3/23/13 with Jason Kovacic) |
| Krishnan et al. [5] | 25 | 28 | 28 | Aspirin | | 1–10 | 0 |
| Loomba et al. [61] | 1 | 1 | 1 | Aspirin | | 3 | 0 |
| Lu et al. [14] | 2 | 2 | 2 | Aspirin | | 7 | 2 cerebrovascular strokes |
| Medeiros et al. [6] | 31 | 31 | 31 | Aspirin | | 7 | 0 |
| Napeñas et al. [10] | 2 | 6 | 6 | Clopidogrel | 1 patient substituted aspirin for clopidogrel on day of 6 extractions; 1 patient stopped clopidogrel 3 days before an oral examination | 1–3 | 0 |
| Omar et al. [9] | 22 | 22 | 376 | 81 or 325 mg aspirin, 75 mg clopidogrel, or dual | | ≥5 | 0 |
| Sadhasivam et al. [46] | 100 | 100 | ≥103 | Aspirin, clopidogrel, and dual | 9 patients had minor bleeding after 1 h | 3–5 | 0 |
| Varghese et al. [7] | 95 | 95 | 95 | Aspirin, clopidogrel, and dual | | 5 | None reported |
| Totals | 702 | ≥752 | | | | | ≥19 (2.7% of patients; 2.5% of cessations) thromboembolic complications |

Adapted and updated from Table 2 in the *American Journal of Medicine,* Vol. 127, "Dental surgery and antiplatelet agents: bleed or die," pages 260–267, Copyright 2014, with permission from Elsevier identified. Of 702 patients undergoing at least 752 interruptions of antiplatelet therapy for dental procedures, there were at least 19 embolic complications (2.5% of cessations). These embolic complications included myocardial infarction, stent thrombosis, coronary artery syndrome, and cerebrovascular strokes. Since the review of the literature of antiplatelet interruption for dental procedures includes some case reports and some studies that were not prospective, randomized, and controlled, it is virtually certain that the actual incidence of embolic complications with antiplatelet interruption for dental procedures is significantly lower than 2.5%, but there certainly is an increased embolic risk, regardless of the reason for the interruption.

Well-controlled studies in the medical literature have repeatedly shown an increased embolic risk in patients whose antiplatelet therapy was interrupted for various medical procedures or as a result of negligence by the patient. In a study of 118 patients in 2013, Derogar et al. found a sevenfold increase in the risk of death or acute cardiovascular event within the first 6 months after low-dose aspirin therapy interruption (after peptic ulcer bleeding) versus those whose aspirin was continued [62].

In a case-control study of 39,513 patients on low-dose aspirin therapy followed for an average of 3.2 years, García Rodríguez et al. [63] found that patients recently interrupting aspirin therapy were significantly more likely to suffer nonfatal myocardial infarction. For every 1000 patients who had recently stopped therapy in the course of a year, there were four more cases of nonfatal myocardial infarction than in those who continued therapy. The authors stated, "Discontinuation of low dose aspirin increases the risk of non-fatal myocardial infarction or death from coronary heart disease by almost 50% in patients in primary care who have a history of ischaemic events." In another analysis of these patients, García Rodríguez et al. [64] showed a 40% increase in the incidence of stroke in those who recently interrupted low-dose aspirin therapy versus those who continued therapy.

In a systematic review and meta-analysis of 50,279 patients on aspirin therapy, Biondi-Zoccai et al. [65] found the risk of major adverse cardiac events three times higher in those whose therapy had been interrupted versus those in whom therapy was continued. The authors concluded that interruption of aspirin therapy has "ominous prognostic implication[s]." Of 289 patients with ischemic stroke studied by Sibon and Orgogozo in 2005 [66], 13 (4.5%) had interrupted antiplatelet therapy within the month before the stroke, either from their own negligence or a physician's recommendation before a surgical procedure, and the authors recommended rethinking the practice of antiplatelet therapy interruption for certain surgical procedures.

In a case-control study by Maulaz et al. of 309 recent stroke patients on aspirin therapy versus 309 control patients on aspirin therapy who had not had a stroke within the previous 6 months, 4.2% study patients had interrupted aspirin within 4 weeks before stroke versus only 1.3% of control patients [67]. Of the 13 stroke patients who had interrupted aspirin therapy within 4 weeks before the stroke, 7 were instructed to do so by a physician for a surgical procedure, leading the authors to conclude that interrupting aspirin therapy for surgical procedures "may not always be the best solution."

In a prospective, randomized, double-blind, placebo-controlled study in 2010, Oscarsson et al. [68] studied 220 patients undergoing noncardiac (nondental) surgery, divided into two groups: 109 receiving aspirin and 111 receiving a placebo for 7 days before and 3 days after the procedure. Ten patients (9%) in the placebo group but only four patients (3.7%) in the aspirin group developed major adverse cardiac events, but there was no significant difference in bleeding complications between the groups. The authors concluded, "In high-risk patients undergoing non-cardiac surgery, perioperative aspirin reduced the risk of major adverse cardiac events without increasing bleeding complications."

In contrast, in a similarly well-controlled 2011 study of 291 patients divided into two groups of 145 patients on aspirin and 146 patients on placebo for 7 days before major noncardiac (nondental) surgery, Mantz et al. showed no differences in bleeding complications or thrombotic complications between the two groups [69]. The Mantz et al. study showed a more favorable outcome in the placebo group than the Oscarsson et al. study did, possibly because aspirin was interrupted for only 7 days in total, whereas in the Oscarsson et al. study, the interruption was for 10 days in total. Although only the former study showed a benefit of decreased thrombotic complications in the interruption group, neither study showed a benefit of decreased risk of bleeding complications in the interruption group. When dental procedures in patients on continuous antiplatelet therapy are considered, it should be noted that there has never been a fatal case of postdental bleeding when antiplatelet medications are continued, but there have been many cases of embolic complications (including at least one fatal embolism) where antiplatelet therapy was interrupted for dental surgery.

In a 2011 study, Broderick et al. [70] found that 114 (5.2%) of 2197 ischemic strokes occurred after antithrombotic medication (either warfarin or antiplatelet medication) interruption, including 53 strokes after antiplatelet medication interruption, either as a result of a physician recommendation or patient negligence. The authors concluded, "The withdrawal of anticoagulant and antiplatelet medications is associated with a substantial number of acute first-ever and recurrent ischemic strokes."

## 12.7 National Medical and Dental Group Statements

National medical and dental groups have recommended against interruption of antiplatelet medication therapy for dental surgery, as the risks of (possibly fatal) thromboembolic complications with interruption exceed the risk of postdental bleeding complications (usually simple to treat with local hemostatic measures) with continuation. In a 2007 joint science advisory statement, the American Heart Association, American College of Cardiology, Society for Cardiovascular Angiography and Interventions, American College of Surgeons, and American Dental Association have stated that single or dual antiplatelet therapy should not be interrupted for dental procedures, concluding "Given the relative ease with which the incidence and severity of oral bleeding can be reduced with local measures during surgery (e.g., absorbable gelatin sponge and sutures) and the unlikely occurrence of bleeding once an initial clot has formed, there is little or no indication to interrupt antiplatelet drugs for dental procedures" [71]. In 2012, the American College of Chest Physicians also recommended continuing aspirin therapy instead of interrupting it for dental procedures [72]. In a systematic literature review and evidence-based practice recommendation, the American Academy of Neurology stated in 2013, "Stroke patients undergoing dental procedures should routinely continue aspirin." [73] In a consensus statement in 2014, the Society for Neuroscience in Anesthesiology and Critical Care stated antiplatelet medication interruption is not required for single dental extractions as the bleeding risk is very low in such patients [74]. In 2015, the American Dental Association stated, "There is general agreement that in most cases, treatment regimens with older anticoagulants (e.g., warfarin) and antiplatelet agents (e.g., clopidogrel, ticlopidine, prasugrel, ticagrelor, and/or aspirin) should not be altered before dental procedures. The risks of stopping or reducing these medication regimens (i.e., thromboembolism, stroke, MI) far outweigh the consequences of prolonged bleeding, which can be controlled with local measures" [75] (see Table 12.5).

**Table 12.5** National medical and dental group statements for dental treatment in patients on antiplatelet medications

| Year | Group | Recommendation |
|---|---|---|
| 2015 [75] | American Dental Association | Continue antiplatelets for dental procedures |
| 2014 [74] | The Society for Neuroscience in Anesthesiology and Critical Care (supported by the American Society of Anesthesiologists) | Continue antiplatelets for single dental extractions |
| 2013 [73] | American Academy of Neurology | Continue aspirin for dental procedures |
| 2012 [72] | American College of Chest Physicians | Continue aspirin for dental procedures |
| 2007 [71] | American Heart Association, American College of Cardiology, Society for Cardiovascular Angiography and Interventions, American College of Surgeons, and American Dental Association | Continue antiplatelets for dental procedures |

## 12.8 Physician Consultation and Informed Consent

If a patient presents for dental treatment while on antiplatelet therapy, then such therapy should generally not be interrupted. Physician consultation is usually not required in such patients. There are occasions that the dentist may require more information about a patient's health condition to aid in a decision and therefore may wish to consult with the patient's physician, but ultimately it is the dentist and not the physician who is responsible for the dental treatment recommendations.

Sometimes a patient on antiplatelet therapy will bring up the idea of an interruption of therapy before a dental procedure, either on his own or because his physician recommended it. In a situation like this, the dentist has an obligation to explain that the issue has been extensively studied, and controlled studies in the medical and dental literature have shown that dental surgery is safe in patients taking antiplatelet medication, but there is an increased embolic risk when such therapy is interrupted. When bleeding complications in patients continuing antiplatelet therapy have been reported in the medical and dental literature, they have never been fatal, but there have been serious, even fatal embolic complications when antiplatelet therapy has been interrupted for dental procedures. The dentist may wish to explain that the literature shows that any patient on antiplatelet drugs who suffered a bleeding complication after dental surgery presumably made a full recovery, while patients with embolic complications after antiplatelet interruption for dental procedures may have suffered permanent disability or even death. Patients have the right to make informed decisions regarding their health, and if a patient decides to interrupt antiplatelet therapy for a dental procedure after being informed of the risks, this decision should be documented, and the treatment can proceed.

A recommendation for antiplatelet therapy alteration should never be made by the dentist; only the physician should make antiplatelet therapy alterations or antiplatelet therapy interruption for dental procedures, and then the dentist has an obligation to inform the patient about the abundance of scientific evidence that dental surgery is safe in patients on antiplatelet therapy and there is an increased risk of embolic complications when such therapy is interrupted. The dentist may wish to share also that national medical and medical group statements confirm that dental treatment is safe while continuing antiplatelet therapy.

## 12.9 Summary

Bleeding complications in patients on continuous antiplatelet medications are rare and are usually simple to treat with local measures for hemostasis. In thousands of cases in the literature, there have been only two nonfatal cases of bleeding complications requiring more than local measures for hemostasis and those two patients presumably made full recoveries. On the other hand, in patients whose antiplatelet medication therapy is interrupted for dental procedures, there have been several reports of serious embolic complications, including at least one fatality. For these patients, the decision has been called "bleed or die." Antiplatelet therapy should not be interrupted for dental procedures.

## References


1. Guyatt GH, Akl EA, Crowther M, et al. for the American College of Chest Physicians Antithrombotic Therapy and Prevention of Thrombosis Panel. Antithrombotic therapy and prevention of thrombosis, 9th ed: American College of Chest Physicians evidence-based practice guidelines. Chest. 2012;141(2 (Suppl)):7S–47S.
2. Ardekian L, Gaspar R, Peled M, et al. Does low-dose aspirin therapy complicate oral surgical procedures? J Am Dent Assoc. 2000;131(3):331–5.
3. Valerin MA, Brennan MT, Noll JL, et al. Relationship between aspirin use and postoperative bleeding from dental extractions in a healthy population. Oral Surg Oral Med Oral Pathol Oral Radiol Endod. 2006;102(3):326.
4. Brennan MT, Valerin MA, Noll JL, et al. Aspirin use and post-operative bleeding from dental extractions. J Dent Res. 2008;87(8):740–4.
5. Krishnan B, Shenoy NA, Alexander M. Exodontia and antiplatelet therapy. J Oral Maxillofac Surg. 2008;66:2063–6.
6. Medeiros FB, deAndrade AC, Angelis GA, et al. Bleeding evaluation during single tooth extraction in patients with coronary artery disease and acetylsalicylic acid therapy suspension: a prospective, double-blinded and randomized study. J Oral Maxillofac Surg. 2011;69(12):2949–55.
7. Varghese KG, Manoharan S, Sadhanandan M. Evaluation of bleeding following dental extraction in patients on long-term antiplatelet therapy: a clinical trial. Indian J Dent Res. 2015;26:252–5.
8. Eapen BV, Baig MF, Avinash S. An assessment of the incidence of prolonged postoperative bleeding after dental extraction among patients on uninterrupted low dose aspirin therapy and to evaluate the need to stop such medication prior to dental extraction. J Maxillofac Oral Surg. 2016. https://doi.org/10.1007/s12663-016-0912-8.
9. Omar HR, Socias SM, Powless RA, et al. Clopidogrel is not associated with increased bleeding complications after full mouth extraction: a retrospective study. JADA. 2015;146(5):303–9.
10. Napeñas JJ, Hong CH, Brennan MT, et al. The frequency of bleeding complications after invasive dental treatment in patients receiving single and dual antiplatelet therapy. J Am Dent Assoc. 2009;140(6):690–5.
11. Lillis T, Ziakas A, Koskinas K, et al. Safety of dental extractions during uninterrupted single or dual antiplatelet treatment. Am J Cardiol. 2011;108(7):964–7.
12. Dudek D, Kuliczkowski W, Kaczmarski J, et al. Response to dual antiplatelet therapy does not impact bleeding risks in patients undergoing oral surgery after acute coronary syndromes. Cardiology. 2015;132(2):119–23.
13. Girotra C, Padhye M, Mandlik G, et al. Assessment of the risk of haemorrhage and its control following minor oral surgical procedures in patients on anti-platelet therapy: a prospective study. Int J Oral Maxillofac Surg. 2014;43:99–106.
14. Lu S-Y, Tsai C-Y, Lin L-H, Lu S-N. Dental extraction without stopping single or dual antiplatelelt therapy: results of a retrospective cohort study. Int J Oral Maxillofac Surg. 2016;45:1293–8.
15. Bajkin BV, Bajkin IA, Petrovic BB. The effects of combined oral anticoagulant-aspirin therapy in patients undergoing tooth extractions. J Am Dent Assoc. 2012;143(7):771–6.
16. Zhao B, Wang P, Dong Y, Zhu Y. Should aspirin be stopped before tooth extraction? A meta-analysis. Oral Surg Oral Med Oral Pathol Oral Radiol. 2015;119:522–30.
17. Nathwani S, Martin K. Exodontia in dual antiplatelet therapy: the evidence. Br Dent J. 2016; 220(5):235–8.
18. Wahl MJ. Dental surgery and antiplatelet agents: bleed or die. Amer J Med. 2014;127:260–7.
19. Bajkin BV, Urosevic IM, Stankov KM, Petrovic BB, Bajkin IA. Dental extractions and risk of bleeding in patients taking single and dual antiplatelet treatment. Br J Oral Maxillofac Surg. 2015;53(1):39–43.
20. Broekema FI, van Minnen B, Jansma J, Bos RRM. Risk of bleeding after dentoalveolar surgery in patients taking anticoagulants. Br J Oral Maxillofac Surg. 2014;52:e15–9.
21. Cañigral A, Silvestre F-J, Cañigral G, et al. Evaluation of bleeding risk and measurement methods in dental patients. Med Oral Patol Oral Cir Bucal. 2010;15(6):e863–8.
22. Cardona-Tortajada F, Sainz-Gómez E, Figuerido-Garmendia J, et al. Dental extractions in patients on antiplatelet therapy. A study conducted by the Oral Health Department of the Navarre Health Service (Spain). Med Oral Patol Oral Cir Bucal. 2009;14(11):e588–92.
23. Clemm R, Neukam FW, Rusche B, Musazada S, Schmitt CM. Management of anticoagulated patients in implant therapy: a clinical comparative study. Clin Oral Impl Res. 2016;27:1274–82.
24. Darawade DA, Kumar S, Desai K, et al. Influence of aspirin on post-extraction bleeding—a clinical study. J Int Soc Prev Community Dent. 2014;4(Suppl 1):S63–7.
25. Dézsi BB, Koritsánszky L, Braunitzer G, et al. Prasugrel versus clopidogrel: a comparative examination of local bleeding after dental extraction in patients receiving dual antiplatelet therapy. J Oral Maxillofac Surg. 2015;73:1894–900.
26. Duygu G, Ozcakir-Tomruk C, Guler N, Sencift K. Assessment of effects of antiplatelet drugs on

bleeding risk after teeth extractions. Biotechnol & Biotechnol Equip. 2010;24(3):2040–3.
27. Flanagan D. Tranexamic acid tamponade to control postoperative surgical hemorrhage. J Oral Implantol. 2015;41(3):e82–9.
28. Garnier J, Truchot F, Quero J, et al. 218 tooth extractions in patients taking platelet aggregation inhibitors. [Article in French. Rev Stomatol Chir Maxillofac. 2007;108(5):407–10.
29. Hanken H, Tieck F, Kluwe L, et al. Lack of evidence for increased postoperative bleeding risk for dental osteotomy with continued aspirin therapy. Oral Surg Oral Med Oral Pathol Oral Radiol. 2015;119:17–9.
30. Hemelik M, Wahl G, Kessler B. Tooth extraction under medication with acetylsalicylic acid. Mund Kiefer Gesichtschir. 2006;10(1):3–6.
31. Hepsö HU, Lökken P, Björnson GHC. Double-blind crossover study of the effect of acetylsalicylic acid on bleeding and post-operative course after bilateral oral surgery. Eur J Clin Pharmacol. 1976;10:217–25.
32. Jimson S, Amaldhas J, Jimson S, Kannan I, Parthiban J. Assessment of bleeding during minor oral surgical procedures and extraction in patients on anticoagulant therapy. J Pharm Bioallied Sci. 2015;7(Suppl 1):S134–7.
33. Kale TP, Singh AK, Kotrashetti SM, Kapoor A. Effectiveness of hemcon dental dressing versus conventional methods of haemostasis in 40 patients on oral antiplatelet drugs. Sultan Qaboos Univ Med J. 2012;12(3):330–5.
34. Lemkin SR, Billesdon JE, Davee JS, et al. Aspirin-induced oral bleeding: correction with platelet transfusion. A reminder. Oral Surg. 1974;37(4):498–501.
35. Madan GA, Madan SG, Madan G, Madan AD. Minor oral surgery without stopping daily low-dose aspirin therapy: a study of 51 patients. J Oral Maxillofac Surg. 2005;63(9):1262–5.
36. McGaul T. Postoperative bleeding caused by aspirin. J Dent. 1978;6(3):207–9.
37. Morimoto Y, Niwa H, Minematsu K. Hemostatic management of tooth extractions in patients on oral antithrombotic therapy. J Oral Maxillofac Surg. 2008;66:51–7.
38. Morimoto Y, Niwa H, Minematsu K. Risk factors affecting postoperative hemorrhage after tooth extraction in patients receiving oral antithrombotic therapy. J Oral Maxillofac Surg. 2011;69:1550–6.
39. Morimoto Y, Niwa H, Minematsu K. Hemostatic management for periodontal treatments in patients on oral antithrombotic therapy: a retrospective study. Oral Surg Oral Med Oral Pathol Oral Radiol Endod. 2009;108:889–96.
40. Nooh N. The effect of aspirin on bleeding after extraction of teeth. Saud Dent J. 2009;21:57–61.
41. Olmos-Carrasco O, Pastor-Ramos V, Espinilla-Blanco R, et al. Hemorrhagic complications of dental extractions in 181 patients undergoing double antiplatelet therapy. J Oral Maxillofac Surg. 2015;73:203–10.
42. Park MW, Her SH, Kwon JB, Lee JB, et al. Safety of dental extractions in coronary drug-eluting stenting patients without stopping multiple antiplatelet agents. Clin Cardiol. 2012;35(4):225–30.
43. Partridge CG, Campbell JH, Alvarado F. The effect of platelet-altering medications on bleeding from minor oral surgery procedures. J Oral Maxillofac Surg. 2008;66:93–7.
44. Pawalk DF, Itkin AB, Lapeyrolerie FM, Zweig B. Clinical effects of aspirin and acetaminophen on hemostasis after exodontics. J Oral Surg. 1978;36:944–7.
45. Pereira CM, Gasparetto PF, Santos Carneiro D, et al. Tooth extraction in patients on oral anticoagulants: prospective study conducted in 108 Brazilian patients. ISRN Dent. 2011;2011:203619.
46. Sadhasivam G, Bhushan S, Chiang KC, Agarwal N, Vasundhar PL. Clinical trial evaluating the risk of thromboembolic events during dental extractions. J Maxillofac Oral Surg. 2016;15(4):506–11.
47. Sammartino G, Maenzi G, Miro A, et al. Local delivery of the hemostatic agent tranexamic acid in chronically anticoagulated patients. J Craniofac Surg. 2012;23(6):e648–52.
48. Sánchez-Palomino P, Sánchez-Cobo P, Rodriguez-Archilla A, et al. Dental extraction in patients receiving dual antiplatelet therapy. Med Oral Patol Oral Cir Bucal. 2015;20(5):e616–20.
49. Shah A, Shah ST, Shah I, Rehman ZU. Post extraction bleeding associated with long-term maintenance dose of aspirin 75–150 mg. Pakistan Oral Dent J. 2012;32(2):199–202.
50. Sung EC, Brar LK, Chung E, et al. Dental treatment in the cardiothoracic intensive care unit for patients with ventricular assist devices awaiting heart transplant: a case series. Oral Surg Oral Med Oral Pathol Oral Radiol. 2014;118:194–201.
51. Svensson R, Hallmer F, Englesson CS, Svensson PJ, Becktor JP. Treatment with local hemostatic agents and primary closure after tooth extraction in warfarin treated patients. Swed Dent J. 2013;37(2):71–7.
52. Thomason JM, Seymour RA, Murphy P, et al. Aspirin-induced post-gingivectomy haemorrhage: a timely reminder. J Clin Periodontol. 1997;24(2):136–8.
53. Wahl MJ, Schmitt MM. Postextraction bleeding in a patient taking antithrombotics: report of a case. Gen Dent. 2016;64(3):60–3.
54. Zirk M, Fienitz T, Edel R, et al. Prevention of post-operative bleeding in hemostatic compromised patients using native porcine collagen fleeces – retrospective study of a consecutive case series. Oral Maxillofac Surg. 2016;20:249–54.
55. Candemir B, Güleç S, Özdemir AO, Kumbasar D. Very late drug-eluting stent thrombosis in a patient with an INR of 4.4. Arch Turk Soc Cardiol. 2010;38:561–3.
56. Collet J-P, Himbert D, Steg PG. Myocardial infarction after aspirin cessation in stable coronary artery disease patients [Letter]. Int J Cardiol. 2000;76:257–8.

57. Ferrari E, Benhamou M, Cerboni P, Marcel B. Coronary syndromes following aspirin withdrawal: a special risk for late stent thrombosis. J Am Coll Cardiol. 2005;45(3):456–9.
58. Ferreira-González I, Marsal JR, Ribera A, et al. Background, incidence, and predictors of antiplatelet therapy discontinuation during the first year after drug-eluting stent implantation. Circulation. 2010;122:1017–25.
59. Gagneja M, Gagneja P, Steelman R, Shaughnessy R, Johannes PW. Oral surgery in a child with a prosthetic aortic valve and pulmonary artery stent at risk for thromboembolism. J Clin Pediatr Dent. 2007;32(2):151–4.
60. Kovacic JC, Lee P, Karjgikar R, et al. Safety of temporary and permanent suspension of antiplatelet therapy after drug eluting stent implantation in contemporary "real world" practice. J Intervent Cardiol. 2012;25:482–92.
61. Loomba A, Loomba K, Bains R, Bains VK. Management of a dentigerous cyst in a medically compromised geriatric patient: a case report. Gerodontology. 2012;29(2):e1190–4.
62. Derogar M, Sandblom G, Lundell L, et al. Discontinuation of low-dose aspirin therapy after peptic ulcer bleeding increases risk of death and acute cardiovascular events. Clin Gastroenterol Hepatol. 2013;11(1):38–42.
63. García Rodríguez LA, Cea-Soriano L, Martín-Merino E, Johansson S. Discontinuation of low dose aspirin and risk of myocardial infarction: case-control study in UK primary care. Brit Med J. 2011;343:d4094.
64. García Rodríguez LA, Cea Soriano L, Hill C, Johansson S. Increased risk of stroke after discontinuation of acetylsalicylic acid: a UK primary care study. Neurology. 2011;76(8):740–6.
65. Biondi-Zoccai GGL, Lotrionte M, Agostoni P, et al. A systematic review and meta-analysis on the hazards of discontinuing or not adhering to aspirin among 50,279 patients at risk for coronary artery disease. Eur Heart J. 2006;27:2667–74.
66. Sibon I, Orgogozo JM. Antiplatelet drug discontinuation is a risk factor for ischemic stroke. Neurology. 2004;62:1187–9.
67. Maulaz AB, Bezerra DC, Michel P, et al. Effect of discontinuing aspirin therapy on the risk of brain ischemic stroke. Arch Neurol. 2005;62(8):1217–20.
68. Oscarsson A, Gupta A, Fredrikson M, et al. To continue or discontinue aspirin in the perioperative period: a randomized, controlled trial. Br J Anaesgth. 2010;104(3):305–12.
69. Mantz J, Samama CM, Tubach F, et al. Impact of preoperative maintenance or interruption of aspirin on thrombotic and bleeding events after elective non-cardiac surgery: the multicentre, randomized, blinded, placebo-controlled STRATAGEM trial. Br J Anaesth. 2011;107(6):899–910.
70. Broderick JP, Bonomo JB, Kissela BM, et al. Withdrawal of antithrombotic agents and its impact on ischemic stroke occurrence. Stroke. 2011;42:2509–14.
71. Grines CL, Bonow RO, Casey DE, et al. Prevention of premature discontinuation of antiplatelet therapy in patients with coronary artery stents: a science advisory from the American Heart Association, American College of Cardiology, Society for Cardiovascular Angiography and Interventions, American College of Surgeons, and American Dental Association, with representation from the American College of Physicians. Circulation. 2007;115:813–8.
72. Douketis JD, Spyropoulos AC, Spencer FA, et al. Perioperative management of antithrombotic therapy: antithrombotic therapy and prevention of thrombosis, 9th ed: American College of Chest Physicians evidence-based clinical practice guidelines. Chest. 2012;141(2 Suppl):e326S–50S.
73. Armstrong MJ, Gronseth G, Anderson DC, et al. Summary of evidence-based guideline: periprocedural management of antithrombotic medications in patients with ischemic cerebrovascular disease. Report of the Guideline Development Subcommittee of the American Academy of Neurology. Neurology. 2013;80(22):2065–9.
74. Mashour GA, Moore LE, Lele AV, Robicsek SA, Gelb AW. Perioperative care of patients at high risk for stroke during or after non-cardiac, non-neurologic surgery: consensus statement from the Society for Neuroscience in Anesthesiology and Critical Care. J Neurosurg Anesthesiol. 2014;26(4):273–85.
75. American Dental Association. Anticoagulant and antiplatelet medications and dental procedures. Available: http://www.ada.org/en/member-center/oral-health-topics/anticoagulant-antiplatelet-medications-and-dental-Accessed January 21, 2017.

# 13 Perioperative Management of Patients on Anticoagulant Medications: General Principles in Medicine and Surgery

Jessica Rimsans and Katelyn W. Sylvester

**Abstract**

Patients on oral anticoagulation (OAC) requiring an invasive procedure or surgery may require interruptions to their anticoagulation regimen depending on patient- and procedure-specific factors. The risks of both thromboembolism and procedural-related bleeding need to be considered as well as provider and patient preferences. Though some dental procedures allow for continuation of OAC, other procedures may require that their anticoagulation regimen be continued at a minimized intensity, held, or switched to a temporary "bridging" agent. A plan specific to each event requires coordination with the patient, the provider overseeing the patient's anticoagulation regimen (e.g., primary care provider, cardiologist, or other specialist) and the provider performing the surgery or invasive procedure. This chapter will focus on the periprocedural management of anticoagulants.

J. Rimsans · K. W. Sylvester (✉)
Brigham and Women's Hospital, Boston, MA, USA
e-mail: jrimsans@bwh.harvard.edu;
Ksylvester3@bwh.harvard.edu

## 13.1 Introduction

For patients on anticoagulation requiring an invasive dental procedure or surgery, providers must consider both the risks of thromboembolism (if anticoagulation is withheld or intensity minimized) and the risk of periprocedural bleeding. This assessment is used to determine if interruption of anticoagulation is required and if so, guides the development of a periprocedural anticoagulation plan to mitigate associated risks. A plan should be developed in conjunction with the patient's primary care provider and/or cardiologist. Most low-risk dental procedures, such as single tooth extractions, will not require interruption of anticoagulation since the procedure itself has minimal risk of bleeding [1, 2]. For other procedures, the risk of bleeding associated with the specific procedure/surgery, patient-specific risk factors for thrombosis and bleeding, and the bleeding risk associated with their current anticoagulation regimen should be considered when evaluating the need to transition to a short-acting parenteral or "bridging" agent. The risks of bleeding and thromboembolism should be weighed to determine if anticoagulation should be continued, continued with minimized intensity, held, or switched to a temporary "bridging" agent. Patient and provider preferences should also be incorporated in the plan. For patients on short-term anticoagulation (e.g., for treatment of a provoked deep vein thrombosis)



R. P. Szumita, P. M. Szumita (eds.), *Hemostasis in Dentistry*, https://doi.org/10.1007/978-3-319-71240-6_13

with a high risk of thromboembolism, the practitioner should consider postponing elective high bleeding risk dental procedures until the risk of thromboembolism is acceptable [3, 4].

## 13.2 Thromboembolism Risk Assessment

Major thromboembolic events, including fatalities, have occurred due to holding anticoagulation for prolonged periods of time around dental procedures, despite there being limited reports of severe bleeding associated with these procedures that cannot be controlled by local hemostatic measures [5, 6]. Prior to a planned procedure, a thorough assessment of the risk of thromboembolism should be completed using a standardized risk stratification tool; when available a tool validated in patients with the same underlying disease state should be utilized [1]. Validated tools include the $CHADS_2$ score (most commonly used in previous clinical trials and current guidelines) and the newer $CHA_2DS_2$-VASc (currently used in clinical practice)—both validated in patients with atrial fibrillation [7]. The American College of Chest Physicians guidelines provide a risk stratification tool to determine if patients are at high, moderate, or low risk for thromboembolism when anticoagulation is interrupted during a perioperative period. Patients categorized as high risk have a greater than 10% annual risk of recurrent thromboembolism [1]. Should anticoagulation be interrupted, factors increasing the risk of an event include a recent thromboembolic event, presence of a mechanical mitral valve, recent stroke/transient ischemic attack (within the past 3 months), and high $CHADS_2$ or $CHA_2DS_2$-Vasc score (Table 13.1) [8]. Other patient-specific factors should be considered such as previous thromboembolic event during interruption of anticoagulation, more than one previous event, or multiple risk factors. Dental procedures/surgeries do not typically increase the risk of thromboembolism above the patient's baseline risk, with the reported incidence of venous thromboembolism in major oral and maxillofacial surgery being less than 0.06% [9].

**Table 13.1** Risk factors for thromboembolic events during interruption of anticoagulation [8]

| |
|---|
| Mitral mechanical valve |
| High-risk prosthetic valve (caged ball, tilting disc) |
| Recent stroke or transient ischemic attack (within 3 months) |
| $CHADS_2$ score 5 or 6 |
| Rheumatic valvular heart disease |
| Recent venous thromboembolism (within 3 months) |
| Severe thrombophilia |

## 13.3 Bleeding Risk Assessment

The risk of periprocedural bleeding must be assessed from multiple viewpoints including (1) the risk associated with the specific intervention; (2) the baseline patient-specific risks including all concurrent medications, bleeding history, and organ function; (3) the risk of the intervention in the presence of anticoagulants; (4) the risks associated with bridging; and (5) the availability of topical hemostatic agents to minimize bleeding and, if needed, emergency agents to address major life-threatening bleeding. Various tools exist to evaluate a patient's risk for bleeding on anticoagulation and should be used where appropriate [10]. It is important to determine the population used to validate the risk assessment tool to ensure it is applicable to the patient being evaluated.

The type of dental procedure is the most important risk factor for post-procedural bleeding. Although there are limited high-quality data published to guide the practitioner, there are published case reports, case series, and extrapolation of data from other fields that provide the baseline for expert opinion guidelines [3–5, 8]. The provider must consider the complexity of the procedure including number of teeth involved, surface area, invasiveness, and expected amount of inflammation when determining the expected risk of bleeding [8]. Procedures that are likely to incur a higher risk of bleeding include multiple extractions or impacted extractions, incisional

**Table 13.2** Patient-specific risk factors for bleeding on anticoagulation

| Patient characteristics | Comorbidities |
|---|---|
| Advanced age (>55 years old) | Diabetes |
| Female gender | Vascular disease |
| Previous history of bleeding | Renal dysfunction |
| Poorly controlled INRs | Heparin dysfunction |
| Alcohol consumption | Congestive heart failure |
| Concomitant drugs | Anemia |
| | Active cancer |
| | Hypotension or hypertension |

biopsies from highly vascular or inflamed tissue, and periodontal grafting [5, 8, 10]. In contrast, dental procedures generally incurring a low risk of bleeding include simple single extractions and routine dental hygiene [10].

Patient-specific considerations include a thorough review of the patient's medication and medical history (Table 13.2) and concomitant medications that may increase the patient's risk of periprocedural bleeding including antiplatelet agents (e.g., aspirin, clopidogrel, ticagrelor, prasugrel) and nonsteroidal anti-inflammatory agents (e.g., ibuprofen, naproxen) [8]. Past medical history should also be reviewed to determine if a patient has had previous dental surgery while on therapeutic anticoagulation, and if so, were there any bleeding complications. Additionally, the provider should evaluate if there is a history of procedures with a similar risk of bleeding, such as dermatological procedures, and if the patient experienced any bleeding events. Finally, the provider should review baseline labs such as coagulation panels with a complete blood count and platelet count to identify predisposing risks for bleeding [8]. For patients on a vitamin K antagonist, an INR should be obtained to ensure anticoagulation is not supratherapeutic at the time of the intervention. For patients on a direct oral anticoagulant (DOAC), serum creatinine and liver function tests should be obtained to evaluate for altered drug clearance.

For patients on vitamin K antagonists with a high risk of thromboembolism whose dental procedure cannot be delayed, the practitioner may decide to hold warfarin and use a short-acting parenteral anticoagulant (once the INR is expected to be less than 2) around the time of the procedure. Registry data demonstrates this is unnecessary for the vast majority of patients and oral anticoagulation with warfarin and may be continued as long as the INR is less than 3 at the time of the procedure [11]. In this case, the risk of bleeding associated with the bridging agent must also be considered. For those receiving a DOAC, bridging is not recommended given the pharamcokinetics of these agents. If interruption of the DOAC is indicated based on evaluation of thrombosis and periprocedural bleeding risk, the time frame for discontinuation should be based on the patient's renal function and risk for bleeding associated with the procedure (see Table 13.3).

**Table 13.3** Management of direct-acting oral anticoagulants if periprocedural interruption of anticoagulation is required [12–17]

| Calculated CrCl (ml/min) | Timing of last dose before surgery | |
|---|---|---|
| | Low risk of bleeding | High risk of bleeding |
| Dabigatran | | |
| >50 | 24 h (PI: discontinue 1–2 days before) | 2 days (PI: consider longer times if major surgery, spinal puncture, spinal or epidural catheter, patients in whom complete hemostasis may be required) |
| 31–50 | 2 days (PI: discontinue 3–5 days before if CrCl <50 ml/min) | 5 days (PI: discontinue 3–5 days before if CrCl <50 ml/min) |
| <30 | 4 days | 5–6 days |
| Rivaroxaban, apixaban, edoxaban | | |
| >50 | 1 day | 2 days |
| 31–50 | 1–2 days | 3–4 days |
| <30 | 2 days | 4 days |

*PI* package insert, *CrCl* creatinine clearance

Regardless of the approach for managing anticoagulation around the time of the procedure, the provider should be aware of the availability of local and system hemostatic agents available should bleeding occur (both of which will be discussed in detail in subsequent chapters).

## 13.4 Periprocedural Management of Anticoagulation

For patients that are deemed high risk for a thromboembolic event and necessitate bridging, use of prophylactic dose low molecular weight heparin (LMWH), therapeutic dose LMWH, or intravenous unfractionated heparin (UFH) may be considered. Other options may include fondaparinux or therapeutic doses of subcutaneous UFH. In those with a mechanical heart valve, continuous infusion UFH is the preferred agent, but LMWH may be utilized in special circumstances. These agents should be started when the INR is less than 2.0, or at the time the next DOAC dose would be due [12–17]. See Fig. 13.1 for details.

Routine monitoring of coagulation assays is not used for determining therapeutic concentrations in those receiving DOACS. Though abnormal coagulation assays may be helpful in deciding if residual effect is circulating, normal assays cannot rule out that the effect has resolved. In patients receiving factor Xa inhibitors (e.g., rivaroxaban, apixaban, edoxaban) undergoing high-risk dental procedures or those with maxillofacial trauma, one may consider using an anti-factor Xa level that is calibrated to LMWH/UFH to exclude any relevant drug concentrations [3]. For those receiving direct thrombin inhibitors (e.g., dabigatran), the activated partial thromboplastin time (aPTT) may be useful in determining residual anticoagulant effect. Though not specific, patients who are anticoagulated will have an elevated aPTT above baseline. Although the ecarin clotting time (ECT) is the most sensitive assay to determine therapeutic levels, it is unavailable for routine use in the United States [3].

If a bridging agent was initiated, it is important to stop this agent prior to the procedure. The exact time to stop the agent is dependent on the bleeding risk of the procedure and patient's renal function. See Tables 13.4 and 13.5 for practical

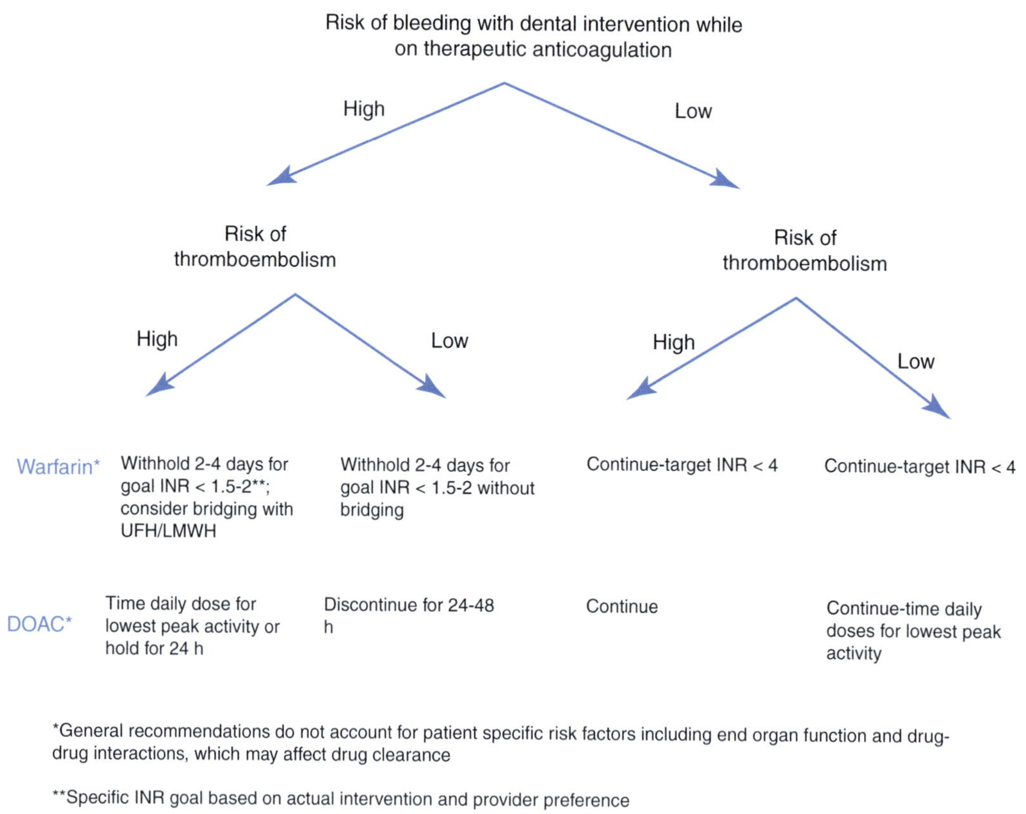


**Fig. 13.1** Periprocedural management of patients on oral anticoagulants

**Table 13.4** Practical considerations for transitioning between various oral anticoagulants and parenteral agents [12–16]

| | To therapeutic dose DOAC | To warfarin | To therapeutic IV UFH | To therapeutic SC LMWH, UFH, or fondaparinux |
|---|---|---|---|---|
| From therapeutic IV UFH | *Considerations*:<br>• $t_{1/2}$ IV UFH = 60 min<br>*Transition*:<br>• Stop IV UFH and administer first dose of DOAC when aPTT <100 s<br>• Continue DOAC based on PI recommendation per indication | *Transition*:<br>• Start warfarin therapy with IV UFH<br>• Discontinue IV UFH when INR ≥2.0 for two consecutive readings | *Transition*:<br>• Restart postoperatively immediately or up to 72 h post-procedure based on hemostasis, renal function, and interventionalist | *Considerations*:<br>• $t_{1/2}$ IV UFH = 60 min<br>*Transition*:<br>• Stop IV UFH and administer first dose of SC LMWH, UFH, or fondaparinux when aPTT <100 s<br>• Hold all subsequent doses of IV UFH |
| From IV DTI (bivalirudin, argatroban) | *Considerations*:<br>• $t_{1/2}$ bivalirudin = 25 min, argatroban = 45 min<br>• Time DOAC dose so that DOAC $t_{max}$ occurs when IV DTI is cleared<br>*Transition*:<br>• Stop IV DTI and administer first dose of DOAC if aPTT <100 s<br>• Evaluate renal and hepatic function; if impaired extend initial interval accordingly<br>• Continue DOAC based on PI recommendation per indication | *Transition*:<br>• Start warfarin therapy with IV DTI<br>• Continue warfarin bridge until INR is ≥4.0 for argatroban or ≥2.5 for bivalirudin<br>• Turn off infusion and recheck INR 4 h later. If INR ≥2.0 resume warfarin alone, if <2.0 resume bridge with IV DTI | *Considerations*:<br>• $t_{1/2}$ bivalirudin = 25 min, argatroban = 45 min<br>• Initial bolus may be utilized to achieve therapeutic aPTT depending on thromboembolic/bleeding risk as determined by interventionalist<br>*Transition*:<br>• Turn off the IV DTI, and start IV UFH +/− bolus<br>• If aPTT >100 s, wait 1 h to start IV UFH infusion | *Considerations*:<br>• $t_{1/2}$ bivalirudin = 25 min, argatroban = 45 min<br>• Time DOAC dose so that DOAC $t_{max}$ occurs when IV DTI is cleared<br>*Transition*:<br>• Stop IV DTI and administer first dose of SC LMWH, UFH, or fondaparinux when aPTT <100 s<br>• Hold all subsequent parenteral DTI doses |
| From therapeutic SC LMWH, UFH, or fondaparinux | *Considerations*:<br>• $t_{1/2}$ LMWH = 6–7 h, fondaparinux = 17–21 h<br>*Transition*:<br>• Administer first dose of DOAC when next SC LMWH/ fondaparinux is due<br>• Hold all subsequent parenteral doses<br>• Continue DOAC based on PI recommendation per indication | *Transition*:<br>• Start warfarin therapy with LMWH, UFH, or fondaparinux<br>• Discontinue the injectable agent when INR ≥2.0 for two consecutive readings | *Considerations*:<br>• $t_{1/2}$ LMWH = 6–7 h, fondaparinux = 17–21 h<br>*Transition*:<br>• Start IV UFH at the next scheduled dose of LMWH, UFH, or fondaparinux | *Transition*:<br>• Restart postoperatively immediately or up to 72 h post-procedure based on hemostasis, renal function, and interventionalist<br>• Hold all subsequent therapeutic doses of LMWH, UFH, or fondaparinux |

(continued)

**Table 13.4** (continued)

| | To therapeutic dose DOAC | To warfarin | To therapeutic IV UFH | To therapeutic SC LMWH, UFH, or fondaparinux |
|---|---|---|---|---|
| From prophylactic dose SC LMWH, UFH, or fondaparinux | *Considerations*:<br>• $t_{1/2}$ LMWH = 6–7 h, fondaparinux = 17–21 h<br>*Transition*:<br>• Administer first dose of DOAC when next SQ LMWH/UFH/ fondaparinux is due<br>• Hold all subsequent parenteral doses<br>• Continue DOAC based on PI recommendation per indication | *Transition*:<br>• Start warfarin therapy with LMWH, UFH, or fondaparinux<br>• Discontinue the injectable agent when INR ≥2.0 for two consecutive readings | *Considerations*:<br>• $t_{1/2}$ LMWH = 6–7 h, fondaparinux = 17–21 h<br>*Transition*:<br>• Start IV UFH at the next scheduled dose of UFH, LMWH, or fondaparinux | *Considerations*:<br>• $t_{1/2}$ LMWH = 6–7 h, fondaparinux = 17–21 h<br>*Transition*:<br>• Administer first dose of SC LMWH, UFH, or fondaparinux when aPTT <100 s<br>• Hold all subsequent prophylactic doses |
| From warfarin | *Considerations*:<br>• For AF patients taking rivaroxaban, consider starting when INR <3.0<br>• For AF patients taking edoxaban, consider starting when INR <2.5<br>*Transition*:<br>• Give final warfarin dose, hold all subsequent doses<br>• Wait 2–3 days or until INR <2.0, give first dose of DOAC | *Considerations*:<br>• Pending thromboembolic risk, a bridging agent may be utilized until a therapeutic INR is reached<br>*Transition*:<br>• Restart postoperatively immediately or up to 72 h post-procedure based on hemostasis, renal function, and interventionalist | *Transition*:<br>• Start IV UFH when the INR is <2.0[a] | *Transition*:<br>• Start SC LMWH, UFH, or fondaparinux doses when the INR <2.0[a] |
| From DOAC | *Transition*:<br>• Restart postoperatively immediately or up to 72 h post-procedure based on hemostasis, renal function, and interventionalist | *Considerations*:<br>• See PI for specific recommendations as differ for each DOAC | *Considerations*:<br>• Initial bolus may be utilized to achieve therapeutic aPTT depending on thromboembolic/bleeding risk as determined by interventionalist<br>*Transition*:<br>• Start IV UFH when the next dose of DOAC is due | *Transition*:<br>• Discontinue the DOAC, and start SC LMWH, UFH, or fondaparinux at the next scheduled dose the DOAC would be due |

Considerations for all transitions:

- Pharmacodynamics including the half-life ($t½$) of the current anticoagulant
- Pharmacokinetics including the time to maximum concentration ($t_{max}$) when transitioning to oral anticoagulants
- Patient-specific factors such as renal and hepatic end-organ function to evaluate for prolonged clearance

*AF* atrial fibrillation; *IV* intravenous; *UFH* unfractionated heparin; *DTI* direct thrombin inhibitor; *DOAC* direct-acting oral anticoagulants including rivaroxaban, dabigatran, edoxaban, and apixaban; *aPTT* activated partial thromboplastin time; *PI* package insert

[a]Note: If INR goal is 2.5–3.5, timing of starting bridge is up to discretion of interventionalist, typically started when INR <2.0

**Table 13.5** Determine when to stop bridging therapy perioperatively

| Bridging therapy | Discontinuation of therapy postoperatively |
|---|---|
| Prophylactic LMWH | Last dose 12–24 h prior to surgery/procedure |
| IV UFH | Discontinue 6 h prior to surgery/procedure |
| Therapeutic LMWH | Last dose 24 h prior to surgery/procedure |

**Table 13.6** Determine when to re-initiate anticoagulation therapy postop [1]

| Surgery/procedure bleeding risk | Anticoagulation re-initiation recommendation |
|---|---|
| Low risk | • Approximately 24 h after (following day)<br>• Warfarin may be initiated the evening of the procedure at the patient's previously determined maintenance dose or a slightly increased dose about 50% higher than previous dose |
| High risk | The following options may be considered:<br>• Therapeutic LMWH/IV UFH re-initiation may be delayed 48–72 h (POD 2 or 3) after procedure<br>• Prophylactic LMWH may be initiated until bleeding risk subsides, and then therapeutic LMWH can be started<br>• All anticoagulant medications may be held<br>• Warfarin may be initiated the evening of surgery (orthopedic surgeries) or delayed until bleeding risk subsides |

considerations for transitioning between various OACs and parenteral anticoagulants [10].

## 13.5 Re-initiation of Anticoagulation

If anticoagulation was held, it is recommended to discuss re-initiation of anticoagulation therapy with the surgeon/proceduralist. Clinicians may prefer to restart anticoagulation once hemostasis is achieved with a shorter-acting parenteral agent, such as continuous infusion UFH to monitor for bleeding. Alternatively, once hemostasis is achieved, the proceduralist may resume the patient's home OAC regimen (Table 13.6).

If the patient was previously on warfarin, a bridge to a therapeutic INR may be considered using a short-acting parenteral agent. This is dependent upon the risk of thromboembolism, where those at high risk may require a bridge [11]. A bridge is not indicated when restarting a DOAC due to their rapid onset of action which is typically between 1 and 4 h depending on the specific agent (refer to Chap. 12 for a more detailed review of the pharmacokinetics of specific oral anticoagulants).

## References

1. Douketis JD, Spyropoulos AC, Spender FA, Mayr M, Jaffer AK, Eckman MH, Dunn AS, Kunz R, American College of Chest Physicians. Perioperative management of antithrombotic therapy: antithrombotic therapy and prevention of thrombosis, 9th ed: American College of Chest Physicians Evidence-Based Clinical Practice Guidelines. Chest. 2012;141(2):e326S–05S.
2. Pototski M, Amenabar JM. Dental management of patients receiving anticoagulation or antiplatelet treatment. J Oral Sci. 2007;49(4):253–8.
3. Steed MB, Swanson MT. Warfarin and newer agents: what the oral surgeon needs to know. Oral Maxillofac Surg Clin North Am. 2016;28:515–21.
4. Martinez M, Tsakiris DA. Management of antithrombotic agents in oral surgery. Dent J. 2015;3:93–101.
5. Ward BB, Smith MH. Dentoalveolar procedures for the anticoagulated patient: literature recommendations versus current practice. J Oral Maxillofac Surg. 2007;65:1454–60.
6. Hong C, Napenas JJ, Brennan M, Furney S, Lockhart P. Risk of postoperative bleeding after dental procedures in patients on warfarin: a retrospective study. Oral Surg Oral Med Oral Pathol Oral Radiol. 2012;114:464–8.
7. Olesen JB, Lip GYH, Hansen ML, Hansen PR, et al. Validation of risk stratification schemes for predicting stroke and thromboembolism in patients with atrial fibrillations: nationwide cohort study. BMJ. 2011;342:d124.
8. Elad S, Marshall J, Meyerowitz C, Connoll G. Novel anticoagulants: general overview and practical considerations for dental practitioners. Oral Dis. 2016;22:23–32.
9. Ramesh Babu MR, Ramesh C, Thirumurugan K, Arun Prasad G. Deep vein thrombosis: a rate complication in oral and maxillofacial surgery: a review of two cases. Contemp Clin Dent. 2013;4(2):236–8.
10. Rimsans J, Sylvester K, Fanikos J. Transitions in care—periprocedural bridging and transitions between agents. In: Dager WE, Gulseth BP, Nutescu EA, editors. ASHP anticoagulation therapy, point of

care. Bethesda, MD: American Society of Health-System Pharmacists. [In Press; expected publication Spring 2017].
11. Douketis JD, Spyropoulos AC, Kaatz S, et al. Perioperative bridging anticoagulation in patients with atrial fibrillation. N Engl J Med. 2015;373:823–33.
12. Dabigatran [package insert]. Ridgefield, CT: Boehringer Ingelheim Pharmaceuticals, Inc; 2015.
13. Rivaroxaban [package insert]. Titusville, NJ: Janssen Pharmaceuticals, Inc; 2015.
14. Apixaban [package insert]. Princeton, NJ: Bristol-Meyers Squibb Company; 2015.
15. Edoxaban [package insert]. Parsippany, NJ: Daiichi Sankyo Inc; 2015.
16. Schulman S, Carrier M, Lee AYY, et al. Perioperative management of dabigatran: a prospective cohort study. Circulation. 2015;132(3):167–73.
17. Spyropoulos AC, Douketis JD. How I treat anticoagulated patients undergoing an elective procedure or surgery. Blood. 2012;120(15):2954–62.

# 14 Perioperative Management of Dental Patients on Anticoagulants

Michael J. Wahl

*The withdrawal of anticoagulant and antiplatelet medications is associated with a substantial number of acute first-ever and recurrent ischemic strokes.*

Broderick et al. Stroke 2011


**Abstract**

When continuously anticoagulated patients present for dental surgery, a decision must be made to continue anticoagulation and risk bleeding complications or to interrupt anticoagulation and risk embolic complication like stroke or heart attack. The incidence and morbidity of postdental bleeding complications in anticoagulated patients have been overestimated, and at the same time the increased embolic risks when anticoagulation has been interrupted have been underestimated. A search of the literature reveals that of more than 7376 anticoagulated patients undergoing 14,879 surgical procedures including 13,703 extractions, there were only about 486 bleeding complications (6% of patient visits), of which only 33 (0.4% of patients and visits) required more than local measures for hemostasis. On the other hand, there have been at least 3278 dental patients whose anticoagulation was interrupted for at least 3380 appointments. A total of 29 of these patients (0.9% of patients or visits) have had embolic complications after interruption, including 7 fatalities (0.2% of patients or visits). As a result, therapeutic anticoagulation levels should not be interrupted for dental surgery.



M. J. Wahl
Christiana Care Health System,
Wilmington, DE, USA


Millions of patients' lives have been prolonged by the discovery of continuous anticoagulant medications, which can prevent embolic complications such as stroke and heart attack. Continuous anticoagulant medications like the vitamin K antagonist warfarin are used to prevent embolic complications including stroke or heart attack in patients with atrial fibrillation, pulmonary embolism, deep vein thrombosis, a history of stroke, and mechanical heart valves. Warfarin's therapeutic effect is measured by the International Normalized Ratio (INR), and for most patients, the therapeutic range for anticoagulation is between INR 2.0 and 3.0, but for patients with mechanical mitral heart valves, the recommended range is between INR 2.5 and 3.5 [1]. Since warfarin's therapeutic effect can be enhanced or diminished by interactions with other medications or food, INR levels are typically checked periodically with blood testing, either at a medical facility or with home testing devices. There are now direct-acting oral anticoagulants (DOACs) that act differently than vitamin K inhibitors like warfarin (Coumadin), including direct thrombin inhibitors like dabigatran (Pradaxa) and direct factor Xa inhibitors like apixaban (Eliquis), rivaroxaban (Xarelto), and edoxaban (Savaysa). Although more expensive than warfarin, the DOACs do not require INR monitoring, have fewer drug interactions, a rapid onset, and a much shorter half-life (5–17 h) than warfarin's 20–60 (mean 40) h. As a result, when



R. P. Szumita, P. M. Szumita (eds.), *Hemostasis in Dentistry*, https://doi.org/10.1007/978-3-319-71240-6_14

DOAC therapy is interrupted, normal coagulation is achieved much faster than when warfarin therapy is interrupted. The standard interruption interval among those recommending interruption of anticoagulation for dental procedures is usually 2 or 3 days for warfarin and 1 day for DOACs.

Dentists see anticoagulated patients on a daily basis and when dental surgery is contemplated must weigh the risks of bleeding complications when anticoagulation is continued versus the risk of embolic complications when anticoagulation is interrupted for surgery. As early as 1956, Askey and Cherry reported on six anticoagulated patients undergoing 14 extractions without bleeding complications and concluded that the embolic risk with anticoagulation interruption for dental extractions exceeded the bleeding risk with continuation [2]. Soon thereafter, however, Ziffer et al. reported in 1957 three cases of "profound" bleeding after dental extractions in two anticoagulated patients and concluded that the risk of excessive bleeding exceeded the risk of thromboembolism in anticoagulated patients and advised a brief interruption in therapy for these patients [3]. Local measures for hemostasis were insufficient, and these patients were given injections of vitamin K to reverse anticoagulation. (It should be noted that anticoagulation in these patients was well above current therapeutic levels.) Ever since these reports, dental surgery in anticoagulated patients has been controversial and the subject of avid interest in the medical and dental literature.

This author and his group have conducted narrative reviews of dental surgery in thousands of anticoagulated patients showing there is a small but significant risk of serious and sometimes fatal embolic complications with anticoagulation interruption for dental procedures, which outweighs the small risk of bleeding complications when anticoagulation is continued [4, 5]. These postdental bleeding complications have never been shown to be fatal and are almost always simple to treat with local measures for hemostasis. Of only 33 cases (0.4%) of bleeding complications requiring more than hemostatic measures, most were in patients with significant comorbidities and/or significantly higher than therapeutic INR levels. Unlike patients suffering embolic complications, who can suffer permanent disabilities or even death, every postdental bleeding complication patient presumably made a full recovery.

These reviews have been updated for this chapter with still more studies of dental surgery in anticoagulated patients (including single, multiple, full mouth, and surgical extractions, as well as other surgical procedures like alveoplasties, gingival surgery, and implant placement) showing that of more than 7376 anticoagulated patients at 7685 visits of more than 14,879 surgical procedures including 13,703 extractions, there were about 486 (6% of patient visits) bleeding complications, of which only 33 (0.4% of patients and visits) required more than local measures for hemostasis [2, 3, 6–11] (see Table 14.1). On the other hand, there have been at least 3278 dental patients whose anticoagulation was interrupted for at least 3380 appointments. Unfortunately, 29 of these patients (0.9% of patients or visits) have had embolic complications after interruption, including 7 fatalities (0.2% of patients or visits) [3, 6, 10, 11, 13, 18, 25, 29, 30, 32, 33, 36, 42, 43, 46, 47, 49, 51, 52, 57, 58, 62, 68, 79, 82, 88, 91, 98, 99, 104, 108, 110–160] (see Table 14.2).

Paradoxically, even though anticoagulation theoretically increases the postoperative bleeding risk, the 6% bleeding complication rate (including both minor bleeding complications requiring additional local hemostatic measures and bleeding complications requiring more than local measures for hemostasis) was the same in both the anticoagulated group and the interruption group, and those bleeding complications requiring more than local measures for hemostasis were actually higher in the interruption group than in the anticoagulation group. Among these embolic complications, 16 (4 fatal) occurred after interruptions of between 1 and 5 days. There is apparently little or no benefit with bleeding complications, but there is increased embolic risk when interrupting anticoagulation for dental procedures.

While these reviews address interruptions only for dental procedures, there have been many more reports of embolic complications after relatively brief periods of anticoagulation

**Table 14.1** Dental surgery in continuously anticoagulated patients

| Source | No. of patients treated (visits) | No. of surgical procedures | No. of extractions | INR for those on vitamin K antagonists like warfarin | Comment | Postop bleeding requiring professional treatment at least with local measures (other than immediately postop) | Bleeding complications requiring more than local measures |
|---|---|---|---|---|---|---|---|
| Abayon et al. 2016 [6] | 3 (3) | 14 | 14 | INR not reported for warfarin patient | Rivaroxaban, dabigatran, or warfarin | 1 | 0 |
| Abdullah and Khalil 2014 [7] | 35 (35) | 35 | 35 | INR 2.0–3.5 | Warfarin | 4 | 0 |
| Al Zoman et al. 2013 [8] | 2 (2) | 2 | 0 | 4.1 and 4.0 on the days of the procedures | | 0 | 0 |
| Al-Belasy and Amer 2003 [9] | 30 (30) | 155 | 155 | 1.7–4.3 | | 5 | 0 |
| Al-Mubarak et al. 2006 [10], 2007 [11] | 110 (110) | >110 | >110 | Mean 2.4–2.7 | | 8 | 0 |
| Alexander et al. 2002 [12] | 15 (15) | 28 | 27 | 1.9–3.6 (mean 2.57) | All 27 extractions were surgical | 0 | 0 |
| Anavi et al. 1981 [13] | 15 (15) | 52 | 52 | PT 19–36%; mean 27.5% [*INR <2.5 to INR >3.0*] | | 7 | 0 |
| Askey and Cherry 1956 [2] | 6 (10) | 14 | 14 | Prothrombin concentration 14–51% [*INR <2.0 to INR >3.5*] | | 0 | 0 |
| Bacci et al. 2010 [14] | 451 (451) | 926 | 926 | 1.8–4.0 (mean 2.14) | 379 extractions were surgical | 7 | 0 |
| Bacci et al. 2011 [15] | 50 (50) | 159 | 0 | 1.8–4.0 | All were single or multiple implant placement | 2 | 0 |
| Bailey and Fordyce 1983 [16] | 25 (25) | 156 | 156 | PT ratio 1.2–4.3; mean PT ratio 2.4 | | 59 | 0 |
| Bajkin et al. 2015 [17] | 125 (125) | 319 | 306 | INR 2.01–4.2 | Warfarin; absorbable collagen, gelatin sponges, oxidized cellulose, and/or suturing | 7 | 0 |
| Bajkin et al. 2009 [18] | 109 (109) | 194 | 194 | 1.68–4.0 (mean 2.45) | | 4 | 0 |
| Bajkin et al. 2012 [19] | 213 (213) | 142 | 235 | Mean 2.43–2.45 | 71 were on combined warfarin-aspirin | 5 (INR 2.32–3.45) | 0 |

(continued)

**Table 14.1** (continued)

| Source | No. of patients treated (visits) | No. of surgical procedures | No. of extractions | INR for those on vitamin K antagonists like warfarin | Comment | Postop bleeding requiring professional treatment at least with local measures (other than immediately postop) | Bleeding complications requiring more than local measures |
|---|---|---|---|---|---|---|---|
| Bajkin et al. 2014 [20] | 90 (90) | >90 | >90 | INR ≤3.0 (mean 2.35–2.43) | Group 1 sutured, group 2 Surgicel, group 3 neither | 5 | 0 |
| Bakathir 2009 [21] | 124 (124) | 157 | 149 | 2.1–3.5 (mean 2.8) | 26 extractions were surgical | 6 | 0 |
| Bal and Hardee 2000 [22] | 50 (50) | 104 | 104 | 2–4.5 | Tranexamic acid | 0 | 0 |
| Bandrowsky et al. 1996 [23] | 1 (1) | 21 | 20 | INR 3.51 preop; INR 9.03 96 h postop | Tranexamic acid | 0 | 1 pt with good hemostasis 72 h after surgery. Amoxicillin 500 mg tid for 7 days postsurgery was prescribed as prophylaxis. On 4th postsurg day, pt was bleeding and INR 9.03. Coumadin withheld, and pt transfused with fresh frozen plasma, then packed red blood cells, and ultimately vit K. Authors conclude the elevated PT was from interaction with amoxicillin and that the amoxicillin was probably unnecessary |

| | | | | | | | |
|---|---|---|---|---|---|---|---|
| Barrero et al. 2002 [24] | 125 (229) | 367 | 367 | 2.0–3.0 | Postop tranexamic acid mouthwash | 1 | 1 required transfusion |
| Behrman and Wright 1961 [25] | 16 (16) | 41 | 31 | PT ratio 1.2–2.5 | | 0 | 0 |
| Benoliel et al. 1986 [26] | >3 <30 (≥3) | 87 | 87 | PT ratio 1.3–2.5 | | 1 | 0 |
| Blinder et al. 1999 [27] | 150 (150) | 359 | 359 | 1.5–4.0 (mean 2.19–2.7) | Some had tranexamic acid mouthwash | 13 | 0 |
| Blinder et al. 2001 [28] | 249 (249) | 543 | 543 | 1.5 to >3.5 (mean ~2.49) | | 30 | 0 |
| Borea et al. 1993 [29] | 15 (15) | 15 | 15 | INR between 3.0 and 4.5; mean INR 3.09 | Tranexamic acid | 1 | 0 |
| Breik et al. 2014 [30] | 4 (4) | 21 | 21 | | Dabigatran | 2 | 1 case of severe bleeding after 18 extractions requiring postoperative interruption of dabigatran |
| Broekema et al. 2014 [31] | 32 (32) | 32 | ≥19 ≤32 | Mean INR 2.6 (1.9–3.4) | Patients instructed to use tranexamic rinse postoperatively | 3 | 0 |
| Brooks 2011 [32] | 1 (1) | 1 | 1 | 2.5 (5.0 at hospital admission) | Preop and postop amoxicillin also prescribed | 1 | 1 fresh frozen plasma transfusion on 11th postop day |
| Campbell et al. 2000 [33] | 12 (12) | 40 | 38 | 1.2–2.9 (mean 2.0) | | 0 | 0 |
| Candemir et al. 2010 [34] | 1 (1) | 1 | 1 | 4.4 10 days after procedure | | 0 | 0 |
| Cañigral et al. 2010 [35] | 19 (19) | 19 | 19 | Not reported | | 1 | 0 |
| Cannon and Dharmar 2003 [36] | 25 (25) | 72 | 70 | 2.1–4.0 (average 3.4) | | 3 | 0 |
| Carter and Goss 2003 [37] | 85 (85) | 152 | 152 | 2.0–4.0 (avg 2.75) | | 3 | 0 |
| Carter et al. 2003 [38] | 1 (1) | 1 | 1 | 3.8 | Fibrin glue used for surg extraction | 0 | 0 |

(continued)

**Table 14.1** (continued)

| Source | No. of patients treated (visits) | No. of surgical procedures | No. of extractions | INR for those on vitamin K antagonists like warfarin | Comment | Postop bleeding requiring professional treatment at least with local measures (other than immediately postop) | Bleeding complications requiring more than local measures |
|---|---|---|---|---|---|---|---|
| Carter et al. 2003 [39] | 49 (49) | 152 | 152 | 2.1–4.0 (mean 3.0–3.1) | | 2 (1 patient INR 3.6 day of surgery and 5.9 7th day postoperatively; 1 patient INR 2.2 day of surgery and 7.9 3rd postoperative day) | 0 |
| Cesar and Itturiaga 2007 [40] | 1 (1) | 1 | 1 | 2.6 | Tranexamic mouthwashes | 1 | 1 transfused with packed red blood cells and administered vitamin K and full anticoagulation with enoxaparin started, and bleeding continued. Finally controlled with desmopressin. The authors theorize that the LMWH caused the bleeding |
| Cieślik-Bielecka et al. 2005 [41] | 40 (≥42) | 186 | 181 | 1.0–4.0 | | 2 | 2 described as “minor bleeding complications” treated with additional sutures and cyclonamine. 1 patient had 3 teeth removed at INR 3.5; 1 patient had 6 teeth removed at INR 3.0 |
| Clemm et al. 2016 [42] | 48 (48) | 48 | 0 | Mean INR 2.62 for warfarin patients | Implant surgeries on patients on warfarin, dabigatran, apixaban, or rivaroxaban | 2 | 0 |

| | | | | | | | |
|---|---|---|---|---|---|---|---|
| Cocero et al. 2014 [43] | ~140 (~200) | 435 | 435 | INR 1.8–2.98 | Warfarin (92%) and acenocoumarin (8%) | 21 | 0 |
| Cone 1993 [44] | 1 (1) | 1 | 1 | INR 1.5 | | 0 | 0 |
| Dantas et al. 2009 [45] | 26 (26) | 47 | 46 | 1.8–3.8 | | 1 | 0 |
| Davies 2003 [46] | ~24 (~24) | ~≥24 | ~≥24 | Not reported | | 0 | 0 |
| Devani et al. 1998 [47] | 33 (33) | 69 | 69 | INR 2.2–3.9 (mean 2.7) | | 1 | 0 |
| Eichhorn et al. 2012 [48] | 637 (637) | 934 | 88 | 1.2–4.2 (mean 2.44) | | 47 | 2 (anticoagulant changed for 6 days) |
| Elad and Findler 2008 [49] | ≥2 ≤498 (≥2) | ≥2 | ≥2 | Not reported | Perio surgery | 2 INR ≥3.5 | 0 |
| Elad et al. 2010 [50] | 2 (2) | 2 | 2 | 1.88–2.0 | | 0 | 0 |
| Erden et al. 2016 [51] | 36 (36) | 36 | 36 | ≤4.0 (mean 2.5) | Warfarin | None reported | 0 |
| Evans et al. 2002 [52] | 57 (57) | 114 | 114 | 1.2–4.7 (mean 2.5) | | 5 | 0 |
| Febbo et al. 2016 [53] | 439 (439) | 1022 | 1022 | 178 cases preop INR <2.2 (mean 1.72); 261 cases preop INR 2–2.r (mean 2.68) | Warfarin; those with INR ≥2.2 received suturing and tranexamic acid rinse | 9 | 1 patient with "multiple severe medical comorbidities," on multiple medications including a single dose of prophylactic antibiotic, awaiting cardiac transplantation presented with oozing 10 days postoperatively, at which time his INR was <5. He was admitted to hospital with a blood transfusion |

(continued)

**Table 14.1** (continued)

| Source | No. of patients treated (visits) | No. of surgical procedures | No. of extractions | INR for those on vitamin K antagonists like warfarin | Comment | Postop bleeding requiring professional treatment at least with local measures (other than immediately postop) | Bleeding complications requiring more than local measures |
|---|---|---|---|---|---|---|---|
| Ferrieri et al. 2007 [54] | 255 (334) | ≥1197 | ≥1177 | 1.3–5.4 (mean 1.4–3.4) | 81 were "complicated" | 5 | 0 |
| Frank et al. 1963 [55] | 11 (11) | 51 | 51 | PT activity from 35% to 15% [*INR <2.5 to INR 3.5*] | | 0 | 0 |
| Gagneja et al. 2007 [56] | 1 (1) | 6 | 6 | 2.97 | Clindamycin prophylaxis | 0 | 0 |
| Gaspar et al. 1997 [57] | 32 (32) | ≥57 | ≥57 | INR 1.9–3.5 (mean 2.5) | Tranexamic acid mouthwash | 2 | 0 |
| Giuffrè et al. 2006 [58] | 156 (156) | ~≥156 | ~≥156 | 2.0–3.5 | Amoxicillin + clavulanic acid prophylaxis; 104 given PRP, 52 given tranexamic acid soaked gauze for hemostasis | 40 | 6 patients in the tranexamic acid group required vitamin K for hemostasis |
| Gómez-Moreno et al. 2016 [59] | 18 (18) | 43 | 0 | | Rivaroxaban patients receiving implants | 1 | 0 |
| Goodchild and Donaldson 2013 [60] | 1 (1) | 6 | 6 | 2.8 | | 1 | 0 |
| Greenberg et al. 1972 [61] | 13 (13) | 27 | 27 | PT activity 28% to 14% [*INR >2.5 to INR >3.5*] | | 0 | 0 |
| Hadziabdic et al. 2011 [62] | 50 (50) | ≥50 | ≥50 | 0.96–2.89 | | 2 | 1 anticoagulant withdrawn for 1 day postoperatively |
| Halfpenny et al. 2001 [63] | 46 (46) | 79 | 79 | 2.0–4.1, mean 2.7–2.9 | 13 were surgical; 1 patient with intermittent bleeding admitted to hospital | 3 | 0 |

| | | | | | | | |
|---|---|---|---|---|---|---|---|
| Hong et al. 2012 [64] | ~105 (105) | 252 | 248 | 1.1–3.3, mean 2.0 | ≥1 surgical | 5 | 1 one patient (post liver transplant, end stage renal disease, and hemodialysis) on combined warfarin-aspirin therapy, who had undergone 5 extractions at INR 2.2. At hospital admission, anticoagulation was INR 5.9. Vitamin K and fresh frozen plasma were administered, and local measures for hemostasis were applied |
| Inchingolo et al. 2011 [65] | 193 (193) | ≥193 | ~≥193 | Not reported | Tranexamic acid | 0 | 0 |
| Iwabuchi et al. 2014 [66] | 496 (496) | 496 | 496 | INR ≤3.0 | Warfarin, data reported by tooth, not by patient so some patients may have been counted more than once | 18 | 0 |
| Jimson et al. 2015 [67] | 3 (3) | ≥3 ≤9 | ≥3 ≤9 | INR 3.0–4.0 | Warfarin | 0 | 0 |
| Karsli et al. 2011 [68] | 13 (13) | 13 | 13 | Mean 2.6 | | 0 | 0 |
| Kataoka et al. 2016 [69] | 258 (258) | 462 | 462 | INR ≤3.0, mean INR 2.0–2.1 | Warfarin, simple and surgical extractions | 21 | 0 |
| Kovács et al. 1976 [70] | 31 (31) | 56 | 53 | Prothrombin level 19 to 49% (avg 33.3%) [*INR <2.0 to INR >3.0 avg INR <2.5*] | | 0 | 0 |
| Kumar et al. 2016 [71] | 30 (30) | 60 | 60 | INR <4.0 | Warfarin HemCon vs. gauze compression | 0 | 0 |

(continued)

**Table 14.1** (continued)

| Source | No. of patients treated (visits) | No. of surgical procedures | No. of extractions | INR for those on vitamin K antagonists like warfarin | Comment | Postop bleeding requiring professional treatment at least with local measures (other than immediately postop) | Bleeding complications requiring more than local measures |
|---|---|---|---|---|---|---|---|
| Kusafuka et al. 2013 [72] | 18 (18) | 35 | 35 | 1.08–2.91 (mean 1.75) | 1 extraction surgical | 0 | 0 |
| Kwapis 1963 [73] | 60 (60) | >85 | >82 | PT ratios not given | | 0 | 3 pts (2 with single exts and PT less than 1.5 the control) had "prolonged bleeding" and administered vit K. (Not known if local measures to control hemostasis were attempted) |
| Martinowitz et al. 1990 [74] | 40 (40) | 63 | 63 | INR 2.5–4.29; avg INR 3.25 | | 1 | 0 |
| Mauprivez et al. 2016 [75] | 51 (51) | 126 | 126 | 2.0–3.0, but those with artificial heart valves or valvulopathy 3.0–4.0 | Apixaban, dabigatran, rivaroxaban, fluindione, or warfarin; 19 extractions were surgical | 9 patients (12 episodes); there was no statistically significant difference between the direct oral anticoagulant group or the VKA group | 0 |
| McBane et al. 2010 [76] | 27 (27) | ≥27 | ≥27 | INR 2.0 | Warfarin was interrupted but only until INR was 2.0 | None reported | 0 |
| McIntyre 1966 [77] | 106 (106) | 636 | 636 | Thrombotest generally 15–7% [*INR 2.1 to INR 3.6*] | | 1 | 1 pt whose thrombotest was 5% [*INR 4.8*] bled for 12 h after 9 exts and administered vit K |
| Mesquita et al. 2017 [78] | 2 (≥2) | 8 | 8 | INR 2.20–3.21 | | 0 | 0 |

| | | | | | | | |
|---|---|---|---|---|---|---|---|
| Morimoto et al. 2008 [79], 2011 [80] | 254 (292) | 533 | 533 | 1.5–2.96 in the 15 patients with postoperative hemorrhage | 18 patients were on combined warfarin-antiplatelet therapy; 68 extractions were surgical | 15 | 1 patient (INR 1.50) on warfarin-antiplatelet combination therapy administered vitamin K because of "markedly prolonged" INR level that was unable to measure 5 days after 3 extractions |
| Morimoto et al. 2009 [81] | ≥36 (≤52) | 52 | 0 | ≤2.97 | 11 patients on combined warfarin-antiplatelet | 1 | 0 |
| Nakasato et al. 1989 [82] | 23 (23) | ≥23 | ≥23 | Not reported | | 0 | 0 |
| Pereira et al. 2011 [83] | 107 (107) | ~214 | ~214 | 0.8–4.9, mean 3.15 | 9 patients on combined warfarin-aspirin | 1 | 0 |
| Pippi et al. 2015 [84] | 20 (20) | 40 | 40 | INR 1.6–3.36 (mean 2.53) | Warfarin, HemCon vs. Collaplug | 0 | 0 |
| Raborn et al. 1990 [85] | 17 (17) | 17 | 17 | Avg (7 pts): PT 15/11.5; (10 pts): 18.4/11.5 | | 0 | 0 |
| Ramli and Rahman 2005 [86] | 21 (30) | 44 | 44 | 1.89–3.5 | Tranexamic acid mouthwash | 1 | 0 |
| Ramstrom et al. 1993 [87] | 89 (89) | ~137 | ~133 | INR 2.1–4.0 | Tranexamic acid or placebo mouthwash | 9 | 1 administered vitamin K (5 mg) after local measures. INR not given |
| Sacco et al. 2007 [88] | 65 (65) | >100 | >100 | Mean 2.89 | | 6 | 0 |
| Salam et al. 2007 [89] | 150 (150) | 279 | 279 | 0.9–4.2 (mean 2.5) | 30 extractions were surgical | 10 | 0 |
| Sammartino et al. 2011 [90] | 50 (50) | 168 | 168 | Mean 3.16 | | 2 | 0 |

(continued)

**Table 14.1** (continued)

| Source | No. of patients treated (visits) | No. of surgical procedures | No. of extractions | INR for those on vitamin K antagonists like warfarin | Comment | Postop bleeding requiring professional treatment at least with local measures (other than immediately postop) | Bleeding complications requiring more than local measures |
|---|---|---|---|---|---|---|---|
| Sammartino et al. 2012 [91] | 53 (≥53) | 173 | 173 | 2.0–4.0 | Tranexamic acid | 2 | 0 |
| Scarano et al. 2014 [92] | 30 (30) | >30 | >30 | 2.0–3.0 | Warfarin | None reported | 0 |
| Schmitt 1960 [93] | 1 (1) | 6 | 6 | PT 39 s (~40%) | | 0 (hematoma) | 0 |
| Shah et al. 2015 [94] | 1 (4) | 9 | 9 | INR 2.04–2.6 | Warfarin, Surgicel, and sutures used for hemostasis; tranexamic acid rinses postoperatively | None | 0 |
| Shira et al. 1962 [95] | 18 (18) | 50 | 45 | PT 16.8–50.7 s [PT ratio 1.4 to 4.225] | Gelfoam and sutures placed for most extractions | 6 | 1: PT 12.5% 35.4 s [PT ratio 2.95] (extraction with suture but no Gelfoam) given vitamin K |
| Sindet-Pedersen et al. 1989 [96] | 39 (39) | 119 | 112 | INR 2.5–4.8 | Tranexamic acid or placebo mouthwash | 10 | 1 pt required hospitalization and fresh frozen plasma. INR not reported |
| Soares et al. 2015 [97] | 38 (38) | 84 | 84 | Mean INR 2.51 | Warfarin patients were in 1 of 3 groups: gauze soaked in tranexamic acid, fibrin sponge, and dry gauze compression | ≥2 ≤4 | 0 |
| Souto et al. 1996 [98] | 153 (156) | ≥153 ≤163 | ≥153 ≤163 | INR 1.5 to INR 5.25 | Tranexamic acid mouthwash for some patients | 7 | 0 (Souto JC, Fontcuberta J. Personal correspondence. August 21, 1996) |

| | | | | | | | |
|---|---|---|---|---|---|---|---|
| Street and Leung 1990 [99] | 12 (12) | 12 | 12 | INR not reported | Tranexamic acid mouthwash | 1 | 0 although 1 patient not compliant with mouthwash who had an impacted infected tooth extraction was admitted to the hospital for observation but not treatment |
| Sung et al. 2014 [100] | 8 (8) | 37 | 37 | INR mean of whole study 2.1 | 6 patients on warfarin and aspirin, argatroban, and/or alteplase; 1 patient on heparin, aspirin, and clopidogrel | 0 | 0 |
| Svensson et al. 2013 [101] | 124 (124) | 194 | 194 | Mean INR 2.4 (1.0–3.5) | | 5 | 0 |
| Throndson and Walstad 1999 [102] | 1 (1) | 1 | 1 | 3.8 | Tranexamic mouthwash postoperatively | 1 | 1 transfusion and argon beam coagulator |
| Tomasi and Wolf 1974 [103] | 1 (1) | 2 | 1 | PT ratio 1.2 | | 0 | 0 |
| Tulloch and Wright 1954 [104] | 1 (1–2) | 1? | 1? | PT ratio 3.3 | | 0 | 0 |
| Wahl and Schmitt 2016 [105] | 1 (1) | 1 | 1 | | Apixaban 10 mg and aspirin 81 mg | 1 | 0 |
| Waldrep and McKelvey 1968 [106] | 20 (20) | 76 | 60 | Prothrombin activity rate 30% or less; avg. 20.3% [*INR 2.5 or more; average INR 3.0*] | | 3 | 2 pts had postop anticoag withdrawn to control postop bleeding |

(continued)

**Table 14.1** (continued)

| Source | No. of patients treated (visits) | No. of surgical procedures | No. of extractions | INR for those on vitamin K antagonists like warfarin | Comment | Postop bleeding requiring professional treatment at least with local measures (other than immediately postop) | Bleeding complications requiring more than local measures |
|---|---|---|---|---|---|---|---|
| Wood and Deeble 1993 [107] | 2 (2) | 7 | 7 | INR 2.3–2.9 preop; INR 4.3–9.1 postop | Sutures and Surgicel | 2 | 2: After bleeding control with local measures, 1 pt (preop INR 2.3) bled 2 days after extraction when his INR was 4.3, possibly from interaction with concomitant erythromycin. Given fresh frozen plasma and blood. 1 pt (preop INR 2.9 for 6 extractions) no bleeding problem until 1 week later (oozing from one socket) when INR was 9.1. Given fresh frozen plasma, blood, and vitamin K |
| Yoshimura et al. 1987 [108] | 13–16 (19) | 19 | 19 | PTR 1.05–2.1 when reported | | 6 | 0 |
| Zanon et al. 2003 [109] | 250 (250) | 525 | 525 | 1.8–4.0 | 236 extractions surgical | 4 | 0 |

| | | | | | | | |
|---|---|---|---|---|---|---|---|
| Ziffer et al. 1957 [3] | 2 (3) | 3 | 3 | PT ratio 2.35–2.8 | | 2 | 2 (3 episodes: PT ratio 2.8 for one patient; PT ratio 2.35 and 2.4 for other patient): vitamin K administered |
| Zirk et al. 2016 [110] | 20(20) | >20 | >20 | INR not reported | Phenprocoumon | 2 | 0 |
| Zusman et al. 1992 [111] | 23 (23) | 61 | 61 | PT 50–19% [*INR <2.0 to INR 3.2*] | | 3 | 0 |
| Totals | >7376 (7685) | >14,879 | >13,703 | | | ~486 (6% of patient visits) | 33 (0.4% of patients and visits) |

Adapted and updated from Table 1 *Oral Surgery Oral Medicine Oral Pathology Oral Radiology*, Vol. 119, "Dental surgery in anticoagulated patients: stop the interruption," pages 136–157, Copyright 2015, with permission from Elsevier

**Table 14.2** Anticoagulation interruption for dental procedures

| Source | No. of patients | No. of interruptions for dental procedures | Presurgical days of cessation or reduction | INR after withdrawal (for warfarin patients) | Bleeding complications treated with local measures by doctor | Thromboembolic complications |
|---|---|---|---|---|---|---|
| Abayon et al. 2016 [6] | 5 | 5 | Rivaroxaban or apixaban interrupted 1 day before extraction and resumed 1 day after; in one case apixaban interrupted 5 days before procedure and restarted 3 days following procedure | | 0 | 0 |
| Akbarian et al. 1968 [112] | 1 | 1 | Not reported | Not reported | 0 | 1 fatal embolism |
| Akopov et al. 2005 [113] | 2 | 2 | 4–6 | Not reported | Not reported | 2: 1 patient withdrawn for 4 days before dental procedure; 1 patient withdrawn for 3 days before cataract surgery and did not restart for the upcoming dental procedure. On the 6th day after withdrawal, a cerebral infarction developed |
| Al-Mubarak et al. 2006, [10] 2007 [11] | 104 | 104 | 2 | Mean 1.8–1.9 | 7 had postoperative bleeding at day 3 | 0 |
| Aldous and Olson 2001 [114] | 1 | 1 | Warfarin withdrawn for 2 days and replaced with heparin | Preop INR not reported, but on postop day 15 INR was 3.5 and on day 18 it was INR 13 | 1 on postop day 15 and eventually on day 18, when INR was 13, transfusion and vitamin K given | 0 |
| Alexander 2003 [115] | 4 | 4 | 1–5 | Not reported | Not reported | 4, 2 fatal |
| Anavi 1981 [13] | 15 | 15 | Until PT level was 50–60% | | 3 | 0 |
| Bajkin et al. 2009 [18] | 105 | 105 | Warfarin or acenocoumarol withdrawn 3–4 days (with LMWH nadroparin-calcium replacement) until INR <1.5 | INR 1.06–1.47 (mean 1.26) | 3 | 0 |
| Baykul et al. 2010 [116] | 2 | 2 | INR reduced, but not reported how | 1.3–1.4 | 1 | 0 |

| | | | | | | |
|---|---|---|---|---|---|---|
| Behrman and Wright 1961 [25] | 1 | 1 | Anticoagulation withdrawn before dental surgery (number of days unreported) | Not reported | 0 | 1 fatal massive cerebral thrombosis 17 days after discontinuing warfarin |
| Behrman and Wright 1961 [25] | 4 | 4 | Warfarin withdrawn day of surgery or 1 day preoperatively | Not reported | 1 | 0 |
| Bloomer 2004 [117] | 1 | 1 | 5 (with enoxaparin substitution but no anticoagulation at all for 12 h) | 1.5 1 day before surgery | 1 (vitamin K administered also) | 0 |
| Borea et al. 1993 [29] | 15 | 15 | Anticoagulation withdrawn or reduced in artificial heart valve patients | Preop INR 1.5–2.5 (mean 1.69) in artificial heart valve patients | 2 | 0 |
| Breik et al. 2014 [30] | 1 | 1 | Dabigatran interrupted 2 days before multiple extractions | | 0 | 0 |
| Broderick et al. 2011 [118] | 1 | 1 | Not reported | Not reported | Not reported | 1 after warfarin cessation for a dental procedure |
| Brooks 2011 [32] | 1 | 1 | 14 (with enoxaparin substitution) | 1.2 (1.4 at hospital admission) | 1 (fresh frozen plasma transfusion) | 0 |
| Campbell et al. 2000 [33] | 13 | 13 | 3–4 | 1.1–3.0 (mean 2.0) | 0 | 0 |
| Campbell et al. 2016 [119] | 4 | 4 | Children with warfarin interrupted and in some but not all cases replaced with LMWH, interval for entire study ranged from 1–9 days (mean 4 days for entire study) | INR <2.0 | 0 | 0 |
| Cannon and Dharmar 2003 [36] | 32 | 32 | 2–4 | <2.0 | 2 | 0 |
| Clemm et al. 2016 [42] | 8 | 8 | Warfarin interrupted and replaced with LMWH, interval not stated | Mean INR 1.95 | 1 | 0 |
| Cocero et al. 2014 [43] | ~26 | ~26 | Patients were switched to heparin | INR 0.92–1.5 (mean INR 1.18) | 0 | 0 |
| Crean et al. 2000 [120] | 1 | 1 | 3 (with heparin substitution on the 3rd day) | 1.3 | 0 | 0 |

(continued)

**Table 14.2** (continued)

| Source | No. of patients | No. of interruptions for dental procedures | Presurgical days of cessation or reduction | INR after withdrawal (for warfarin patients) | Bleeding complications treated with local measures by doctor | Thromboembolic complications |
|---|---|---|---|---|---|---|
| Davies 2003 [46] | 1 | 1 | 2 (anticoagulant reduced) | Not reported | 0 | 1 TIA |
| Davis and Sczupak 1979 [121] | 28 | 28? | Up to 2 weeks for "dental or surgical procedures" | Not reported | Not reported | 0 |
| Della Valle et al. 2003 [122] | 40 | 40 | 1.5 | 1.5–3.0 | 17 | 0 |
| Devani et al. 1998 [47] | 32 | 32 | Warfarin withdrawn 2 days preoperatively until INR 1.5–2.1 | INR 1.2–2.1 (mean 1.6) | 1 | 0 |
| Douketis et al. 2004 [123] | 3 | 3 | 5–6 days (LMWH dalteparin replacement); stop dalteparin at least 12 h before surgery) | Not reported | 0 (but rectus sheath hematoma) | 0 |
| Dunn et al. 2007 [124] | 26 | 26 | Warfarin interrupted for 5 days before dental procedure and replaced with enoxaparin | INR <1.8 | ≤26 | 0 |
| Dunn et al. 2007 [124] | 22 | ≥22 | 5 days (LMWH enoxaparin replacement; stop enoxaparin day of procedure) | <1.8 | 0 | 0 |
| Elad and Findler 2008 [49] | 2 | 2 | Not reported; warfarin replaced with LMWH | Not reported | 2 | 0 |
| Erden et al. 2016 [51] | 36 | 36 | 5 days with LMWH replacement bridging | Mean 1.1 | None reported | 0 |
| Evans et al. 2002 [52] | 52 | 52 | 2 | 1.2–2.3 (mean 1.6) | 0 | 0 |
| Finn and Schow 1993 [125] | 1 | 1 | 4 (with heparin substitution) | PT 12.8 secs (INR not reported) | 0 | 0 |
| Garcia et al. 2008 [126] | 257 | 323 | 1–10 in larger study | Not reported | Not reported | 1 after a 7 day interruption for oral surgery |
| Gaspar et al. 1997 [57] | 15 | 15 | Warfarin withdrawn for 3 days | INR 1.25–1.9 (mean 1.45) | 1 | 0 |

| | | | | | | |
|---|---|---|---|---|---|---|
| Giuffrè et al. 2006 [58] | 52 | 52 | Until PT, PTT, and INR values reached 50% (heparin replacement) | 1.0–1.75 | 0 | 0 |
| Hadziabdic et al. 2011 [62] | 21 | 21 | For 1 day, anticoagulation reduced in 4 and withdrawn in 17 patients | Not reported | 0 | 0 |
| Jaffer et al. 2005 [127] | 1 | 1 | Warfarin interrupted 5 or 6 days before dental procedure and replaced with enoxaparin | INR typically <1.5 | 0 | 0 |
| Johnson-Leong and Rada 2002 [128] | 1 | 1 | 4 (with enoxaparin substitution but no anticoagulation at all for 24 h) | 1.1 | 0 | 0 |
| Karsli et al. 2011 [68] | 21 | 26 | 3 days with LMWH or UFH bridging | Mean 1.6 | 0 | 0 |
| Kovacs et al. 2004 [129] | 25 | 25 | Warfarin interrupted 5 days before dental extraction and replaced with dalteparin | INR ≤1.4 | None reported | 1 stroke 42 days after interrupting warfarin for bridging therapy with LMWH for tooth extraction. Warfarin had been restarted the day after surgery but then stopped again on day 36 because of GI bleeding |
| Lund et al. 2002 [130] | 6 | ≥6 | Heparin replacement to reach PTT 55–65 s (all patients were on mechanical circulatory support) | Not reported | 3 patients had minor hemorrhage 4 days after surgery | 2 transient ischemic events |
| Marshall 1963 [131] | 1 | 1 | Anticoagulation withdrawn 9 days preoperatively | Not reported | 0 | 1 fatal myocardial infarction 19 days after interruption of therapy of 9 days duration |
| Mehra et al. 2000 [132] | 20 | 20 | 1–2 days with heparin replacement | Not reported | 1 | 0 |
| Miclotte et al. 2016 [133] | 26 | 26 | Dabigatran, rivaroxaban, or apixaban interrupted on morning of procedure | Morning dose of anticoagulant skipped, last dose on average 30.5 h before extraction | 7 | 0 |

(continued)

**Table 14.2** (continued)

| Source | No. of patients | No. of interruptions for dental procedures | Presurgical days of cessation or reduction | INR after withdrawal (for warfarin patients) | Bleeding complications treated with local measures by doctor | Thromboembolic complications |
|---|---|---|---|---|---|---|
| Milligan et al. 2003 [134] | ≥1 | 1 | 4–5 | 1.2–1.8 (mean INR 1.5 for entire study, which included nondental surgeries) | Not reported | 0 |
| Morimoto et al. 2008 [79] | 4 | 7 | 2 days warfarin reduction with LMWH (dalteparin) replacement | 1.2–2.36 | 1 (compression and warfarin discontinuation 6 days postop due to high INR and oozing) | 0 |
| Mulligan 1987 [135] | 17 | 44 | Anticoagulation withdrawn 2–7 days preoperatively | PTR 1.13–1.93 | 0 | 0 |
| Nakasato et al. 1989 [82] | 28 | 28 | Warfarin discontinued until thrombin test level raised from 40 to 50% | Mean thrombin test value 49.8 ± 14.5% | 0 | 0 |
| O'Donnell et al. 2007 [136] | 1 | 1 | Warfarin interrupted 4 or 5 days before dental extraction and bridged with enoxaparin twice daily with last dose evening before surgery; warfarin restarted evening after surgery | Not reported | None | 0 |
| Ogiuchi et al. 1985 [137] | 128 | 128 | Warfarin dose decreased 3–7 days preoperatively, then discontinued the day of the procedure and restarted afterward | Thrombotest values 10–100% | 0 | 1 fatal cerebral thromboembolia 5 days postoperatively |
| Palomäki et al. 2016 [138] | 2 | 2 | Warfarin or dabigatran; interval not reported | Not reported | Not reported | 2 ischemic strokes; for entire study, median interval between procedure and stroke 4 days |
| Pávek and Bigl 1993 [139] | 11 | 11 | Anticoagulation reduced for 1 day and then withdrawn for 1 day with heparin replacement | ≤1.87 | 0 | 0 |
| Pearce et al. 1975 [140] | 1 | 1 | Warfarin withdrawn for unknown days | Not reported | 0 | 0 |

| | | | | | | |
|---|---|---|---|---|---|---|
| Picard et al. 2010 [141] | 1 | 1 | 5 days | INR 1.3 in emergency room (36 h after restarting warfarin just after extraction) | None reported | 1 ischemic stroke 2 days after procedure |
| Prudoff and Stratigos 1972 [142] | 2 | 2 | Warfarin withdrawn 2 days preoperatively | Protime 13/13 and 22/14 | 0 | 0 |
| Roberts 1961 [143] | 3 | 3 | 3–4 | PT 25–33 s; 24; 21 | 1 After 2 days of postoperative bleeding, intravenous estrogen was administered for hemostasis | 0 |
| Roberts 1966 [144] | ≥40 | ≥40 | 3 days | PT up to 25 s | 0 | 0 |
| Romond et al. 2013 [145] | 1 | 1 | Dabigatran 2 days: interrupted the night before and restarted the day after surgery | Dabigatran | None | 0 |
| Russo et al. 2000 [146] | 104 | 104 | 2 | 1.18–3.4 (mean INR 1.87) | 2 | 0 |
| Sacco et al. 2007 [88] | 66 | 66 | 3 (dosages reduced until for target INR 1.8) | Mean 1.77 | 10 | 0 |
| Sammartino et al. 2012 [91] | 31 | ≥31 | Warfarin withdrawn "some days" before procedure until INR <2.0 | Preop INR <2.0 | 4 treated with local measures 2–4 days postoperatively | 0 |
| Saour et al. 1994 [147] | 212 | 212 | Warfarin withdrawn 2 days or until INR ≤1.5 | INR ≤1.5 | 0 | 0 |
| Scheitler et al. 1988 [148] | 1 | 1 | 1 day; heparin replacement until 6 h before surgery | PT 13.0/10.2 s | 0 | 0 |
| Schofield 1984 [149] | ~168 | ~168 | Warfarin withdrawn 6 days preoperatively | Thrombotest >25% | 0 | 0 |
| Sheller and Tong 1994 [150] | 1 | 1 | Warfarin withdrawn for 2 days | Not reported | 0 | 0 |
| Somma et al. 2010 [151] | 80 | ≥80 | 3 days | Not reported | 0 | 2 thromboembolic complications |
| Somma et al. 2010 [151] | 800 | ≥800 | Warfarin dosage adjusted | 1.6–1.8 | 82 | 0 |

(continued)

**Table 14.2** (continued)

| Source | No. of patients | No. of interruptions for dental procedures | Presurgical days of cessation or reduction | INR after withdrawal (for warfarin patients) | Bleeding complications treated with local measures by doctor | Thromboembolic complications |
|---|---|---|---|---|---|---|
| Souto et al. 1996 [98] | 39 | 39 | Anticoagulation reduced for 2 days and replaced with heparin | INR 1.25–5.0 | 13 | 0 |
| Spandorfer et al. 1999 [152] | 3 | 3 | Warfarin interrupted 5 or 6 days before oral surgery and replaced with dalteparin | Not reported | None reported | 0 |
| Spyropoulos et al. 2004 [153] | 6 | 6 | Warfarin interrupted 4 days before dental extraction and replaced with enoxaparin | INR <1.5 | 2 | 0 |
| Steinberg et al. 2015 [154] | 182 | 182 | Warfarin or dabigatran (166 with no bridging; 16 with bridging); interruption interval not reported | Not reported | 0 | 1 embolic complication ≤30 days after procedure for interruption (without bridging) |
| Street and Leung 1990 [99] | 2 | 2 | Not reported | Not reported | 0 | 0 |
| Tinmouth et al. 2001 [155] | 2 | 2 | Warfarin interrupted 4 days before dental extractions and replaced with dalteparin | INR <1.5 | None reported | 0 |
| Todd 2001 [156] | 1 | 1 | Anticoagulant withdrawn until INR normalized | Not reported | 0 | 0 |
| Tulloch and Wright 1954 [104] | 12 | 13 | Anticoagulant withdrawn for 4 days in most cases | Not reported | 0 | 1 pt whose therapy was withdrawn for 8 days developed cerebral and brachial nonfatal emboli |
| Wilson et al. 2001 [157] | 6 | 6 | Warfarin discontinued 5 days before procedure with LMWH (dalteparin) substitution | ≤1.5 | 1 | 0 |
| Won et al. 2014 [158] | 165 | 165 | Warfarin interrupted 4 days preprocedure and replaced with enoxaparin or unfractionated heparin | | 11 instances of "major bleeding," defined as ≥2 g/dL hemoglobin decrease, packed red blood cell transfusion, bleeding requiring surgery, or "life-threatening bleeding" | 2 (1 stroke, 1 fatal embolism) within 30 days |
| Wood and Conn 1954 [159] | 5 | 5 | Anticoagulation withdrawn "dental extraction or surgical procedure" 7–37 days | Not reported | 0 | 0 |

| | | | | | | |
|---|---|---|---|---|---|---|
| Yasaka et al. 2006 [160] | 4 | 4 | 3–6 | 0.94–2.5 on admission | Not reported | 4 cardioembolic strokes: interrupted at 3, 4, 5, and 6 days before dental extractions |
| Yoshimura et al. 1987 [108] | 4 | 4 | Anticoagulant withdrawn or reduced 1–2 days preoperatively | Not reported | 0 | 0 |
| Ziffer et al. 1957 [3] | 1 | 1 | 9 days | | 0 | 0 |
| Zirk et al. 2016 [110] | 84 | 84 | Phenprocoumon interrupted and bridged with LMWH or unfractionated heparin, interval not reported | INR not reported | 6 | 0 |
| Zusman et al. 1993 [111] | 23 | 23 | 2 | Not reported | 0 | 0 |
| Totals | ≥3278 | ≥3380 | | | 214 (6% of visits), including ≤16 (≤0.5%) administered more than local measures | 29 (0.9% of patients or visits); 7 (0.2% of patients or visits) fatal |

Adapted and updated from Table 2 *Oral Surgery Oral Medicine Oral Pathology Oral Radiology*, Vol. 119, "Dental surgery in anticoagulated patients: stop the interruption," pages 136–157, Copyright 2015, with permission from Elsevier interruption when considering all types of medical procedures. Wysokinski et al. found a 1.1% embolic complication rate in 345 patients whose anticoagulation was interrupted for 4 or 5 days with or without bridging therapy [161]. In a study of 984 patients whose anticoagulation was interrupted for 5 days or fewer, Garcia et al. reported 4 embolic complications, an incidence of 0.4% [126]. In a 2011 study, Broderick et al. [118] found that 114 (5.2%) of 2197 ischemic strokes occurred after antithrombotic medication (either warfarin or antiplatelet medication) interruption, including 61 strokes after warfarin interruption, either as a result of a physician recommendation or patient negligence. The authors concluded, "The withdrawal of anticoagulant and antiplatelet medications is associated with a substantial number of acute first-ever and recurrent ischemic strokes."

Based on a close look at the studies in anticoagulation of dental patients, there is overwhelming evidence that therapeutic levels of anticoagulation should not be interrupted for dental procedures as the increased (but low) risk of serious and possibly fatal embolic complications or death with interruption exceeds the (low) risk of nonfatal and fully recoverable bleeding complications with anticoagulation. No wonder continuing anticoagulation without interruption for dental surgery has been called the "gold standard in the perioperative management of anticoagulation" [75].

## 14.1 Direct-Acting Oral Anticoagulants (DOACs)

Although their safety and efficacy appear to be similar to that of vitamin K inhibitors like warfarin [162, 163], there have been very few studies on dental surgery in patients on DOACs. Some advocate interrupting DOAC therapy before dental surgery. In a 2016 study by Miclotte et al. [133] of 26 patients on dabigatran, rivaroxaban, or apixaban, patients skipped their morning dose before a dental extraction and restarted the normal regimen at least 4 h after the procedure. These patients were compared with 26 matched control healthy patients not on antithrombotic therapy. Although all bleeding was controlled with local hemostatic methods and there was no difference in early bleeding events, there was more delayed bleeding in the study group (seven patients versus none in the control group). The authors concluded, "Skipping the morning dose of new oral anticoagulants avoids excess bleeding during and early after the procedure. However, anticoagulated patients had an increased risk of delayed bleedings. Further study is needed to determine the optimal postprocedural management." A problem with this study is there was not a third group of patients whose anticoagulation was continued. It is conceivable that an anticoagulation continuation group would have had a similar frequency of delayed bleeding, controlled with local hemostatic measures. Some delayed bleeding controlled with local measures for hemostasis with anticoagulation seems a small price to pay versus a small chance of a serious embolic complication or death when skipping a dose.

In a pilot study of anticoagulated patients undergoing extractions, 31 patients taking direct oral anticoagulants were matched with 20 taking vitamin K anatagonists, and there was no significant difference in the incidence of postoperative bleeding events; all of which were treated with local measures for hemostasis [75]. In a study of anticoagulated implant surgical patients including 30 with vitamin K inhibitors, 16 with DOACs, and a control group of 447 patients, there were 2 bleeding complications in the vitamin K inhibitor group, 3 in the control group, but none in the DOAC group, though all bleeding complications were minor and simple to treat with local hemostatic methods [42]. In a study of 18 rivaroxaban patients undergoing implant surgery and 39 matched control patients, there was no significant difference in bleeding episodes after surgery [59]. The authors of these studies have each independently concluded that anticoagulation therapy should be continued for dental surgery. Most authorities agree that

DOACs should be continued for dental extractions or minor oral surgery, but that for "major" oral surgery (including >5 extractions, surgical extractions with ostectomy, multiple implant placement, or torus removal), recommend interrupting anticoagulation 24 h before the procedure and restarting at least 24 h after the procedure [164]. Although there has been one report of "severe bleeding" after 18 extractions in a patient on continuous dabigatran requiring postoperative interruption of dabigatran" [30], until there is more evidence of serious bleeding risks among these patients, it appears more prudent to continue anticoagulation rather than subject these patients to an increased embolic risk with interruption.

## 14.2 To Bridge or Not to Bridge?

In the past, bridging anticoagulation with replacement has been advocated as an alternative to anticoagulation continuation or anticoagulation interruption without replacement. Rather than go without any anticoagulation during the entire interruption period, a long-acting anticoagulant like warfarin (half-life ~40 h) is interrupted 4 or 5 days before the procedure and then replaced with a short-acting anticoagulant like heparin (half-life ~60 min), until just before the medical or dental procedure, at which time no anticoagulant would be given, and the patient would not be anticoagulated at all. Warfarin dosing resumes shortly after the procedure (and depending on the procedure, possibly heparin also), and after 2 days, once the patient's INR levels are therapeutic, then the heparin dosing stops and warfarin continues as before the bridging. Although bridging is theoretically a reasonable alternative to anticoagulation interruption without any replacement, in practice it has been shown to cause "excessive bleeding, longer length of hospital stay, and other significant morbidities, while providing no clear prevention of [embolic complications]" [165]. A systematic review and meta-analysis of 7118 heparin bridged patients and 5160 nonbridged anticoagulated patients concluded, "Vitamin K antagonist-treated patients receiving periprocedural heparin bridging appear to be at increased risk of overall and major bleeding and at similar risk of thromboembolic events compared to nonbridged patients" [166]. Erden et al. showed that there was less total blood loss in dental extraction patients whose anticoagulation was continued versus those whose therapy was interrupted with low molecular weight heparin bridging [51]. Bridging anticoagulation is both unnecessary and unwise in dental patients as dental surgery in anticoagulated patients without interruption has been shown to be safe.

## 14.3 Physician Consultation

Physician consultation is sometimes advocated as a method to protect patients from harm and dentists from potential lawsuits. In the early twentieth century, dentists often blindly followed physicians' recommendations to extract mouthfuls of salvageable and/or healthy teeth to treat or prevent all kinds of maladies such as arthritis, psychiatric illness, kidney disease, and colitis, based on the focal infection theory [167]. Since such treatment would usually have no beneficial effect, after such extractions, an arthritic patient, for example, would now end up with two maladies—both arthritis and edentulousness. In 1920, C. Edmund Kells, a pioneer in the use of dental X-rays and the inventor of surgical suction, spoke about blindly following such physician recommendations as "The Crime of the Age" and wrote, "The time will come, however,—the time must come—when no exodontist of *standing* will extract a tooth upon the orders of a physician. A dentist, and no one but a dentist, should sign the death certificate of a tooth. The Lord only knows why physicians should want to sign such certificates. Don't they sign enough such certificates in their own legitimate line?" [168]. Nearly 100 years later, the editor of the *Journal of the American Dental Association* stated that although physician consultation can be a helpful tool, it should not be a "crutch" [169]. If anticoagulation is interrupted for a dental extraction as a result of physician consultation, and the patient suffers a stroke even though dental extractions carry very minimal bleeding risks and national medical and dental groups recommend against interruption in such cases, then physician consultation protects neither the patient from harm nor the dentist (and presumably the physician) from a lawsuit. The Division of Legal Affairs of the American Dental Association has stated, "[T]he dentist who blindly follows the physician's recommendation, even though it conflicts with the dentist's professional judgment, will not be able to defend himself or herself by claiming 'the devil made me do it' if the patient sues. The courts recognize that each independent professional is ultimately responsible for his or her own treatment decisions" [170]. Cases where a dentist who does not know how to proceed therefore follows the advice of a physician (who also does not know how to proceed but advises nonetheless) have been called "the blind leading the blind" [171].

There may be some physicians who recommend clinically acceptable amalgam restoration removal and replacement with nonamalgam materials as a cure for multiple sclerosis, but there is no credible evidence amalgam restorations cause or amalgam removal cures multiple sclerosis, and a dentist who follows such advice to his patient's detriment could be liable for any harm caused by such negligent treatment. Physician consultation for dental surgery in anticoagulated patients is similar.

Physicians have been shown to overestimate bleeding risks associated with dental surgery in anticoagulated patients and underestimate embolic risks. For example, many physicians recommend anticoagulation interruption for procedures like dental cleanings, which should never cause postoperative bleeding significant enough to interrupt anticoagulation [172]. In a 1996 survey, more physicians recommended interruption for root canal therapy than for professional cleanings, even though root canal therapy would rarely cause any bleeding at all (and certainly less than cleanings), neither of which would warrant anticoagulation interruption [173]. In a 2011 survey of 1648 anticoagulated patients, about half of the respondents had been asked to interrupt warfarin anticoagulation for dental or medical procedures. Of those asked to interrupt warfarin anticoagulation, about half were for procedures specifically contraindicated for interruption by national medical or dental guidelines, including many who were asked to interrupt warfarin for dental cleanings [172].

Just like most medications dental patients may be taking, anticoagulants may be safely continued for dental treatment. As a result, as long as recent INR levels are known for warfarin-based medications and there are no other contraindications in the patient's medical history, the dentist may proceed with treatment. But many dentists request a physician consultation before an extraction for an anticoagulated patient, and the physician often recommends anticoagulation interruption. If such a patient suffers a stroke after anticoagulation interruption, a lawsuit may be filed against the dentist (and most likely, the physician also). The dentist may try to use the defense that he or she simply followed the advice of the physician to interrupt anticoagulation for a patient undergoing a dental procedure, but there was no need to expose the patient to an increased embolic risk (with interruption) without any evidence of a significant bleeding risk (with anticoagulation) and in spite of national dental and medical group recommendations to the contrary.

In a case like this, it is likely that *both* the dentist and the physician may be liable. Once a physician consultation is requested (and regardless of the physician's opinion), the dentist has the obligation to inform the patient that the relevant medical and dental literature show that the procedure can be performed safely without interrupting anticoagulation and with minimal bleeding risk and that in the unlikely event of postoperative bleeding, the complication can be treated simply without long-term effects. The patient should also be informed that if anticoagulation is interrupted, there is a small but significant embolic risk; the consequence of which is possibly catastrophic and even fatal.

There have been at least four cases of serious embolic complications; two of which were fatal, after physician consultation and anticoagulation interruption for dental extractions [115]. In each of these cases, a lawsuit was filed against the dentist. Alexander stated, "Consulting with the patient's physician certainly did not help in [these] cases....These cases did not go to the literature, only to litigation. Medical consultation is a process by which the requesting doctor gathers information about a patient's condition. After gathering this information, the treating doctor, as captain of the ship, must decide on the appropriate course of therapy based on information provided by the consultant."

There are valid reasons for physician consultation. The dentist may need to consult the physician for recent INR levels if the patient does not know them. If INR levels are known and not within the therapeutic range—too high or too low—then the dentist may wish to consult for that. Dental treatment is safe when INR levels are slightly above therapeutic levels up to INR 4.0, within therapeutic levels (INR 2.0–3.0 for most conditions and INR 2.5–3.5 for mechanical mitral valves), or below therapeutic levels but can be deferred if INR levels are well above therapeutic levels. Ultimately, however, dental treatment decisions should not be deferred to nondentists, even if the nondentists are physicians. It is the dentist and not the physician who is ultimately responsible for such decisions. There is no substitute for good clinical judgment, experience, and education.

## 14.4 Informed Consent

Patients have a right to make an informed decision if anticoagulation interruption for dental surgery is considered, including the potential risks and benefits. Although patients can be anxious about potential bleeding problems when continuing anticoagulation, it should be explained that such problems are uncommon, but when they occur, they are usually simple to treat. No bleeding complications in anticoagulated patients have ever been documented in the medical and dental literature to be fatal, but patients should also be informed of the increased risk of embolic complications if anticoagulation is interrupted. Although such embolic complications are also uncommon, they often create devastating long-term consequences or can even lead to death. A physician once commented that upon contemplation, after considering the risks and benefits of anticoagulation interruption, many patients say they may actually prefer death to the long-term consequences of surviving a stroke. When properly informed, most patients would choose to continue anticoagulation for dental surgery. If anticoagulation is to be interrupted, it is only the physician (and never the dentist) who should direct the patient to do so. The physician prescribes the medication; the dentist does the dentistry. Whether anticoagulation is interrupted or not, the dentist can safely proceed with the dental surgery, provided the levels are not above INR 4.0 for warfarin anticoagulation. If the physician or patient volunteers that anticoagulation should be interrupted for a dental procedure, then the dentist is obligated to explain why it should be continued, including the risks and benefits of interruption versus continuation. The dentist may wish to share national medical and dental group recommendations with the patient and the physician as well. If anticoagulation is interrupted before dental surgery, it should be restarted as soon as possible after the procedure.

## 14.5 National Medical and Dental Group Recommendations

There are at least seven national medical or dental group statements on dental surgery in anticoagulated patients [174–180]. They all recommend continuing anticoagulation without interruption for most or all anticoagulated patients. The American College of Chest Physicians issued statements in 2001 [181], 2004 [182], and 2008 [183] recommending continuing anticoagulation for dental procedures but in 2012 added a 2- to 3-day interruption option with a prohemostatic agent (although this option has been criticized for various reasons) [5, 184, 185] (see Table 14.3).

**Table 14.3** National medical and dental group statements

| Year | Group | Recommendation |
|---|---|---|
| 2016 [174] | American Academy of Oral Medicine | Continue warfarin anticoagulation with INR testing within a few days of the procedure |
| 2015 [175] | American Dental Association | Continue warfarin or DOAC for most patients |
| 2014 [176] | The Society for Neuroscience in Anesthesiology and Critical Care (supported by the American Society of Anesthesiologists) | Continue anticoagulation for single dental extractions |
| 2013 [177] | American Academy of Neurology | Continue warfarin anticoagulation |
| 2012 [178] | American College of Chest Physicians | Continue warfarin anticoagulation with oral prohemostatic agent or interrupt anticoagulation for 2–3 days before dental surgery |
| 2007 [179] | The Haemostasis and Thrombosis Task Force of the British Committee for Standards in Haematology | Continue warfarin anticoagulation, checking INR levels within 72 h of dental surgery |
| 2003 [180] | American Heart Association and American College of Cardiology | Continue warfarin with antifibrinolytic mouthwash |

## 14.6 Specialist Versus Generalist

The majority of dentists in a 2016 survey in Germany did not perform extractions on patients anticoagulated with warfarin [186], perhaps partly because some authors have recommended that dental extractions in anticoagulated patients be performed by specialists (e.g., oral surgeons) in hospitals. Many controlled comparative studies have shown that bleeding complications and/or blood loss are not significantly different in anticoagulated patients versus non-anticoagulated (those whose anticoagulation was interrupted or reduced) patients [11, 15, 16, 28, 29, 33, 36, 47, 52, 57, 59, 68, 77]. Bleeding complications can occur in both anticoagulated patients and healthy patients. When they occur, they are usually simple to treat with additional local measures for hemostasis. These measures include gauze compression, biting on tea bags, oxidized cellulose (Surgicel), absorbable gelatin, sutures, and antifibrinolytic rinses like tranexamic acid. The normal protocol for postextraction bleeding complications for any other patient will suffice for anticoagulated patients. As a result, no special training or special facilities are necessary for these procedures in anticoagulated patients. Both general dentists and dental specialists familiar with postextraction hemostatic methods can safely perform dental surgery in such patients.

## 14.7 Interruption Arguments

Although the evidence is overwhelming that dental surgery is safe in anticoagulated patients, there are still a few authorities who recommend a brief (2- or 3-day) interruption in some cases. A 2010 “decision-tree analysis” purported to show that anticoagulation interruption is slightly favored over continuation for dental surgery [187], but the analysis was widely discredited for various reasons [184, 188–190]. The author of the decision-tree analysis used a grossly overestimated fatal bleeding incidence of 1% although the literature has failed to document a single case of fatal bleeding in anticoagulated patients (a 0% incidence). Dental surgery is different than other types of surgery in that major blood vessels are unlikely to be encountered, and perioperative and postoperative bleeding complications are usually simple to treat with local measures instead of additional surgeries.

It was also asserted in the decision-tree analysis that “there has been no reported case of a dental extraction causing a cardiovascular accident (CVA) in a patient whose warfarin was temporarily discontinued” [187], but there had in fact been many documented cases of postdental embolic complications, including several deaths, after anticoagulation interruption, at least five documented in the 1998 review and now, at least 29. The embolic complication rate used in the decision-tree analysis was 0.059%, much lower than rates of 1.1% [161] and 0.4% [126] shown in relatively large prospective studies with brief (≤5-day) interruption periods. An embolic rate of 0.9% after anticoagulation interruption for dental procedures is more than 15 times the 0.059% used in the decision analysis. Even if the 0.059% is accepted as accurate, it is still not worth the increased risk of a debilitating or even fatal stroke without any attendant benefit when interrupting anticoagulation. Bleeding complications are uncommon and have never been shown to be fatal in anticoagulated patients. To understand risk, a comparison has been made with airplane flights. Of 87,000 daily airplane flights in the United States, there would be 51 crashes every day if the crash rate were 0.059% [184]. Few people would choose to fly with such a high incidence of crashes. So it is with anticoagulation interruption—if patients and practitioners fully understand the increased embolic risk with interruption and the safety of dental procedures with anticoagulation, then very few would choose interruption.

Some advocating interruption also point out that bleeding complications can cause "anxiety and distress" [178] and can be "troublesome" [191], but surely, these bleeding complications, usually simple to treat with simple local measures and never fatal, are not nearly as troublesome as embolic complications, which often cause permanent disability or even death. Finally, another reason given for interrupting anticoagulation has been the unavailability of "prohemostatic agents" [192], apparently defined as any local hemostatic measures other than gauze, used for compression. Specific examples of prohemostatic agents have been antifibrinolytic rinses (like tranexamic acid) and sutures. While it is true that antifibrinolytic rinses may not be widely available to dental practitioners in the United States, sutures are readily available to any dentist performing extractions, on anticoagulated patients and any other patients. In addition, oxidized cellulose, absorbable gelatin, and other forms of local hemostatic aids are readily available to practitioners. Fortunately, although additional hemostatic aids should be available when performing dental surgery, compressed gauze is usually all that is needed for hemostasis [7, 20, 97].

**Conclusion**

When anticoagulated patients require dental surgery, a decision must be made whether to continue anticoagulation and risk bleeding complications or interrupt anticoagulation and risk embolic complications. Fortunately, dental surgery is unlike surgery in other parts of the body. Major vessels are unlikely to be encountered, and bleeding complications can usually be directly addressed either perioperatively or postoperatively without additional surgery. In studies and reports on thousands and thousands of anticoagulated patients, there has never been a fatal bleeding complication, and only 0.4% suffered bleeding complications requiring more than local measures for hemostasis. On the other hand, among thousands of patients whose anticoagulation was interrupted for dental procedures, 0.9% suffered embolic complications, including many who died. The decision should be very simple: anticoagulation should not be interrupted for dental surgery.

## References

1. Guyatt GH, Akl EA, Crowther M, et al. Executive summary: antithrombotic therapy and prevention of thrombosis, 9th ed: American College of Chest Physicians Evidence-Based Clinical Practice Guidelines. Chest. 2012;141(2 Suppl):7S–47S.
2. Askey JM, Cherry CB. Dental extraction during dicumarol therapy. Calif Med. 1956;84:16–7.
3. Ziffer AM, Scopp IW, Beck J, Baum J, Berger AR. Profound bleeding after dental extractions during dicumarol therapy. N Engl J Med. 1957;256:351–3.
4. Wahl MJ. Dental surgery in anticoagulated patients. Arch Intern Med. 1998;158:1610–6.
5. Wahl MJ, Pintos A, Kilham J, Lalla RV. Dental surgery in anticoagulated patients: stop the interruption. Oral Surg Oral Med Oral Pathol Oral Radiol. 2015;119(2):136–57.
6. Abayon M, Kolokythas A, Slu H, Elad S. Dental management of patients on direct oral anticoagulants: case series and literature review. Quintessence Int. 2016;47(8):687–96.

7. Abdullah WA, Khalil H. Dental extraction in patients on warfarin treatment. Clin Cosmet Investig Dent. 2014;6:65–9.
8. Al Zoman H, Al Jetaiy S, Robert AA, et al. Flapless dental implant surgery for patients on oral anticoagulants – the "WarLess Procedure": a report of 2 cases. J Oral Implantol. 2013;39(Spec Issue):264–70.
9. Al-Belasy FA, Amer MZ. Hemostatic effect of n-butyl-2-cyanoacrylate (Histoacryl) glue in warfarin-treated patients undergoing oral surgery. J Oral Maxillofac Surg. 2003;61:1405–9.
10. Al-Mubarak S, Rass MA, Alsuwyed A, et al. Thromboembolic risk and bleeding in patients maintaining or stopping oral anticoagulant therapy during dental extraction. J Thromb Haemost. 2006;4:689–91.
11. Al-Mubarak S, Al-Ali N, Abou Rass M, et al. Evaluation of dental extractions, suturing and INR on postoperative bleeding of patients maintained on oral anticoagulant therapy. Br Dent J. 2007;203:E15.
12. Alexander R, Ferretti AC, Sorensen JR. Stop the nonsense not the anticoagulants: a matter of life and death. N Y State Dent J. 2002;68(9):24–6.
13. Anavi Y, Sharon A, Gutman D, Laufer D. Dental extractions during anticoagulant therapy. Isr J Dent Med. 1981;28(4):9–12.
14. Bacci C, Maglione M, Favero L, et al. Management of dental extraction in patients undergoing anticoagulant treatment. Results from a large, multicenter, prospective, case-control study. Thromb Haemost. 2010;104(5):972–5.
15. Bacci C, Berengo M, Favero L, Zanon E. Safety of dental implant surgery in patients undergoing anticoagulation therapy: a prospective case-control study. Clin Oral Implants Res. 2011;22:151–6.
16. Bailey BMW, Fordyce AM. Complications of dental extractions in patients receiving warfarin anticoagulant therapy: a controlled clinical trial. Br Dent J. 1983;155:308–10.
17. Bajkin BV, Vujkov SB, Milekic BR, Vuvkovic BA. Risk factors for bleeding after oral surgery in patients who continued using oral anticoagulant therapy. J Am Dent Assoc. 2015;146(6):375–81.
18. Bajkin BV, Popovic SL, Selakovic SDJ. Randomized, prospective trial comparing bridging therapy using low-molecular-weight heparin with maintenance of oral anticoagulation during extraction of teeth. J Oral Maxillofac Surg. 2009;67(5):990–5.
19. Bajkin BV, Bajkin IA, Petrovic BB. The effects of combined oral anticoagulant-aspirin therapy in patients undergoing tooth extractions: a prospective study. J Am Dent Assoc. 2012;143(7):771–6.
20. Bajkin BV, Selaković SD, Mirković SM, et al. Comparison of efficacy of local hemostatic modalities in anticoagulated patients undergoing tooth extractions. Vojnosanit Pregl. 2014;71(12):1097–101.
21. Bakathir AA. Minor oral surgery procedures in patients taking warfarin: a 5-year retrospective study at Sultan Qaboos University Hospital, Sultanate of Oman. Sultan Qaboos Univ Med J. 2009;9(3):279–86.
22. Bal BJ, Hardee PS. Efficacy and cost effectiveness of tranexamic acid mouthrinse for oral surgery in warfarinised patients [Abstract]. Br J Oral Maxillofac Surg. 2000;38(4):390.
23. Bandrowsky T, Vorono AA, Borris TJ, Marcantoni HW. Amoxicillin-related postextraction bleeding in an anticoagulated patient with tranexamic acid rinses. Oral Surg Oral Med Oral Pathol Oral Radiol Endod. 1996;82:610–2.
24. Barrero MV, Knezevic M, Martín MT, et al. Oral surgery in patients undergoing oral anticoagulant therapy. Med Oral. 2002;7(1):63–70.
25. Behrman SJ, Wright IS. Dental surgery during continuous anticoagulant therapy. J Am Dent Assoc. 1961;62:172–80.
26. Benoliel R, Leviner E, Katz J, Tzukert A. Dental treatment for the patient on anticoagulant therapy: prothrombin time value – what difference does it make? Oral Surg Oral Med Oral Pathol. 1986;62:149–51.
27. Blinder D, Manor Y, Martinowitz U, Taicher S. Dental extractions in patients maintained on continued oral anticoagulant: comparison of local hemostatic modalities. Oral Surg Oral Med Oral Pathol Oral Radiol Endod. 1999;88:137–40.
28. Blinder D, Manor Y, Martinowitz U, Taicher S. Dental extractions in patients maintained on oral anticoagulant therapy: comparison of INR value with occurrence of postoperative bleeding. Int J Oral Maxillofac Surg. 2001;30(6):518–21.
29. Borea G, Montebugnoli L, Capuzzi P, Magelli C. Tranexamic acid as a mouthwash in anticoagulant-treated patients undergoing oral surgery: an alternative method to discontinuing anticoagulant therapy. Oral Surg Oral Med Oral Pathol. 1993;75:29–31.
30. Breik O, Cheng A, Sambrook PJ, Goss AN. Protocol in managing oral surgical patients taking dabigatran. Aust Dent J. 2014;59:296–301.
31. Broekema FI, van Minnen B, Jansma J, Bos RRM. Risk of bleeding after dentoalveolar surgery in patients taking anticoagulants. Br J Oral Maxillofac Surg. 2014;52:e15–9.
32. Brooks AS. Delayed complications of tooth extractions in patients taking warfarin, antibiotics, and other medications. J Oral Maxillofac Surg. 2011;69:977–9.
33. Campbell JH, Alvarado F, Murray RA. Anticoagulation and minor oral surgery: should the anticoagulation regimen be altered? J Oral Maxillofac Surg. 2000;58:131–5.
34. Candemir B, Güleç S, Özdemir AO, Kumbasar D. Very late drug-eluting stent thrombosis in a patient with an INR of 4.4. Arch Turk Soc Cardiol. 2010;38:561–3.
35. Cañigral A, Silvestre F-J, Cañigral G, et al. Evaluation of bleeding risk and measurement methods in dental patients. Med Oral Patol Oral Cir Bucal. 2010;15(6):e863–8.

36. Cannon PD, Dharmar VT. Minor oral surgical procedures in patients on oral anticoagulants – a controlled study. Aust Dent J. 2003;48(2):115–8.
37. Carter G, Goss A. Tranexamic acid mouthwash – a prospective randomized study of a 2-day regimen *vs* 5-day regimen to prevent postoperative bleeding in anticoagulated patients requiring dental extractions. Int J Oral Maxillofac Surg. 2003;32:504–7.
38. Carter G, Goss AN, Lloyd J, Tocchetti R. Local haemostasis with autologous fibrin glue following surgical enucleation of a large cystic lesion in a therapeutically anticoagulated patient. Br J Oral Maxillofac Surg. 2003;41:275–6.
39. Carter G, Goss A, Lloyd J, et al. Tranexamic acid mouthwash verses autologous fibrin glue in patients taking warfarin under-going dental extractions: a randomized prospective clinical study. J Oral Maxillofac Surg. 2003;61:1432–5.
40. Cesar JM, Iturriaga TM. Correction by desmopressin of bleeding following dental extraction in a patient under antithrombotic therapy. [Letter]. Oral Surg Oral Med Oral Pathol Oral Radiol. 2007;104(2):151.
41. Cieślik-Bielecka A, Pelc R, Cieślik T. Oral surgery procedures in patients on anticoagulants. Preliminary report. Kardiol Pol. 2005;63:137–40.
42. Clemm R, Neukam FW, Rusche B, Musazada S, Schmitt CM. Management of anticoagulated patients in implant therapy: a clinical comparative study. Clin Oral Impl Res. 2016;27:1274–82.
43. Cocero N, Mozzati M, Ambrogio M, Bisi M, Morello M, Bergamasco L. Bleeding rate during oral surgery of oral anticoagulant therapy patients with associated systemic pathologic entities: a prospective study of more than 500 extractions. J Oral Maxillofac Surg. 2014;72:858–67.
44. Cone A. Dental abscess in an anticoagulated patient with ankylosing spondylitis. Br J Hosp Med. 1993;49:190.
45. Dantas AK, Deboni MC, Peratininga JL. Dental surgery in patients on oral anticoagulation therapy. Rev Bras Hematol Hemoter. 2009;31(5):337–40.
46. Davies D. Minor oral surgical procedures in patients on oral anticoagulants. [Letter]. Aust Dent J. 2003;48(4):267.
47. Devani P, Lavery M, Howell CJT. Dental extractions in patients on warfarin: is alteration of anticoagulation regime necessary? Br J Oral Maxillofac Surg. 1998;36:107–11.
48. Eichhorn W, Burkert J, Vorwig O, et al. Bleeding incidence after oral surgery with continued oral anticoagulation. Clin Oral Invest. 2012;16:1371–6.
49. Elad S, Findler M. Periodontal surgery for patients receiving anticoagulant therapy. [Letter]. Arch Intern Med. 2008;168(15):1719.
50. Elad S, Zadik Y, Kaufman E, et al. A new management approach for dental treatment after a cerebrovascular event: a comparative retrospective study. Oral Surg Oral Med Oral Pathol Oral Radiol Endod. 2010;110:145–50.
51. Erden I, Erden EÇ, Aksu T, et al. Comparison of uninterrupted warfarin and bridging therapy using low-molecular weight heparin with respect to the severity of bleeding after dental extractions in patients with prosthetic valves. Anatol J Cardiol. 2016;16:467–73.
52. Evans IL, Sayers MS, Gibbons AJ, et al. Can warfarin be continued during dental extraction? Results of a randomized controlled trial. Br J Oral Maxillofac Surg. 2002;40(3):248–52.
53. Febbo A, Cheng A, Stein B, Goss A, Sambrook P. Postoperative bleeding following dental extractions in patients anticoagulated with warfarin. J Oral Maxillofac Surg. 2016;74:1518–23.
54. Ferrieri GB, Castiglioni S, Carmagnola D, et al. Oral surgery in patients on anticoagulant treatment without therapy interruption. J Oral Maxillofac Surg. 2007;65:1149–54.
55. Frank BW, Dickhaus DW, Claus EC. Dental extractions in the presence of continual anticoagulant therapy. Ann Intern Med. 1963;59:911–3.
56. Gagneja M, Gagneja P, Steelman R, Shaughnessy R, Johannes PW. Oral surgery in a child with a prosthetic aortic valve and pulmonary artery stent at risk for thromboembolism. J Clin Pediatr Dent. 2007;32(2):151–4.
57. Gaspar R, Brenner B, Ardekian L, Peled M. Use of tranexamic acid mouthwash to prevent postoperative bleeding in oral surgery patients on oral anticoagulant medication. Quintessence Int. 1997;28:375–9.
58. Giuffrè G, Caputo G, Misso S, Peluso F. Platelet-rich plasma treatment and hemostasis in patients with hemorrhagic risk. Minerva Stomatol. 2006;55:599–609.
59. Gómez-Moreno G, Aguilar-Salvatierra A, Fernández-Cejas E, et al. Dental implant surgery in patients in treatment with the anticoagulant oral rivaroxaban. Clin Oral Implants Res. 2016;27:730–3.
60. Goodchild JH, Donaldson M. A clinically significant drug interaction between warfarin and amoxicillin resulting in persistent postoperative bleeding in a dental patient. Gen Dent. 2013;61(4):50–4.
61. Greenberg MS, Miller MF, Lynch MA. Partial thromboplastin time as a predictor of blood loss in oral surgery patients receiving coumarin anticoagulants. J Am Dent Assoc. 1972;84:583–7.
62. Hadziabdic N, Sulejmanagic H, Haracic M, et al. Recommended INR values for performing oral-surgical interventions. HealthMED. 2011;5(6 Suppl 1):2243–51.
63. Halfpenny W, Fraser JS, Adlam DM. Comparison of 2 hemostatic agents for the prevention of postextraction hemorrhage in patients on anticoagulants. Oral Surg Oral Med Oral Pathol Oral Radiol Endod. 2001;92(3):257–9.
64. Hong C, Napenas JJ, Brennan M, et al. Risk of postoperative bleeding after dental procedures in patients on warfarin: a retrospective study. Oral Surg Oral Med Oral Pathol Oral Radiol. 2012;114(4):464–8.

65. Inchingolo F, Tatullo M, Abenavoli FM, et al. Odontostomatologic management of patients receiving oral anticoagulant therapy: a retrospective multicentric study. Ann Surg Innov Res. 2011;5(1):5.
66. Iwabuchi H, Imai Y, Asanami S, et al. Evaluation of postextraction bleeding incidence to compare patients receiving and not receiving warfarin therapy: a cross-sectional, multicentre, observational study. BMJ Open. 2014;4:e005777. https://doi.org/10.1136/bmjopen-2014-005777.
67. Jimson S, Amaldhas J, Jimson S, Kannan I, Parthiban J. Assessment of bleeding during minor oral surgical procedures and extraction in patients on anticoagulant therapy. J Pharm Bioallied Sci. 2015;7(Suppl 1):S134–7.
68. Karsli ED, Erdogan O, Esen E, Acartürk E. Comparison of the effects of warfarin and heparin on bleeding caused by dental extraction: a clinical study. J Oral Maxillfac Surg. 2011;69:2500–7.
69. Kataoka T, Hoshi K, Ando T. Is the HAS-BLED score useful in predicting post-extraction bleeding in patients taking warfarin? A retrospective cohort study. BMJ Open. 2016;6(3):e010471. https://doi.org/10.1136/bmjopen-2015-010471.
70. Kovács B, Tóth K, Kerényi G. Post-extraction hemostasis during coumarin anticoagulant therapy with a locally applied coagulation-active substance. Int J Oral Surg. 1976;5:3–7.
71. Kumar KRA, Kumar J, Sarvagna J, Gadde P, Chikkaboriah S. Hemostasis and post-operative care of oral surgical wounds by hemocon dental dressing in patients on oral anticoagulant therapy: a split mouth randomized controlled clinical trial. J Clin Diagn Res. 2016;10(9):ZC37–40.
72. Kusafuka Y, Kurita H, Sakurai S, et al. Effect of single-dose extended-release oral azithromycin on anticoagulation status in warfarinized patients. Oral Surg Oral Med Oral Pathol Oral Radiol. 2013;115:148–51.
73. Kwapis BW. Anticoagulant therapy and dental practice. J Am Dent Assoc. 1963;66:172–5.
74. Martinowitz U, Mazar AL, Taicher S, et al. Dental extraction for patients on oral anticoagulant therapy. Oral Surg Oral Med Oral Pathol. 1990;70:274–7.
75. Mauprivez C, Khonsari RH, Razouk O, et al. Management of dental extraction in patients undergoing anticoagulant oral direct treatment: a pilot study. Oral Surg Oral Med Oral Pathol Oral Radiol. 2016;122(5):e146–55.
76. McBane RD, Wysokinski WE, Daniels PR, et al. Periprocedural anticoagulation management of patients with venous thromboembolism. Arterioscler Thromb Vasc Biol. 2010;30(3):442–8.
77. McIntyre H. Management, during dental surgery of patients on anticoagulants. Lancet. 1966;2:99–100.
78. Mesquita KC, Teófilo CR, Perdigão JP, et al. Dental care in patients with antiphospholipid syndrome: two case reports. Gen Dent. 2017;65(1):e9–e13.
79. Morimoto Y, Niwa H, Minematsu K. Hemostatic management of tooth extractions in patients on oral antithrombotic therapy. J Oral Maxillofac Surg. 2008;66:51–7.
80. Morimoto Y, Niwa H, Minematsu K. Risk factors affecting postoperative hemorrhage after tooth extraction in patients receiving oral antithrombotic therapy. J Oral Maxillofac Surg. 2011;69(6):1550.
81. Morimoto Y, Niwa H, Minematsu K. Hemostatic management for periodontal treatments in patients on oral antithrombotic therapy: a retrospective study. Oral Surg Oral Med Oral Pathol Oral Radiol Endod. 2009;108:889–96.
82. Nakasato S, Okamura S, Osaka H, et al. Management of dental surgery problems for outpatients with cardiovascular diseases. Anesth Prog. 1989;36:140–9.
83. Pereira CM, Gasparetto PF, Santos Carneiro D, et al. Tooth extraction in patients on oral anticoagulants: prospective study conducted in 108 Brazilian patients. ISRN Dent. 2011;2011:203619.
84. Pippi R, Santoro M, Cafolla A. The effectiveness of a new method using an extra-alveolar hemostatic agent after dental extractions in older patients on oral anticoagulation treatment: an intrapatient study. Oral Surg Oral Med Oral Pathol Oral Radiol. 2015;120:15–21.
85. Raborn GW, Hohn FI, Grace MGA, Arora BK. Tisseel, a two component fibrin tissue sealant system: report of a trial involving anticoagulated dental patients. J Can Dent Assoc. 1990;56(8):779–81.
86. Ramli R, Rahman RA. Minor oral surgery in anticoagulated patients: local measures alone are sufficient for haemostasis. Singap Dent J. 2005;27(1):13–6.
87. Ramstrom G, Sindet-Pedersen S, Hall G, Blomback M, Alander U. Prevention of postsurgical bleeding in oral surgery using tranexamic acid without dose modification of oral anticoagulants. J Oral Maxillofac Surg. 1993;51:1211–6.
88. Sacco R, Sacco M, Carpenedo M, Mannucci PM. Oral surgery in patients on oral anticoagulant therapy: a randomized comparison of different intensity targets. Oral Surg Oral Med Oral Pathol Oral Radiol Endod. 2007;104:e18-e21.
89. Salam S, Yusuf H, Milosevic A. Bleeding after dental extractions in patients taking warfarin. Br J Oral Maxillofac Surg. 2007;45(6):463.
90. Sammartino G, Ehrenfest DMD, Carile F, Tia M, Bucci P. Prevention of hemorrhagic complications after dental extractions into open heart surgery patients under anticoagulant therapy: the use of leukocyte- and platelet-rich fibrin. J Oral Implantol. 2011;37(6):681–90.
91. Sammartino G, Maenzi G, Miro A, et al. Local delivery of the hemostatic agent tranexamic acid in chronically anticoagulated patients. J Craniofac Surg. 2012;23(6):e648–52.
92. Scarano A, Sinjari B, Murmura G, et al. Hemostasis control in dental extractions in patients receiving oral anticoagulant therapy: an approach with calcium sulfate. J Craniofac Surg. 2014;25(3):843–6.
93. Schmitt J, Ingram RC, Harpole HJ. Hematoma following dental extractions in a patient receiving

unreported anticoagulant therapy. Oral Surg Oral Med Oral Pathol. 1960;13:791–4.
94. Shah AH, Khalil HS, Kola MZ. Dental management of a patient fitted with subcutaneous Implantable Cardioverter Debfibrillator device and concomitant warfarin treatment. Saud Dent J. 2015;27(3):165–70.
95. Shira RB, Hall RJ, Guernsey LH. Minor oral surgery during prolonged anticoagulant therapy. J Oral Surg. 1962;20:93–9.
96. Sindet-Pedersen S, Ramstrom G, Bernvil S, Blomback M. Hemostatic effect of tranexamic acid mouthwash in anticoagulant-treated patients undergoing oral surgery. N Engl J Med. 1989;320:840–3.
97. Soares ECS, Costa FWG, Bezerra TP, et al. Postoperative hemostatic efficacy of gauze soaked in tranexamic acid, fibrin sponge, and dry gauze compression following dental extractions in anticoagulated patients with cardiovascular disease: a prospective, randomized study. Oral Maxillofac Surg. 2015;19:209–16.
98. Souto JC, Oliver A, Zuazu-Jausoro I, Vives FJ. Oral surgery in anticoagulated patients without reducing the dose of oral anticoagulant: a prospective randomized study. J Oral Maxillofac Surg. 1996;54:27–32.
99. Street AM, Leung W. Use of tranexamic acid mouthwash in dental procedures in patients taking oral anticoagulants. Med J Aust. 1990;153:630.
100. Sung EC, Brar LK, Chung E, et al. Dental treatment in the cardiothoracic intensive care unit for patients with ventricular assist devices awaiting heart transplant: a case series. Oral Surg Oral Med Oral Pathol Oral Radiol. 2014;118:194–201.
101. Svensson R, Hallmer F, Englesson CS, Svensson PJ, Becktor JP. Treatment with local hemostatic agents and primary closure after tooth extraction in warfarin treated patients. Swed Dent J. 2013;37(2):71–7.
102. Throndson RR, Walstad WR. Use of the argon beam coagulator for control of postoperative hemorrhage in an anticoagulated patient. J Oral Maxillofac Surg. 1999;57:1367–9.
103. Tomasi NJ, Wolf JE. Presurgical management of a patient receiving anticoagulant therapy: report of case. J Am Dent Assoc. 1974;88:1028–9.
104. Tulloch J, Wright IS. Long-term anticoagulant therapy: further experiences. Circulation. 1954;9:823–34.
105. Wahl MJ, Schmitt MM. Postextraction bleeding in a patient taking antithrombotics: report of a case. Gen Dent. 2016;64(3):60–3.
106. Waldrep AC, McKelvey LE. Oral surgery for patients on anticoagulant therapy. J Oral Surg. 1968;26:374–80.
107. Wood GD, Deeble T. Warfarin: dangers with antibiotics. Dent Update. 1993;20:350–3.
108. Yoshimura Y, Oka M, Kishimoto H, Matsuura R, Mishima K. Hemodynamic changes during dental extraction and post-extraction bleeding in patients with prosthetic heart valves. Int J Oral Maxillofac Surg. 1987;16:425–31.
109. Zanon E, Martinelli F, Bacci C, et al. Safety of dental extraction among consecutive patients on oral anticoagulant treatment managed using a specific dental management protocol. Blood Coagul Fibrinolysis. 2003;14(1):27–30.
110. Zirk M, Fienitz T, Edel R, et al. Prevention of postoperative bleeding in hemostatic compromised patients using native porcine collagen fleeces – retrospective study of a consecutive case series. Oral Maxillofac Surg. 2016;20:249–54.
111. Zusman SP, Lustig JP, Nun GB. Cost evaluation of two methods of post tooth extraction hemostasis in patients on anticoagulant therapy. Community Dent Health. 1993;10:167–73.
112. Akbarian M, Austen WG, Yurchak PM, Scannell JG. Thromboembolic complications of prosthetic cardiac valves. Circulation. 1968;37:826–31.
113. Akopov SE, Suzuki S, Fredieu A, et al. Withdrawal of warfarin prior to a surgical procedure: time to follow the guidelines? Cerbrovasc Dis. 2005;19(5):337–42.
114. Aldous JA, Olson CJ. Managing patients on warfarin therapy: a case report. Spec Care Dentist. 2001;21(3):109–12.
115. Alexander R. More nonsense. N Y State Dent J. 2003;69(4):11.
116. Baykul T, Alanoglu EG, Kocer G. Use of Ankaferd Blood Stopper as a hemostatic agent: a clinical experience. J Contemp Dent Pract. 2010;11(1):1–7.
117. Bloomer CR. Excessive hemorrhage after dental extractions using low-molecular-weight heparin (Lovenox) anticoagulation therapy. J Oral Maxillofac Surg. 2004;62:101–3.
118. Broderick JP, Bonomo JB, Kissela BM, et al. Withdrawal of antithrombotic agents and its impact on ischemic stroke occurrence. Stroke. 2011;42(9):2509–14.
119. Campbell S, Monagle P, Newall F. Oral anticoagulant therapy interruption in children: a single Centre experience. Thromb Res. 2016;140:89–93.
120. Crean SJ, Sivarajasingam V, Muhammed J, Sharma V, Fardy M. Thrombophilia and dental surgery: a report of dental extraction in a patient with protein S deficiency. Dent Update. 2000;27:302–5.
121. Davis FB, Sczupak CA. Outpatient oral anticoagulation: guidelines for long-term management. Postgrad Med. 1979;66:100–9.
122. Della Valle A, Sammartino G, Marenzi G, et al. Prevention of postoperative bleeding in anticoagulated patients undergoing oral surgery: use of platelet-rich plasma gel. J Oral Maxillofac Surg. 2003;61:1275–8.
123. Douketis JD, Johnson JA, Turpie AG. Low-molecular-weight heparin as bridging anticoagulation during interruption of warfarin: assessment of a standardized periprocedural anticoagulation regimen. JAMA Intern Med. 2004;164(12):1319–26.
124. Dunn AS, Spyropoulos AC, Turpie AGG. Bridging therapy in patients on long-term oral anticoagulants who require surgery: the Prospective perio-perative

Enoxaparin Cohort Trial (PROSPECT). J Thromb Haemost. 2007;5(11):2211–8.
125. Finn MD, Schow SR. Sugical management of a protein S-deficient patient. J Oral Maxillofac Surg. 1993;51:181–3.
126. Garcia DA, Regan S, Henault LE, et al. Risk of thromboembolism with short-term interruption of warfarin therapy. Arch Intern Med. 2008;168(1):63–9.
127. Jaffer AK, Ahmed M, Brotman DJ, et al. Low molecular weight heparins as periprocedural anticoagulation for patients on long-term warfarin therapy: a standardized bridging therapy protocol. J Thromb Thrombolysis. 2005;20(1):11–6.
128. Johnson-Leong C, Rada RE. The use of low-molecular-weight heparins in outpatient oral surgery for patients receiving anticoagulation therapy. J Am Dent Assoc. 2002;133:1083–7.
129. Kovacs MJ, Kearon C, Rodger M, et al. Single-arm study of bridging therapy with low-molecular-weight heparin for patients at risk of arterial embolism who require temporary interruption of warfarin. Circulation. 2004;110:1658–63.
130. Lund J-P, Drews T, Hetzer R, Reichart PA. Oral surgical management of patients with mechanical circulatory support. Int J Oral Maxillofac Surg. 2002;31:629–33.
131. Marshall J. Rebound phenomena after anticoagulant therapy in cerebrovascular disease. Circulation. 1963;28:329–32.
132. Mehra P, Cottrell DA, Bestgen SC, Booth DF. Management of heparin therapy in the high-risk, chronically anticoagulated, oral surgery patient: a review and a proposed nomogram. J Oral Maxillofac Surg. 2000;58:198–202.
133. Miclotte I, Vanhaverbeke M, Agbaje JO. Pragmatic approach to manage new oral anticoagulants in patients undergoing dental extractions: a prospective case-control study. Clin Oral Investig. 2016;21:2183. https://doi.org/10.1007/s00784-016-2010-1.
134. Milligan PE, Banet GA, Gage BF. Perioperative reduction of the warfarin dose. [Letter]. Am J Med. 2003;115:741–2.
135. Mulligan R. Response to anticoagulant withdrawal. JADA. 1987;115:435–8.
136. O'Donnell MJ, Kearon C, Johnson J, et al. Brief communication: preoperative anticoagulant activity after bridging low-molecular-weight heparin for temporary interruption of warfarin. Ann Intern Med. 2007;146:184–7.
137. Ogiuchi H, Ando T, Tanaka M, Kuwasawa T, Sangu Y, Abe H, Kawanishi I. Clinical reports on dental extraction from patients undergoing oral anticoagulant therapy. Bull Tokyo Dent Coll. 1985;26(4):205–12.
138. Palomäki A, Kiviniemi T, Hartikainen JE, et al. Postoperative strokes and intracranial bleeds in patients with atrial fibrillation: the FibStroke study. Clin Cardiol. 2016;39(8):471–6.
139. Pávek V, Bigl P. Stomatological treatment of patients with artificial heart valves: coagulation control and antibiotic cover. Int Dent J. 1993;43:59–61.
140. Pearce RL, Summers L, Herrmann RP. The management of patients with the Kasabach-Merritt Syndrome. Br J Oral Surg. 1975;13:188–95.
141. Picard A, Zwetchkenbaum S, Morganstern LB. Dental implications of acute stroke therapy and anticoagulation for stroke prevention. Compend Contin Educ Dent. 2010;31(3):190–5.
142. Prudoff SH, Stratigos GT. Successful management of patients with cardiac valvular prostheses. N Y State Dent J. 1972;38:207–10.
143. Roberts HJ. Control of bleeding after dental extraction during anticoagulation therapy: with particular reference to estrogenic prophylaxis. J Am Med Assoc. 1961;175(11):962–6.
144. Roberts HJ. Anticoagulants during dental surgery. Lancet. 1966;288(7464):639.
145. Romond KK, Miller CS, Henry RG. Dental management considerations for a patient taking dabigatran etexilate: a case report. Oral Surg Oral Med Oral Pathol Oral Radiol. 2013;116:e191–5.
146. Russo G, Corso LD, Biasolo A, et al. Simple and safe method to prepare patients with prosthetic heart valves for surgical dental procedures. Clin Appl Thromb Hemost. 2000;6(2):90–3.
147. Saour JN, Ali HA, Mammo LARF, Sieck JO. Dental procedures in patients receiving oral anticoagulation therapy. J Heart Valve Dis. 1994;3:315–7.
148. Scheitler LE, Hart N, Phillips G, Weinberg JB. Hematologic and surgical management of the dental patient with plasminogen activator deficiency. Oral Surg Oral Med Oral Pathol. 1988;66:680–2.
149. Schofield JJ. Complications of dental extractions in patients receiving anticoagulant therapy. [Letter]. Br Dent J. 1984;156(6):200.
150. Sheller B, Tong D. Dental management of a child on anticoagulant therapy and the International Normalized Ratio: case report. Pediatr Dent. 1994;16(1):56–8.
151. Somma F, Grande NM, Plotino G, Camelli G, Pameijer CH. Conservative approach to dental extractions in patients on anticoagulant therapy: a clinical study. Gen Dent. 2010;58(1):e30–5.
152. Spandorfer JM, Lynch S, Weitz HH, Fertel S, Merli GJ. Use of enoxaparin for the chronically anticoagulated patient before and after procedures. Am J Cardiol. 1999;84:478–80.
153. Spyropoulos AC, Jenkins P, Bornikova L. A disease management protocol for outpatient perioperative bridge therapy with enoxaparin in patients requiring temporary interruption of long-term oral anticoagulation. Pharmacotherapy. 2004;24(5):649–58.
154. Steinberg BA, Peterson ED, Kim S, et al. Use and outcomes associated with bridging during anticoagulation interruptions in patients with atrial fibrillation: findings from the Outcomes Registry for

a Better Informed Treatment of Atrial Fibrillation (ORBIT-AF). Circulation. 2015;131:488–94.
155. Tinmouth AH, Morrow BH, Cruickshank MK, Moore PM, Kovacs MJ. Dalteparin as periprocedure anticoagulation for patients on warfarin and at high risk of thrombosis. Ann Pharmacother. 2001;35:669–74.
156. Todd DW. Outpatient use of low-molecular weight heparin in an anticoagulated patient requiring oral surgery: report of a case. J Oral Maxillofac Surg. 2001;59:1090–2.
157. Wilson SJ, Morgan J, Gray L, Newman V, Anderson DR. A model of perioperative outpatient management of anticoagulation in high-risk patients: an evaluation of effectiveness and safety. Can J Hosp Pharm. 2001;54:269–77.
158. Won K-B, Lee S-H, Chang H-J, et al. Safety and cost-effectiveness of bridge therapies for invasive dental procedures in patients with mechanical heart valves. Yonsei Med J. 2014;55(4):937–43.
159. Wood JC, Conn HL. Prevention of systemic arterial embolism in chronic rheumatic heart disease by means of protracted anticoagulant therapy. Circulation. 1954;10:517–23.
160. Yasaka M, Naritomi H, Minematsu K. Ischemic stroke associated with brief cessation of warfarin. [Letter]. Thromb Res. 2006;118(2):290–3.
161. Wysokinski WE, McBane RD, Daniels PR, et al. Periprocedural anticoagulation management of patients with nonvalvular atrial fibrillation. Mayo Clin Proc. 2008;83(6):639–45.
162. Halperin JL, Hankey GJ, Wojdyla DM, et al. Efficacy and safety of rivaroxaban compared with warfarin among elderly patients with nonvalvular atrial fibrillation in the Rivaroxaban Once Daily, Oral, Direct Factor Xa Inhibition Compared with Vitamin K Antagonism for Prevention of Stroke and Embolism Trial in Atrial Fibrillation (ROCKET AF). Circulation. 2014;130(2):L138–46.
163. Pelliccia F, Rosanio S, Marazzi G, et al. Efficacy and safety of novel anticoagulants versus vitamin K antagonists in patients with mild and moderate to severe renal insufficiency: focus on apixaban. Int J Cardiol. 2016;225:77–81.
164. Costantinides F, Rizzo R, Pascazio L, Maglione M. Managing patients taking novel oral anticoagulants (NOAs) in dentistry: a discussion paper on clinical implications. BMC Oral Health. 2016;16:5.
165. Rechenmacher SJ, Fang JC. Bridging anticoagulation: primum non nocere. J Am Coll Cardiol. 2015;66(12):1392–403.
166. Siegal D, Yudin J, Kaatz S, et al. Periprocedural heparin bridging in patients receiving vitamin K antagonists: systematic review and meta-analysis of bleeding and thromboembolic rates. Circulation. 2012;126:1630–9.
167. Pallasch TJ, Wahl MJ. Focal infection: new age or ancient history? Endod Topics. 2003;4:32–45.
168. Kells CE. The X-ray in dental practice: the crime of the age. J Nat Dent Assoc. 1920;7(3):241–72.
169. Gary CJ, Glick M. Medical clearance: an issue of professional autonomy, not a crutch. J Am Dent Assoc. 2012;143(11):1180–1.
170. American Dental Association Division of Legal Affairs. An updated legal perspective on antibiotic prophylaxis. JADA. 2003;134(9):1260.
171. Wahl MJ. Myths of dental-induced endocarditis. Arch Intern Med. 1994;154:137–44.
172. Skolarus LE, Morgenstern LB, Froehlich JB, Lisabeth LD, Brown DL. Guideline-discordant periprocedural interruptions in warfarin therapy. Circ Cardiovasc Qual Outcomes. 2011;4:206–10.
173. Wahl MJ, Howell J. Altering anticoagulation therapy: a survey of physicians. J Am Dent Assoc. 1996;127(5):625–34.
174. Lockhart PB. AAOM clinical practice statement. Subject: management of patients on warfarin therapy. Oral Surg Oral Med Oral Pathol Oral Radiol. 2016;122(6):702–4.
175. American Dental Association. Anticoagulant and antiplatelet medications and dental procedures. Available: http://www.ada.org/en/member-center/oral-health-topics/anticoagulant-antiplatelet-medications-and-dental. Last updated 22 Oct 2015. Accessed 12 Nov 2016.
176. Mashour GA, Moore LE, Lele AV, Robicsek SA, Gelb AW. Perioperative care of patients at high risk for stroke during or after non-cardiac, non-neurologic surgery: consensus statement from the Society for Neuroscience in Anesthesiology and Critical Care. J Neurosurg Anesthesiol. 2014;26(4):273–85.
177. Armstrong MJ, Gronseth G, Anderson DC, et al. Summary of evidence-based guideline: periprocedural management of antithrombotic medications in patients with ischemic cerebrovascular disease. Report of the Guideline Development Subcommittee of the American Academy of Neurology. Neurology. 2013;80(22):2065–9.
178. Douketis JD, Spyropoulos AC, Spencer FA, et al. Perioperative management of antithrombotic therapy. Antithrombotic therapy and prevention of thrombosis, 9th ed: American College of Chest Physicians Evidence-Based Clinical Practice Guidelines. Chest. 2012;141(2 Suppl):e326–e350S.
179. Perry DJ, Noakes TJC, Helliwell PS. Guidelines for the management of patients on oral anticoagulants requiring dental surgery. Br Dent J. 2007;203:389–93.
180. Hirsh J, Fuster V, Ansell J, Halperin JL. American Heart Association/American College of Cardiology Foundation guide to warfarin therapy. Circulation. 2003;107:1692–711.
181. Ansell J, Hirsh J, Dalen J, et al. Managing oral anticoagulant therapy. Chest. 2001;119:22S–38S.
182. Ansell J, Hirsh J, Poller L, et al. The pharmacology and management of the vitamin K antagonists: The Seventh AACP Conference on

Antithrombotic and Thrombolytic Therapy. Chest. 2004;126:204S–33S.
183. Douketis JD, Berger PB, Dunn AS, et al. The perioperative management of antithrombotic therapy. American College of Chest Physicians Evidence-Based Clinical Practice Guidelines (8th Edition). Chest. 2008;133:299–339S.
184. Wahl MJ. Anticoagulation in dental surgery: is it rude to interrupt? Cleve Clin J Med. 2016;83(6):409–13.
185. Wahl MJ, Pintos A, Lalla RV. Interruption of warfarin anticoagulation for dental surgery [Letter]. Chest. 2013;144(4):1424.
186. Ringel R, Maas R. Dental procedures in patients treated with antiplatelet or anticoagulation therapy – an anonymous survey. Gerodontology. 2016;33(4):447–52.
187. Balevi B. Should warfarin be discontinued before a dental extraction? A decision-tree analysis. Oral Surg Oral Med Oral Pathol Oral Radiol Endod. 2010;110(6):691–7.
188. Wahl MJ. Bleed or die? A bloody simple decision. [Letter]. Oral Surg Oral Med Oral Pathol Oral Radiol. 2011;113(2):147–8.
189. Lalla RV, Peterson DE, Aframian DJ. Should warfarin be discontinued before a dental extraction? [Letter]. Oral Surg Oral Med Oral Pathol Oral Radiol. 2012;113(2):149–50.
190. Miller CS. Evidence does not support the discontinuation of warfarin before a dental extraction. [Letter]. Oral Surg Oral Med Oral Pathol Oral Radiol. 2012;113(2):148–9.
191. Todd DW. Anticoagulated patients and oral surgery [letter]. Arch Intern Med. 2003;163:1242.
192. Kunz R, Spyropoulos AC, Spencer FA, et al. Response [to letter]. Chest. 2013;144(4):1424–6.

# Local Techniques and Pharmacologic Agents for Management of Bleeding in Dentistry

15

Richard P. Szumita and Paul M. Szumita

**Abstract**

In surgical or traumatic wounds, the cessation of bleeding ranges from spontaneous hemostasis, where no intervention is required, to complex multidisciplinary management requiring multiple systemic and local therapies. Effective management begins with understanding bleeding has diverse causes. Generally, the causes of bleeding can be local, systemic, or a combination. Local factors include injured vessel(s) size and type (large versus small; arterial versus venous versus capillary) and fragility of capillaries and perivascular tissues due to age, disease, or medications. Systemic factors include drug-induced coagulopathies and underlying hematologic defects. Obtaining hemostasis is interdependent on the cause(s) of bleeding and event-specific factors such as size of wound, type of procedure/surgery performed, degree of inflammation at the wound site, and response to pharmacologic interventions.

R. P. Szumita (✉)
Department of Dentistry/Oral and Maxillofacial Surgery, St. Joseph's University Medical Center, Paterson, NJ, USA

Private Practice, Little Falls, NJ, USA
e-mail: Szumita@northeastoralsurgerycenter.com

P. M. Szumita
Department of Pharmacy Services, Brigham and Women's Hospital, Boston, MA, USA
e-mail: pszumita@partners.org

In oral hemostasis, the dental practitioners' goal for patient management should be to minimize and control local bleeding and minimize the risk of systemic thrombosis. Accomplishing this goal begins with understanding pathologic bleeding can occur due to many diverse factors. Local factors include injured vessel size and type, fragility of capillaries and perivascular tissues. Systemic causes include bleeding disorders and drug-induced coagulopathies [1–5]. This understanding should help in obtaining a thorough and effective patient history. Key elements of a hematologic history include ascertaining previously diagnosed bleeding diatheses, bleeding tendencies, or diseases of organ systems intimately involved in hemostasis—bone marrow suppression and liver disease. Ascertaining a complete list of medications and supplements taken is also a critical portion of the history. When necessary, clarification of patient's history and quantification of disease should be discussed with the patient's primary care physician and/or hematologist.

With information obtained from the history, the dental practitioner should then consider the following patient-specific issues: etiology of bleeding, impact of antithrombotic medication(s) on local bleeding versus systemic thrombosis risk, impact of hematologic disease on bleeding risk, and therapeutic modalities available to help control bleeding.





R. P. Szumita, P. M. Szumita (eds.), *Hemostasis in Dentistry*, https://doi.org/10.1007/978-3-319-71240-6_15

In evaluating and managing patients, one method the author finds helpful is to stratify patients in terms of bleeding risk as follows: no pathology of hemostasis, pharmacologic alteration of hemostasis, and pathology of hemostasis (i.e., von Willebrand disease, hemophilia A). Patients with absence of a bleeding disorder and no unusual bleeding tendencies are at the lowest risk for bleeding and will likely require minimal local techniques to control procedural or postoperative bleeding.

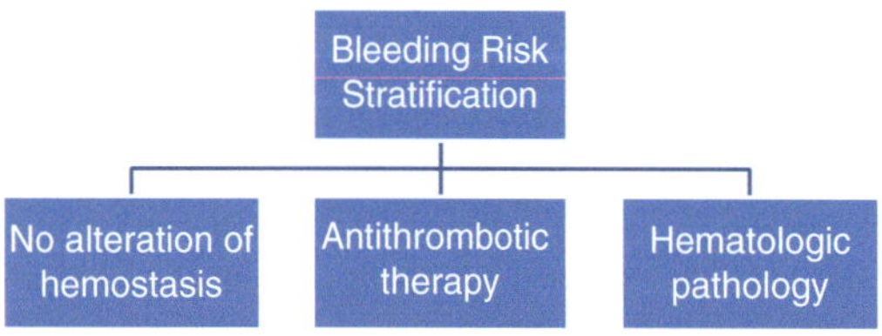


Patients on antithrombotic medications have been reviewed extensively in this book. If within therapeutic ranges, most patients on anticoagulant or antiplatelet medications do carry a slight increase in surgical site bleeding. However, bleeding is well controlled with local treatments, and alteration of medications is usually not indicated. (The reader is directed to Chaps. 12 and 14 in this book and the extensive bibliography provided.)

Generally, patients with diseases of hemostasis have the highest risk for bleeding. As discussed in several of the chapters of this book, management depends on disease severity and often includes pre-procedural systemic optimization by a hematologist, intraoperative local therapy, and postoperative local and systemic interventions. In this patient population, local procedures alone will often be insufficient to control procedural and postoperative bleeding. Management of these patients should be coordinated with patient's hematologist. The hematologist directs and prescribes the systemic management as directed by the patient's disease. The dentist directs and employs local therapies which, combined with systemic management, provide the optimum conditions to overcome the defects in hemostasis.

Procoagulant therapeutic modalities are medical and surgical interventions which help the patient's physiologic clotting—especially when clotting is insufficient. The interventions are divided into local (surgical) and systemic (medical). Local modalities include procedures and products that are applied locally to help stop bleeding. Systemic interventions include systemic administration of pharmacologic agents, pharmacologic reversal agents, and transfusions. Employment of the appropriate therapies is based on the suspected etiology and severity of bleeding. Systemic therapies are associated with various disease processes and have been reviewed throughout this book.

The remainder of this chapter reviews the local therapies or "local measures" to help with obtaining hemostasis in dental patients. When needed, a number of these local "tools" are available to the dental practitioner to employ at the site of bleeding or potential bleeding. Each of these therapies varies in efficacy, complexity, availability, price, adverse reactions, and degree of patient compliance needed. All of these factors should be considered prior to implementing into practice.

Local measures can be divided into:

1. Surgical techniques
2. Local pressure
3. Hemostatic wound dressings
4. Local pharmacologic agents
5. Tissue adhesives
6. Energy-based treatments

## 15.1 Surgical Techniques

Properly employed surgical techniques along with appropriate and immediate wound care are essential in minimizing posttreatment hemorrhage. Each dental/oral surgical procedure, ranging from dental prophylaxis and dental extractions to soft and hard tissue reconstruction of the dentition and maxillofacial skeleton, is associated with unique challenges to hemostasis. In the performance of procedures, there are several key elements to consider to minimize intraoperative hemorrhage and to manage postoperative bleeding. Central to all surgical procedures is the proper handling of the tissues—soft and hard tissues. Proper soft tissue management decreases excessive soft tissue injury and increases the efficacy of post-procedural wound maintenance. Effective soft tissue management includes avoidance of tearing, excessive stretching, and crushing. These can extend microtrauma to vessels and tissues beyond the immediate incision sites creating increased tissue inflammation. Well-planned soft tissue surgical design, sharp incisions, careful control of tissue elevation in the proper tissue plane, and gentle retraction create less soft tissue trauma. The appropriate use and placement of releasing incisions further helps in preventing tearing and maceration of tissue. Of course, avoidance of direct injury to the larger vascular structures of the oral cavity is important. These structures include the mental, inferior alveolar, greater palatine, and lingual vessels.

Hard tissue management to decrease local bleeding includes thorough debridement of chronic inflammatory (granulation) tissue from bone and roots of teeth, reduction of sharp and loose areas of bone, and identification of bleeding vessels in bone. Granulation tissue tends to bleed with manipulation. Clinical experience shows thorough debridement of granulation tissue from the alveolar bone and roots of teeth decreases intraoperative bleeding and leads to better local hemostasis. Reduction of sharp edges of bone and removal of grossly mobile spicules of bone from the surgical field allow for less tissue trauma and inflammation and allow for application of surface pressure (gauze) with increased comfort.

Suturing is an important surgical skill to utilize for both wound management and hemostasis. Indications for suturing oral wounds include immobilization of soft tissue after mobilization (flap elevation), repositioning of soft tissue to new location (flap advancement), securing soft tissue grafts, minimizing dead space in multilayer wounds, and aid in hemostasis. Of course, not all oral wounds require suturing. Use of suture and implementation of suturing techniques vary based on procedure performed. When needed to assist in hemostasis, sutures are employed in several ways. First, sutures can be used to directly ligate a soft tissue vessel not controlled by other techniques. Suture ligation is often needed to control bleeding from an injured artery. If the vessel is accessible, the vessel is clamped with a hemostat, and a suture is used to tie around the vessel. If the point of bleeding is identified but the vessel cannot be isolated, a figure "8" suture can be placed around the bleeding point. Vessel ligation is often performed with 3-0 silk suture. More commonly in dentoalveolar surgery, sutures placed in the gingiva are useful for applying adequate pressure on the soft tissues surrounding extraction sockets and the alveolar ridge.

## 15.2 Local Pressure

Application of pressure to a bleeding site is elementary to first aid. In dentistry, application of pressure to a surgical area comes in several forms. Pressure can be divided into digital (direct) pressure, superficial (external) wound packing, and application of oral stents.

Digital (direct) pressure will be most often applied to bleeding site that may be encountered with injury to one of the larger blood vessels (arteries/veins) of the oral cavity. Disruption of an artery produces a brisk and voluminous bleeding. This bleeding can be complicated in the oral cavity if the bleeding is in the depth of a bony crypt as in the extraction socket of a mandibular third molar or the access bony cavity in endodontic apical surgery. Immediate pressure is needed and best supplied with digital pressure, with or without intervening gauze, to quell the amount of bleeding. Application of topical medicaments at this stage is often insufficient to slow bleeding. The use of cautery is also unlikely to stop the bleeding and greatly increases the chance of neural injury. Once the bleeding is reduced from direct pressure, placement of wound dressings and medicaments can be used as discussed below. In the case of persistent bleeding after release of pressure, gauze pack can be compressed into the socket, and the gauze help in place with figure "8" or mattress sutures for 24–48 h. Close follow-up with the patient is recommended.

Packing of surgical wounds to aid in hemostasis is well known. A ubiquitous method used in dentistry to apply superficial pressure is the placement of gauze pads over oral wounds and utilizing firm continuous biting pressure to help in local hemostasis. This method is safe, efficacious, and cost-effective. Additionally, tea bags are also empirically used if gauze packing is ineffective. Although the literature is scant with studies on the efficacy of tea bag use, the physical properties allow for contouring to the wound and biting pressure similar to gauze packing. Tea bags are also safe and relatively cost-effective. Additionally, tea leaves have been proposed to contain substances to aid in hemostasis. Tannins, present in tea and many other plants, have astringent properties. Tannins in tea extracts have implicated in antifibrinolysis through inhibition of plasmin [6–8]. Whether tea leaves contained in commercial tea bags exert significant procoagulant properties topically is not clear, the use of tea bags as a superficial pressure dressing is safe and has empiric efficacy.

There are several deficiencies to the use of superficial pressure packs. The primary drawback is the need for patient compliance. Young children and patients with certain neurologic pathologies may be unable to keep the gauze in the proper position and apply continuous pressure. In addition, the use of a pressure dressing is also often ineffective in patients with "liver" clots. "Liver" clots have also been referred to in the dental literature as "currant jelly" clots due to their physical appearance. The pathophysiology of liver clots is not clear. However, clinically patients often described postsurgical bleeding which persists and often increases despite the diligent application of surface gauze pressure. Upon presentation, an exuberant mass of clot is present extruding from the surgical wound. A persistent ooze of blood is noted from around the mass. The mass is often soft and compressible. Manipulation can cause increase in local bleeding [9, 10] (Fig. 15.1).

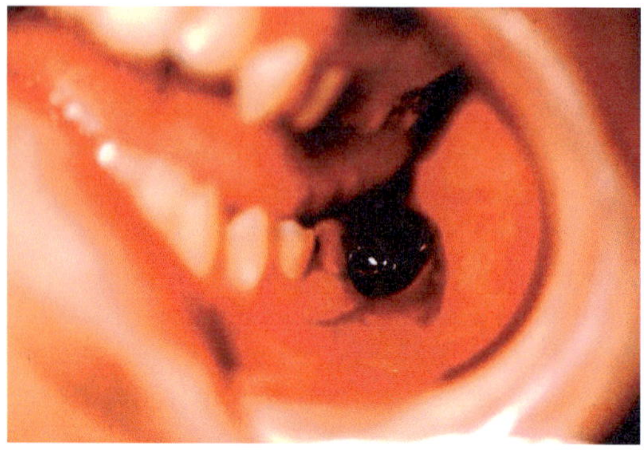

**Fig. 15.1** "Liver" clot from molar extraction site

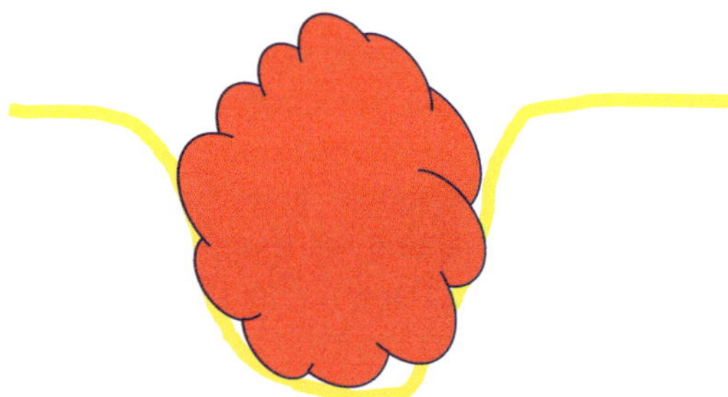

**Fig. 15.2** "Normal" clot adherent to the sockets walls

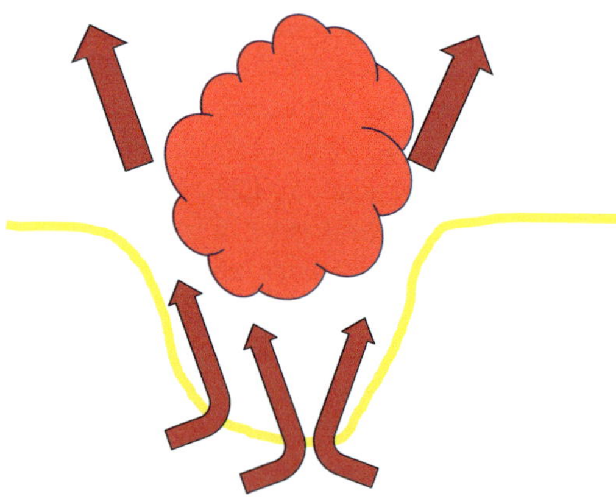

**Fig. 15.3** "Liver" clot dislodged from socket walls. Bleeding occurs around the clot

The following diagrams illustrate why surface pressure with gauze may be insufficient to obtain hemostasis (Figs. 15.2, 15.3, and 15.4).

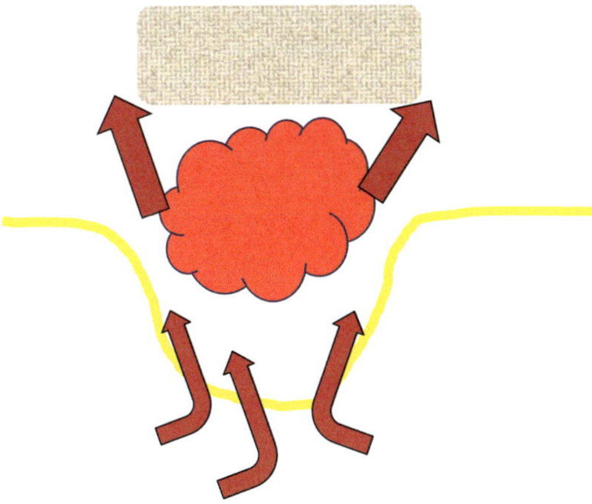

**Fig. 15.4** Gauze pressure compresses exuberant clot without applying pressure to bleeding socket

Management of this condition includes reassessment of patient's bleeding risk by review of the patient's medical, medication, and bleeding history. If multiple surgical sites are present, bleeding at only one of the sites will confirm bleeding is a local issue. If multiple sites are bleeding, suspicion of an underlying coagulopathy should be entertained. Hemostasis is obtained by complete debridement of all exuberant clot from the surgical wound, irrigation of the area, and reapplication of direct gauze pressure. Use of wound dressings and suturing is up to the discretion of the practitioner.

Superficial pressure dressings may also be ineffective when used alone in the management of patient with systemic bleeding disorders. Pressure dressings are almost always indicated but may need to be used in conjunction with other local and systemic therapies.

Direct wound pressure can also be obtained through the use of custom intraoral splints. This is especially effective if the splint is made in preparation for intraoral surgical procedures. A surgical splint can be designed to be more comfortable than pressure packing and decrease the need for patient compliance in the proper placement of gauze pads. Splints can also act as carriers for prohemostatic material and medicaments if needed [11–13]. Fabrication of splints is safe, cost-effective, efficacious, and easily performed by dental professionals.

## 15.3 Hemostatic Wound Dressings

Hemostatic wound dressings consist of materials placed within the confines of a traumatic or surgically created wound to assist the patient's physiology in the cessation of bleeding. The first two commercially available hemostatic wound dressings, which became commercially available in the 1940s, were oxidized cellulose, Oxycel (Becton Dickinson), and gelatin, Gelfoam (Pfizer) [14]. Since then, many more wound dressings have become available for use in the oral cavity.

The hemostatic wound dressings are divided into:

1. Oxidized cellulose
2. Gelatin
3. Collagen products
4. Chitosan products

### 15.3.1 Oxidized Cellulose

Oxidized cellulose is composed of polyanhydroglucuronic acid. The material has a low pH. Its prohemostatic properties are related to providing a scaffold for clot formation, denaturation of blood proteins, and contact activation of the clotting cascade. Oxidized cellulose has been shown to be bacteriostatic likely related to its acidic properties. The acidity may also be irritating and possibly damaging if in close proximity to vital structures like the inferior alveolar nerve [15]. Although it is reported to completely resorb in 4–8 weeks, there have been several case reports of residue of oxidized cellulose (used outside of the oral cavity) present on reoperation. Biodegradability may be influenced by quantity used and site of implantation [14, 16–19]. The material is easy to work with and easily cut to size and placed into wounds.

### 15.3.2 Gelatin

Commercially available gelatin products are derived from porcine or bovine sources and are available in granular or sponge forms. Gelatin dressings can provide a mechanical matrix for which a clot can form. These products will conform to irregular wounds and expand up to 200% of its initial volume providing a tamponade effect. They also likely initiate contact activation of the clotting. Gelatin products produce minimal to no tissue reaction and completely resorbs 4–6 weeks [14, 17, 19].

### 15.3.3 Collagen Products

Absorbable collagen products are derived from bovine source and are available in several forms: sheets, sponges, plugs (for extraction sockets), and powder-like. Collagen dressings help promote hemostasis via two mechanisms: contact activation of clotting and promotion of platelet aggregation [16, 17, 20].

### 15.3.4 Chitosan Products

Chitosan is a derivative of chitin (*N*-acetyl-D-glucosamine) which is ubiquitous natural biopolymer. Despite chitin forming the bulk of the exoskeleton of shellfish, there have been no reactions reported of using chitosan in shellfish-sensitive patients. Chitosan is positively charged and attracts negatively charged red blood cells forming a viscous clot and seals the wound promoting hemostasis. This mechanism functions independent of the coagulation factors. Chitosan is completely biodegradable and usually resorbs in approximately 48 h.

Chitosan has also shown to enhance the release of PDGF and TGF-β aiding in wound healing [16, 21–24].

## 15.4 Local Pharmacologic Agents

Locally applied pharmacologic agents are divided into:

1. Bone wax
2. Caustic agents
3. Antifibrinolytic agents
4. Epinephrine
5. Thrombin

### 15.4.1 Bone Wax

Bone wax is composed primarily of beeswax with isopropyl palmitate (wax-like substance) and/or paraffin wax. Bone wax's mechanism of action is to provide a physical barrier in the area of bleeding bone causing a tamponade effect. There is no interaction with platelets or coagulation factors. Its use is primarily limited to areas of low-flow bleeding bone. High-flow bleeding (from an artery) may displace from the bone rendering the bone wax ineffective. Bone wax is easily malleable and can be readily molded and adapted to the intended area.

The disadvantage to the use of bone wax is its inhibition to new bone growth. Bone wax is insoluble in the body and remains indefinitely. Its presence prevents ingrowth of the soft tissue and bone. It can also induce a foreign body granuloma, become infected, and induce local inflammation and pain [25–29].

A synthetic substance with similar handling properties to bone wax is now available which does not inhibit osteogenesis. The product is an alkylene oxide copolymer which is applied to the bleeding bone in the same manner as bone wax. However, this polymer is water soluble, absorbed within approximately 48 h, and has no adverse tissue interactions. Since the material is resorbed, bone growth and normal healing progress. One product commercially available is Ostene® (Baxter International Inc.) [5, 27].

### 15.4.2 Caustic Agents

Caustic agents induce local hemostasis by causing a degree of superficial destruction of the tissue it contacts and interacting with the proteins at the site of bleeding. These substances have also been classified as styptics and astringents. There effect is best seen in minor, superficial bleeding [26, 30].

The caustic agents are divided into:

1. Silver nitrate
2. Ferric compounds
3. Aluminum compounds

#### 15.4.2.1 Silver Nitrate

Silver nitrate exerts its hemostatic effect by releasing free silver ions topically which bind to and precipitate tissue proteins causing obstruction of small vessels. Application of silver nitrate is most commonly performed with sticks although a solution is available. Application should be with light pressure at the site of minor bleeding. Initially, there is temporary black discoloration of the tissue which disappears. Adverse reactions can include local tissue irritation, possible tattoo formation due to the impregnated silver particles, and discomfort during application [26].

#### 15.4.2.2 Ferric Compounds

Ferric compounds have been used in topical hemostasis: ferric chloride, ferric sulfate, and ferric subsulfate. The iron-containing solutions are dark and have the ability to stain tissues and teeth.

Ferric chloride reacts with blood proteins causing them to coagulate. This reaction seals the openings of small vessels and capillaries. This effect occurs independent of the hemostatic system [26, 30, 31].

Ferric subsulfate is also known as Monsel's salt and, when combined with distilled water, Monsel's solution. Historically, it has been used for topical hemostasis of minor wounds in dermatology and surgery, including oral surgery and dentistry. This compound is acidic and the subsulfate group acts as an oxidant. Both of these properties catalyze protein precipitation which causes occlusion of small vessels [26, 30].

Today, commercially available products for dentistry usually contain a combination of ferric sulfate with and without subsulfate along with a buffer due to its acidity [32]. Ferric local hemostatics have been shown to be irritating to tissues and have caused delay in osseous and soft tissue healing. When used, they should be completely removed from the tissue by curettage and reestablishing bleeding bone. Their use in close proximity to neural structures and the sinus and nasal cavities is not advised [33, 34].

#### 15.4.2.3 Aluminum Compounds

Three aluminum compounds are available for use in dentistry: aluminum chloride, aluminum potassium sulfate, and aluminum sulfate. Aluminum chloride has been used in medicine and surgery as a topical hemostatic agent. Aluminum chloride is thought to hydrolyze to hydrogen chloride which exerts its hemostatic effects by protein coagulation, vasoconstriction, and/or activation of the extrinsic coagulation pathway. Aluminum chloride can result in tissue irritation and dysesthesias [26, 35]. In dentistry, aluminum chloride is available in solution and found in certain brands of gingival retraction cord. Aluminum chloride has also been reported to be used successfully for hemostasis in periapical surgery [36–41]. Aluminum chloride can lead to tissue irritation and delayed bone healing. When it is used for hemostasis during periapical surgery, all of the product should be removed and the bone edges freshened prior to wound closure [37].

Aluminum potassium sulfate and aluminum sulfate have been used in gingival retraction in prosthetic dentistry [38, 41]. The product alum, marketed to dentists, refers to aluminum potassium sulfate [42].

### 15.4.3 Antifibrinolytic Agents

Antifibrinolytic agents used in dentistry are aprotinin, aminocaproic acid, and tranexamic acid. These agents have primarily been used systemically but have also been reported to be efficacious when used topically in the oral cavity. In the USA, aprotinin is no longer available for systemic use; however, it is still a component of some topical fibrin sealants [43–46]. Aminocaproic acid and tranexamic acid have been used topically as oral rinses and placed onto gauze packs and wound dressings as an aid in achieving topical hemostasis. Tranexamic acid is believed to be a more powerful antifibrinolytic. However, in the USA, tranexamic acid is often difficult to obtain in the outpatient setting.

Therefore, aminocaproic acid has been used [47–57].

The mechanism of action of antifibrinolytic agents is the inhibition of the conversion of plasminogen to plasmin. Plasmin is a proteolytic enzyme that hydrolyzes fibrin [58]. Both aminocaproic acid and tranexamic acid block the conversion of plasminogen to plasmin, thereby stabilizing the forming clot.

Aminocaproic acid is supplied as tablets (500 and 1000 mg) and syrup (250 mg/cc) for oral use and an intravenous formulation (5 g/20 cc). Tranexamic acid is supplied as 600 mg tablets and an intravenous formulation of 1000 mg/10 cc [59]. The mouth rinses are compounded from the systemic formulations (Figs. 15.5 and 15.6).

### 15.4.4 Epinephrine

The use of epinephrine in dentistry is well known and well established. The two main forms of epinephrine employed in dental practice are in conjunction with local anesthetics and in gingival retraction. Epinephrine provides vasoconstriction of peripheral tissues due to its agonist activity on α-adrenergic receptors. When local anesthesia with epinephrine is infiltrated into local tissues, decrease in

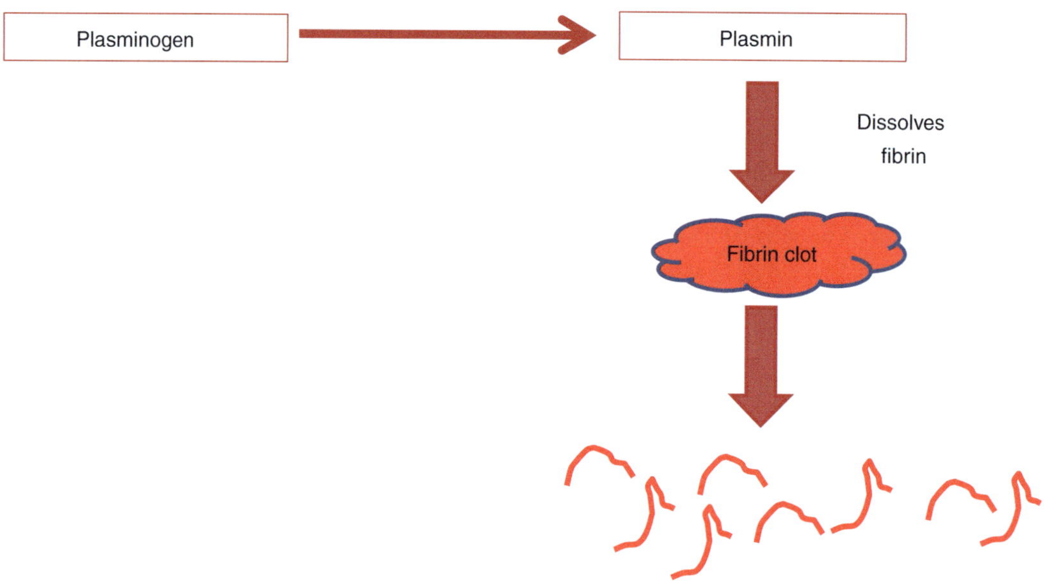


**Fig. 15.5** Fibrinolysis with plasmin

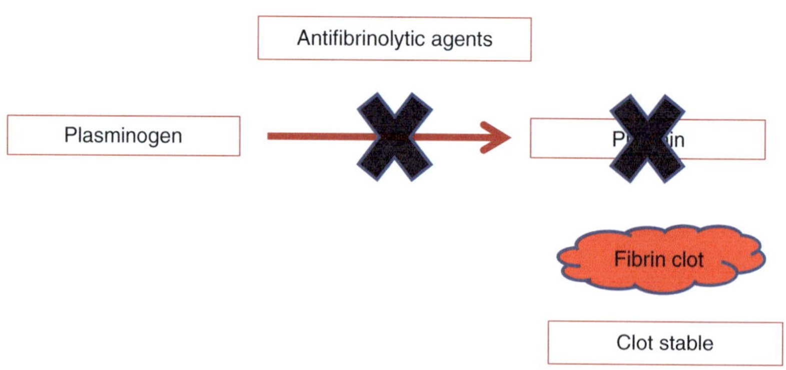


**Fig. 15.6** Site of action of antifibrinolytics

blood flow is noted, but the length of vasoconstriction is finite. Rebound (postoperative) bleeding is possible [60, 61]. There should be consideration given for the use of additional adjuncts when treating patients at a higher risk for bleeding.

For gingival retraction, retraction cord impregnated with racemic epinephrine and solutions of racemic epinephrine are available for use. The solution of racemic epinephrine (2.2%) placed on gauze or collagen has also been reported to be effective for intraoperative bleeding during periapical surgery [62, 63].

### 15.4.5 Thrombin

Thrombin, which is an activated factor II (fIIa), is available for topical application. Thrombin stimulates platelets, converts fibrinogen to fibrin, and activates factor XIII, promoting clot stabilization [16].

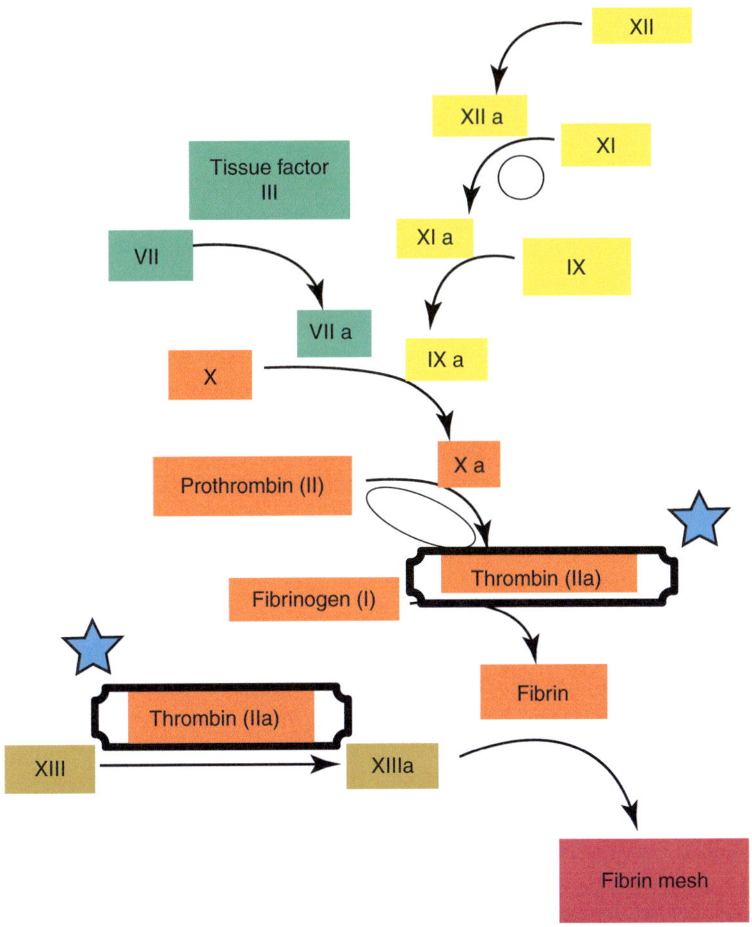


Commercially available thrombin is obtained from one of three sources: bovine thrombin, pooled human plasma thrombin, or recombinant thrombin. Bovine and recombinant thrombin are supplied as a powder, stored at room temperature, and reconstituted with saline when ready for use. These properties allow for consideration for use in dental practice. Pooled human thrombin is the most expensive and supplied as liquid which requires refrigeration [20].

There are well-documented significant risks with the use of thrombin products. Bovine thrombin has been associated with development of immunologic reaction related to factor V which increases the risk of patients developing a coagulopathy when reexposed to the product. A significant percentage of patients also develop antibodies to the product. Recombinant thrombin is manufactured using cells from hamsters and snakes. Allergic reactions have occurred in patients allergic to hamster or snake proteins. Pooled human thrombin carries risk of viral disease transmission [20, 26]. In addition, great care is needed to avoid entrance of any of the thrombin products into systemic circulation via large diameter vessels in the wound as there is a risk of disseminated intravascular coagulation and death [26].

## 15.5 Tissue Adhesives

Tissue adhesives are defined as substances which polymerize and serve to hold tissues together and/or provide a barrier to leakage [64]. Tissue adhesives now encompass a large group of substances used for wound closure, flap and graft adhesion, and wound hemostasis. In addition, many terms are used to classify these various "tissue glues" available in medicine and surgery. This section will primarily review tissue adhesives that have applications to dentistry.

Tissue adhesives can be generally classified into two categories: alloplastic and biologic adhesives. The alloplastic tissue adhesives are represented by cyanoacrylates. Generally, cyanoacrylates are divided into three groups based on the length of their side chains: short (ethyl), intermediate (butyl), and long (octyl). Short-chain cyanoacrylates are sold as household and construction glues such as Krazy Glue® (Elmer's Products) and Super Glue® (3M). These substances are more toxic to tissues than the longer-chain cyanoacrylates and are not marketed for medical use. The intermediate- and long-chain cyanoacrylates are available for medical use. Their use is primarily in superficial wound closure [26, 64]. The effectiveness of cyanoacrylate in local hemostasis is likely due to its ability to maintain wound closure [65].

The biologic tissue adhesives available are divided into fibrin sealants, albumin-glutaraldehyde compounds, hydrogels (polyethylene glycol polymers), and gelatin-thrombin products [5, 16, 17, 64]. Unlike the alloplastic (cyanoacrylate) adhesives, the biologic adhesives contain components which actively promote hemostasis. These products are also referred to as "flowable" sealants or hemostatic agents. Of the biologic adhesives, fibrin sealants have had the most applicability to dentistry.

There are three basic categories of fibrin adhesives: autologous, allogeneic (homologous), and commercial [46]. Autologous fibrin sealants are prepared from blood drawn from the patient immediately prior to treatment. Various preparation methods have been described, including the incorporation of platelet concentrations [66].

Allogeneic fibrin sealants are derived from cryoprecipitate. Cryoprecipitate is prepared from plasma drawn from either a single donor or pooled donors. Cryoprecipitate contains fibrinogen, factor VIII, v WF, and fibronectin. Each bag of cryoprecipitate is approximately 15–20 ml. Adding bovine thrombin to cryoprecipitate yields approximately 10 ml of fibrin sealant [46].

Commercial forms of fibrin sealants represent the third category of fibrin sealants. They are also referred to as synthetic sealants; however, this is a misnomer as these products are not synthesized but rather are produced primarily from human donor plasma. The principal ingredients are pooled human fibrinogen and thrombin. Calcium chloride and trace levels of human albumin are also present [46, 67]. Four commercial fibrin sealants have FDA approval in the USA: TISSEEL® (Baxter), RAPLIXA® (The Medicines Company), ARTISS® (Baxter), and Evicel® (OMRIX Biopharmaceuticals). TISSEEL, RAPLIXA, and Evicel are approved to aid in local hemostasis [68].

ARTISS is approved for use in enhancing tissue adhesion in autologous skin grafting in burn patients and in flap adhesion in facial rhytidectomy. It is *not* approved as an aid in local hemostasis [69].

Non-fibrin-containing tissue adhesives are divided into albumin-based compounds, hydrogels (polyethylene glycol polymers), and gelatin-thrombin products. These have been used in various hospital-based surgical procedures. At this time, their use in dentistry is limited.

## 15.6 Energy-Based Treatments

Energy-based treatments refer to the use of electrocautery, radiofrequency, or laser energy to assist in obtaining hemostasis. Each of these modalities imparts energy to the tissue causing physical changes to seal vessels. Care needs to be taken to prevent damage to adjacent tissues.

## References


1. De Paepe A, Malfait F. Bleeding and bruising in patients with Ehlers-Danlos syndrome and other collagen vascular disorders. Br J Haematol. 2004;127(5):491–500.
2. Malfait F, De Paepe A. Bleeding in the heritable connective tissue disorders: mechanisms, diagnosis and treatment. Blood Rev. 2009;23(5):191–7.
3. Farage MA, Miller KW, Berardesca E, Maibach HI. Clinical implications of aging skin: cutaneous disorders in the elderly. Am J Clin Dermatol. 2009;10(2):73–86.
4. da Rosa RS, Garcia RC, Cury AA, Faot F. Management of the oral manifestations of senile purpura in an edentulous patient: a case report. Spec Care Dentist. 2011;31(3):111–3.
5. Ogle OE, Swantek J, Kamoh A. Hemostatic agents. Dent Clin N Am. 2011;55(3):433–439, vii.
6. Song JS, Lim KM, Kang S, et al. Procoagulant and prothrombotic effects of the herbal medicine, Dipsacus asper and its active ingredient, dipsacus saponin C, on human platelets. J Thromb Haemost. 2012;10(5):895–906.
7. Pereira B, Brazon J, Rincon M, Vonasek E. Browplasminin, a condensed tannin with anti-plasmin activity isolated from an aqueous extract of Brownea grandiceps Jacq. flowers. J Ethnopharmacol. 2017;198:282–90.
8. Soltani R, Haghighat A, Fanaei M, Asghari G. Evaluation of the effect of green tea extract on the prevention of gingival bleeding after posterior mandibular teeth extraction: a randomized controlled trial. Evid Based Complement Alternat Med. 2014;2014:857651.
9. Druckman RF, Fowler EB, Breault LG. Post-surgical hemorrhage: formation of a "liver clot" secondary to periodontal plastic surgery. J Contemp Dent Pract. 2001;2(2):62–71.
10. Pandya D, Manohar B, Mathur LK, Shankarapillai R. "Liver clot" - a rare periodontal postsurgical complication. Indian J Dent Res. 2012;23(3):419–22.
11. Adornato MC, Penna KJ. Hemostatic technique. Using a splint in oral bleeding. N Y State Dent J. 2001;67(6):24–5.
12. Im-erbsin T, Suwannuraks M. Local hemostatic technic using a celluloid splint in bleeding disorders. Southeast Asian J Trop Med Public Health. 1993;24(Suppl 1):167–8.
13. Gupta A, Epstein JB, Cabay RJ. Bleeding disorders of importance in dental care and related patient management. J Can Dent Assoc. 2007;73(1):77–83.
14. Gabay M. Absorbable hemostatic agents. Am J Health Syst Pharm. 2006;63(13):1244–53.
15. Loescher AR, Robinson PP. The effect of surgical medicaments on peripheral nerve function. Br J Oral Maxillofac Surg. 1998;36(5):327–32.
16. Barnard J, Millner R. A review of topical hemostatic agents for use in cardiac surgery. Ann Thorac Surg. 2009;88(4):1377–83.
17. Samudrala S. Topical hemostatic agents in surgery: a surgeon's perspective. AORN J. 2008;88(3):S2–11.
18. Tomizawa Y. Clinical benefits and risk analysis of topical hemostats: a review. J Artif Organs. 2005;8(3):137–42.
19. Kamoh A, Swantek J. Hemostasis in oral surgery. Dent Clin N Am. 2012;56(1):17–23, vii.
20. Schreiber MA, Neveleff DJ. Achieving hemostasis with topical hemostats: making clinically and economically appropriate decisions in the surgical and trauma settings. AORN J. 2011;94(5):S1–20.
21. Gustafson SB, Fulkerson P, Bildfell R, Aguilera L, Hazzard TM. Chitosan dressing provides hemostasis in swine femoral arterial injury model. Prehosp Emerg Care. 2007;11(2):172–8.
22. Malmquist JP, Clemens SC, Oien HJ, Wilson SL. Hemostasis of oral surgery wounds with the HemCon Dental Dressing. J Oral Maxillofac Surg. 2008;66(6):1177–83.
23. Azargoon H, Williams BJ, Solomon ES, Kessler HP, He J, Spears R. Assessment of hemostatic efficacy and osseous wound healing using HemCon dental dressing. J Endod. 2011;37(6):807–11.
24. Waibel KH, Haney B, Moore M, Whisman B, Gomez R. Safety of chitosan bandages in shellfish allergic patients. Mil Med. 2011;176(10):1153–6.
25. Finn MD, Schow SR, Schneiderman ED. Osseous regeneration in the presence of four common hemostatic agents. J Oral Maxillofac Surg. 1992;50(6):608–12.
26. Palm MD, Altman JS. Topical hemostatic agents: a review. Dermatol Surg. 2008;34(4):431–45.
27. Magyar CE, Aghaloo TL, Atti E, Tetradis S. Ostene, a new alkylene oxide copolymer bone hemostatic material, does not inhibit bone healing. Neurosurgery. 2008;63(4 Suppl 2):373–378; discussion 378.
28. Ibarrola JL, Bjorenson JE, Austin BP, Gerstein H. Osseous reactions to three hemostatic agents. J Endod. 1985;11(2):75–83.
29. Bruckner T, Schamel M, Kubler AC, Groll J, Gbureck U. Novel bone wax based on poly(ethylene glycol)-calcium phosphate cement mixtures. Acta Biomater. 2016;33:252–63.
30. Thoma KH. Oral surgery. 3rd ed. St. Louis: Mosby; 1958.
31. Nouri S, Sharif MR, Sahba S. The effect of ferric chloride on superficial bleeding. Trauma Mon. 2015;20(1):e18042.

32. Ultradent Products, Inc. Safety data sheet for Astringedent, Astringedent X, and Viscostat (Registered trademarks). South Jordan, UT: Ultradent Products, Inc.; 2015. p. 7.
33. Niemczyk SP. Essentials of endodontic microsurgery. Dent Clin N Am. 2010;54(2):375–99.
34. Jang Y, Kim H, Roh BD, Kim E. Biologic response of local hemostatic agents used in endodontic microsurgery. Restor Dent Endod. 2014;39(2):79–88.
35. Larson PO. Topical hemostatic agents for dermatologic surgery. J Dermatol Surg Oncol. 1988;14(6):623–32.
36. Felpel LP. A review of pharmacotherapeutics for prosthetic dentistry: Part II. J Prosthet Dent. 1997;77(3):293–305.
37. Menendez-Nieto I, Cervera-Ballester J, Maestre-Ferrin L, Blaya-Tarraga JA, Penarrocha-Oltra D, Penarrocha-Diago M. Hemostatic agents in periapical surgery: a randomized study of gauze impregnated in epinephrine versus aluminum chloride. J Endod. 2016;42(11):1583–7.
38. Donovan TE, Gandara BK, Nemetz H. Review and survey of medicaments used with gingival retraction cords. J Prosthet Dent. 1985;53(4):525–31.
39. Penarrocha-Diago M, Maestre-Ferrin L, Penarrocha-Oltra D, von Arx T, Penarrocha-Diago M. Influence of hemostatic agents upon the outcome of periapical surgery: dressings with anesthetic and vasoconstrictor or aluminum chloride. Med Oral Patol Oral Cir Bucal. 2013;18(2):e272–8.
40. Polat NT, Ozdemir AK, Turgut M. Effects of gingival retraction materials on gingival blood flow. Int J Prosthodont. 2007;20(1):57–62.
41. Ahmed SN, Donovan TE. Gingival displacement: survey results of dentists' practice procedures. J Prosthet Dent. 2015;114(1):81–85 e81–82.
42. Gurney BF. Chemotherapy in dental practice. Topical antihemorrhagic agents. 1. Dent Dig. 1966;72(4):173–4.
43. US Food and Drug Administration. Aprotinin injection (marketed and Trasylol) information. 2008. https://www.fda.gov/Drugs/DrugSafety/PostmarketDrugSafetyInformationforPatientsandProviders/ucm142720.htm.
44. Forcillo J, Perrault LP. Armentarium of topical hemostatic products in cardiovascular surgery: an update. Transfus Apher Sci. 2014;50(1):26–31.
45. Mangano DT, Tudor IC, Dietzel C, Multicenter Study of Perioperative Ischemia Research Group, Ischemia Research and Education Foundation. The risk associated with aprotinin in cardiac surgery. N Engl J Med. 2006;354(4):353–65.
46. Fattahi T, Mohan M, Caldwell GT. Clinical applications of fibrin sealants. J Oral Maxillofac Surg. 2004;62(2):218–24.
47. Borea G, Montebugnoli L, Capuzzi P, Magelli C. Tranexamic acid as a mouthwash in anticoagulant-treated patients undergoing oral surgery. An alternative method to discontinuing anticoagulant therapy. Oral Surg Oral Med Oral Pathol. 1993;75(1):29–31.
48. Carter G, Goss A, Lloyd J, Tocchetti R. Tranexamic acid mouthwash versus autologous fibrin glue in patients taking warfarin undergoing dental extractions: a randomized prospective clinical study. J Oral Maxillofac Surg. 2003;61(12):1432–5.
49. Frachon X, Pommereuil M, Berthier AM, et al. Management options for dental extraction in hemophiliacs: a study of 55 extractions (2000–2002). Oral Surg Oral Med Oral Pathol Oral Radiol Endod. 2005;99(3):270–5.
50. Ramstrom G, Sindet-Pedersen S, Hall G, Blomback M, Alander U. Prevention of postsurgical bleeding in oral surgery using tranexamic acid without dose modification of oral anticoagulants. J Oral Maxillofac Surg. 1993;51(11):1211–6.
51. Sindet-Pedersen S, Stenbjerg S. Effect of local antifibrinolytic treatment with tranexamic acid in hemophiliacs undergoing oral surgery. J Oral Maxillofac Surg. 1986;44(9):703–7.
52. Sindet-Pedersen S. Distribution of tranexamic acid to plasma and saliva after oral administration and mouth rinsing: a pharmacokinetic study. J Clin Pharmacol. 1987;27(12):1005–8.
53. Sindet-Pedersen S, Ramstrom G, Bernvil S, Blomback M. Hemostatic effect of tranexamic acid mouthwash in anticoagulant-treated patients undergoing oral surgery. N Engl J Med. 1989;320(13):840–3.
54. Sindet-Pedersen S, Ingerslev J, Ramstrom G, Blomback M. Management of oral bleeding in haemophilic patients. Lancet. 1989;1(8633):325.
55. Patatanian E, Fugate SE. Hemostatic mouthwashes in anticoagulated patients undergoing dental extraction. Ann Pharmacother. 2006;40(12):2205–10.
56. Soares EC, Costa FW, Bezerra TP, et al. Postoperative hemostatic efficacy of gauze soaked in tranexamic acid, fibrin sponge, and dry gauze compression following dental extractions in anticoagulated patients with cardiovascular disease: a prospective, randomized study. Oral Maxillofac Surg. 2015;19(2):209–16.
57. Aldridge E, Cunningham LL Jr. Current thoughts on treatment of patients receiving anticoagulation therapy. J Oral Maxillofac Surg. 2010;68(11):2879–87.
58. O'Reilly RA. Anticoagulant, antithrombotic, and thrombolytic drugs. In: Gilman AGG, Louis S, Rall TW, Murad F, editors. Goodman and Gilman's the pharmacological basis of therapeutics. 7th ed. New York: MacMillan Publishing Company; 1985. p. 1338–62.
59. Hamilton R. Tarascon pocket pharmacopoeia. Burlington, MA: Jones & Bartlett Publishing; 2015. 2015
60. Sisk AL. Vasoconstrictors in local anesthesia for dentistry. Anesth Prog. 1992;39(6):187–93.
61. Baker TF, Torabinejad M, Schwartz SF, Wolf D. Effect of intraosseous anesthesia on control of hemostasis in pigs. J Endod. 2009;35(11):1543–5.
62. Cle-Ovejero A, Valmaseda-Castellon E. Haemostatic agents in apical surgery. A systematic review. Med Oral Patol Oral Cir Bucal. 2016;21(5):e652–7.

63. Vy CH, Baumgartner JC, Marshall JG. Cardiovascular effects and efficacy of a hemostatic agent in periradicular surgery. J Endod. 2004;30(6):379–83.
64. Reece TB, Maxey TS, Kron IL. A prospectus on tissue adhesives. Am J Surg. 2001;182(2 Suppl):40S–4S.
65. Al-Belasy FA, Amer MZ. Hemostatic effect of n-butyl-2-cyanoacrylate (histoacryl) glue in warfarin-treated patients undergoing oral surgery. J Oral Maxillofac Surg. 2003;61(12):1405–9.
66. Soffer E, Ouhayoun JP, Anagnostou F. Fibrin sealants and platelet preparations in bone and periodontal healing. Oral Surg Oral Med Oral Pathol Oral Radiol Endod. 2003;95(5):521–8.
67. Silvergleid A, Peralta E. Fibrin sealants - UpToDate. UpToDate 2017. www.uptodate.com.
68. FDA. Vaccines, blood & biologics: licensed biologic products with supporting documents. 2017. https://www.fda.gov/BiologicsBloodVaccines/ucm133705.htm.
69. Baxter Healthcare Corporation. Package insert for ARTISS [Fibrin Sealant (Human)]. Westlake Village, CA: Baxter Healthcare Corporation; 2011. p. 14.

# Index




R. P. Szumita, P. M. Szumita (eds.), *Hemostasis in Dentistry*, https://doi.org/10.1007/978-3-319-71240-6

MIX
Papier aus verantwortungsvollen Quellen
Paper from responsible sources
FSC® C105338

If you have any concerns about our products,
you can contact us on
**ProductSafety@springernature.com**

In case Publisher is established outside the EU,
the EU authorized representative is:
**Springer Nature Customer Service Center GmbH**
**Europaplatz 3, 69115 Heidelberg, Germany**

Printed by Libri Plureos GmbH
in Hamburg, Germany